BASIC ARRHYTHMIAS

Second Edition, Revised

Gail Walraven

A BRADY BOOK

PRENTICE-HALL, INC.

ENGLEWOOD CLIFFS, NEW JERSEY 07632

Library of Congress Cataloging-in-Publication Data

Walraven, Gail, [date]
    BASIC ARRHYTHMIAS.

    ''A Brady book.''
    Includes index.
        1. Arrhythmia—Diagnosis—Programmed instruction.
    2. Electocardiography—Programmed instruction.
    I. Title. [DNLM: 1. Arrhythmia—programmed instuction.
    2. Electrocardiography—programmed instruction.
    WG 18 W221b]
    RC685.A65W33   1986   616.1′ 2807543   86–8882
    ISBN 0–13–057092–3

Editorial supervision: Serena Hoffman
Cover design: Ben Santora
Manufacturing buyer: Barbara Kelly Kittle
Page makeup: Frances M. Kasturas

Printed in the United States of America

10 9 8 7 6 5 4 3

ISBN   0-13-057092-3   025

PRENTICE-HALL INTERNATIONAL (UK) LIMITED, *London*
PRENTICE-HALL OF AUSTRALIA PTY. LIMITED, *Sydney*
PRENTICE-HALL CANADA INC., *Toronto*
PRENTICE-HALL HISPANOAMERICANA, S.A., *Mexico*
PRENTICE-HALL OF INDIA PRIVATE LIMITED, *New Delhi*
PRENTICE-HALL OF JAPAN, INC., *Tokyo*
PRENTICE-HALL OF SOUTHEAST ASIA PTE. LTD., *Singapore*
EDITORA PRENTICE-HALL DO BRASIL, LTDA., *Rio de Janeiro*
WHITEHALL BOOKS LIMITED, *Wellington, New Zealand*

Contents

Preface v

Directions vii

Chapter 1 — Electrophysiology 1
Self-Instructional Unit
  Electrical activity vs. mechanical activity; initiation of electrical flow (polarization depolarization, repolarization); conduction system; inherent rates; pacemaker principles; irritability/escape; innervation
Key Points 14
Self-Test 16

Chapter 2 — Waves and Measurements 19
Self-Instructional Unit
  Electrodes; flow of electricity; monitoring; leads; electrode placement; graph paper markings; cardiac cycle; wave identification; measurements; artifact and interference; refractoriness
Key Points 37
Self-Test 39
Practice Sheet 1 44
Practice Sheet 2 49

Chapter 3 — Analyzing EKG Rhythm Strips 53
Self-Instructional Unit
  Interpreting vs. pattern recognition; organization of approach; regularity of rhythm; rate determination; P waves and other waves; relationships; PRI and QRS measurements; interpretation of data; learning rules of arrhythmias; categorization of arrhythmias; understanding findings
Key Points 64
Self-Test 66
Practice Sheet 3 70
Practice Sheet 4 73

Chapter 4 — Sinus Rhythms 77
Self-Instructional Unit
  Normal Sinus Rhythm; Sinus Bradycardia; Sinus Tachycardia; Sinus Arrhythmia
Key Points 86
Self-Test 87
Practice Sheet 5 90

Chapter 5 — Atrial Rhythms 101
Self-Instructional Unit
  Premature Atrial Contraction; Atrial Flutter; Atrial Fibrillation; Atrial Tachycardia; Wandering Pacemaker
Key Points 115
Self-Test 117
Practice Sheet 6 123

Chapter 6 — Junctional Rhythms   135

Self-Instructional Unit
   Premature Junctional Contraction; Junctional Escape Rhythm; Accelerated Junctional Rhythm; Junctional Tachycardia; Supraventricular Tachycardia
Key Points   151
Self-Test   153
Practice Sheet 7   160

Chapter 7 — Heart Blocks   167

Self-Instructional Unit
   First Degree Heart Block; Classical Second Degree Heart Block; Wenckebach; Complete Heart Block
Key Points   186
Self-Test   188
Practice Sheet 8   195

Chapter 8 — Ventricular Rhythms   205

Self-Instructional Unit
   Premature Ventricular Contractions; Ventricular Tachycardia; Ventricular Fibrillation; Idioventricular Rhythm; Asystole
Key Points   224
Self-Test   227
Practice Sheet 9   236

Chapter 9 — Practice Makes Perfect   253

Introduction
Practice Sheet 10   255

Answer Keys   365

Practice Sheets: Answers

Practice Sheet 1   367
Practice Sheet 2   370
Practice Sheet 3   376
Practice Sheet 4   377
Practice Sheet 5   378
Practice Sheet 6   381
Practice Sheet 7   385
Practice Sheet 8   388
Practice Sheet 9   392
Practice Sheet 10   398

Appendix A — Clinical Effects of Arrhythmias   436

Appendix B — Treatment Concepts   437

Appendix C — Arrhythmia Significance and Treatments   440

Glossary   445

Index   452

Flash Cards   457

Preface

There are many ways to learn electrocardiography, and many levels of expertise within this complex field. For ease of reference, the various levels of knowledge/ability can be outlined as below:

SINGLE-LEAD RHYTHM INTERPRETATION

Level I: Ability to recognize a limited number of familiar patterns, usually the major life—threatening rhythms. No understanding of rules or mechanisms.

Level II: Basic understanding of the rules and mechanisms of common arrhythmias according to pacemaker sites. No familiarity with more sophisticated features that complicate basic arrhythmias.

Level III: Ability to interpret arrhythmias which include more sophisticated features such as sinus arrest, pacemakers, aberrancy, and blocked beats.

12-LEAD EKGS

Level IV: Familiarity with 12—lead EKGs, e.g., bundle branch block, infarction location, axis deviation.

Level V: Ability to distinguish subtle EKG findings, e.g., concealed conduction, reciprocal conduction, trifascicular block, His bundle recordings.

Levels I—III are concerned with interpretation of patterns; these categories address only arrhythmias, and do not delve into the meanings of each of the individual wave forms. Levels IV and V include arrhythmias, but also discuss the complexities of 12—lead interpretation and auxiliary diagnostic mechanisms.

It is usual for a student to proceed through these levels in a relatively logical progression from simple to complex. Unfortunately, it is also common for a potential student to be prevented from entering this fascinating field for lack of the initial training upon which to build more sophisticated understanding. *Basic Arrhythmias* is designed to provide a sound base of understanding for those interested individuals who have been unable to receive other forms of training. Its primary area of concentration is Level II, the area of basic understanding of the common, uncomplicated rhythms. It is hoped that *Basic Arrythmias* will provide an enjoyable and interesting way for people to develop the framework which will later support continued learning in the area of electrocardiography.

This self-instructional program is targeted toward several groups of people:

- those who have previously approached EKGs with "pattern recognition"
- those who have been unable to participate in more conventional EKG training
- those who are involved in a formal EKG training program and will use this program concurrently, to solidify their learning experience.

Because the nature of the book is to provide a foundation for future learning, great care was taken to instill simple, basic concepts without giving the student any misconceptions or erroneous impressions. To this end, some information may have been eliminated or lightly passed over because it was considered to be more sophisticated than necessary, and thus might leave the reader confused and without immediate access to an instructor's tutelage. It is hoped that *Basic Arrhythmias* will open the door for new learners, and will provide instructors with more class time for the critical area of reinforcement and refinement.

Acknowledgments

I would like to thank the following people for their assistance with preparation of *Basic Arrhythmias:*

Mary Barrett, RN, Newport Beach, CA
Dave Bergerson, PhD, VA
Chris Breu, RN, UCLA, Los Angeles, CA
Eleanor Dimick, EMT-1, Birmingham, Alabama
Leonard Evans, PhD, University of Southern California
Marion Kavanaugh, RN, Long Beach, CA
Julie Lawler, RN, Sharp Hospital, San Diego, CA
Sally LeBoeuf, MD, University of Southern California
Sylvia Micik, MD, La Jolla, CA
Barbara Pierce, RN, Long Beach, CA
Linda Pierog, RN, Laguna Beach, CA
Vicki Schreckengost, RN, Sharon, PA
Elaine Serra, RN, Newport Beach, CA
Sharp Hospital ICU Staff, San Diego, CA
Nancy Smith, RN, Charlottesville, VA
Nancy Varah, RN, University Hospital, San Diego, CA
St. Joseph's Hospital Arrhythmia Monitoring Staff, Omaha, NE
Millie Walraven, Sharp Hospital, San Diego, CA
Jan Rydell Williams, RN, Mercy Hospital, San Diego, CA
Muriel Wolkow, EdD, University of Southern California

This is admittedly a partial list, so I offer a broad thank you to the dozens of anonymous contributors whose comments and suggestions improved the usefulness of the final product. And I extend heartfelt appreciation to my family and friends for their endless encouragement and support along the way.

Gail Walraven

Directions

This self-instructional EKG course is designed to be a complete self-contained learning package. The only additional materials you will require are a pencil and a set of EKG calipers, which are available at most medical supply houses and medical bookstores. Everything else is provided here in a format designed to make this learning an enjoyable and worthwhile process.

Before you start the program, you should know something about the format of the chapters. Most of the material has been organized into learning units of approximately similar time frames, so that you can pace yourself as you go along. The first three chapters prepare you with the basic principles of electrocardiography, and explain many of the theories and concepts that are the foundation of arrhythmia interpretation. Starting with Chapter 4 you will begin systematically learning arrhythmias according to their site of origin within the heart. Finally, you will be given supplemental practice material to ensure retention of your learning. The internal structure of each individual chapter is essentially the same:

Self-Instructional Unit

This programmed narrative will teach you any rules and explanatory materials that you will need to know to interpret arrhythmias. As you read the text, you will be asked to respond to incomplete sentences or direct questions. The answers are given in the right-hand margin directly across from the question. Get into the habit of covering the margin with a slip of paper before reading the text, then as you are asked to respond, write your answer in the blank space provided, and slide the paper down the page to reveal the desired response. If you have trouble with an answer, go back over the preceding frames to find the solution.

Flash Cards

Some of the chapters will ask you to take time out from the program to memorize material such as specific rules for each arrhythmia. For your convenience, any material that must be committed to memory has been printed on the flash cards that were provided with this book. This is an effective method of memorizing material in a short period of time. Whenever you are directed to memorize information, stop working on the program and use the flash cards to accomplish this task. Then return to the text.

Key Points

Near the end of each chapter you will find a brief summary of each of the key points contained in that chapter. This is provided for your review as you complete the chapter, and also a reference should you need to look up a point in the future.

Self-Tests

Each chapter is closed with a self-test of the important information contained in that chapter. The format of the self-tests is very similar to the format of the text, except that each question is keyed back to the frames in the chapter that specifically provide the answer to the question. Since the self-test is intended to tell you whether or not you learned the material in the chapter, you will want to let a little time pass between completing the chapter and beginning the self-test. If you take the test immediately after finishing the chapter, you might be simply recognizing familiar terms, rather than truly understanding the information. So, once you finish the chapter, take a break from the subject for an hour or two. Then come back to take the test. If you do well on the test, go on to the next chapter, but if your results indicate that you did not really learn the material, do not proceed until you remedy that. To do so will merely confuse you, and may eventually prevent you from learning the subject well.

Practice Sheets

Most of the chapters include at least one Practice Sheet of EKG rhythm strips for you to develop skill in analyzing and interpreting arrhythmias. All of the answers to the Practice Sheets are included at the end of the book. Since practice is probably the single most important element in developing skill at arrhythmia interpretation, it is critical that you take advantage of the practice time provided.

    This book is designed to enable you to teach yourself arrhythmia interpretation. However, your learning will be greatly expedited if you have access to an instructor who will guide your learning and stimulate your thinking. If possible, identify a potential instructor before you begin the program, and arrange for tutorial help should you require it. Then your questions can be answered and your horizons expanded as you progress within this self-instructional course.

This is a revised printing of the second edition of this text, in which certain design modifications were made and material reorganized in better sequence.

1

Electrophysiology

1. The human heart is intended to pump blood to the rest of the body. This process has two distinct components:
    - The *electrical* impulse that tells the heart to beat; and
    - The *mechanical* beating of the heart in response to the electrical stimulation, resulting in pumping of blood.

To perform these two functions, the heart has two distinct types of cells. There are electrical (conductive) cells, which initiate electrical activity and conduct it through the heart, and there are mechanical (contracting) cells, which respond to the electrical stimulus and contract to pump blood. After the _____ cells initiate the impulse and conduct it through the heart, the _____ cells respond by contracting the heart and pumping blood.

electrical
mechanical

2. The heart will only respond with contraction if it is stimulated by electrical activity. Thus, you cannot have a mechanical response if there is no _____ stimulus.

electrical

3. After the electrical cells have discharged their stimuli, the mechanical cells are expected to respond by _____.

contracting

4. Without _____ stimulus, the mechanical cells can't be expected to contract.

electrical

5. Since it is not practical to see inside a living patient's heart, we must rely on external evidence to evaluate the status of both electrical and mechanical cardiac function. For a complete assessment of cardiac status we must evaluate both _____ and _____ functions.

electrical
mechanical

6. As part of our assessment of mechanical function, we use blood pressure, pulses, and other perfusion parameters to determine whether or not the heart is pumping adequately. We must also look for external evidence to evaluate the heart's electrical activity. The best way to do this is to monitor the electrocardiogram (EKG). An EKG tracing is used to evaluate the _____ activity of the heart, while the mechanical activity is evaluated by assessing _____ and _____ _____.

electrical
pulses;
blood pressure

7. You might occasionally encounter a situation in which the heart muscle is not able to contract in response to the electrical stimulus. In this case, you could have electrical activity but with no _____ response. If you had a functioning electrical system but a failing heart muscle, you could very likely see a viable EKG tracing but the patient might not have palpable _____ or blood pressure.

mechanical

pulses

8. To evaluate a patient's cardiac function, you must assess the mechanical function by examining _____ and _____ _____, and evaluate electrical function by analyzing the _____ tracing.

pulses; blood
pressure
EKG

9. An EKG tracing is designed to give a graphic display of the electrical activity in the heart. The pattern displayed on the EKG is called the heart rhythm. Technically, the word "arrhythmia" refers to an abnormal heart rhythm, although the term is often used more generally to refer to all cardiac electrical patterns. The term "dysrhythmia" is synonymous with arrhythmia; both are used to refer to patterns of _____ activity within the heart.

electrical

10. An EKG can't tell you about the heart's mechanical activity— you have to assess the patient's pulse and blood pressure to determine that. But an EKG can tell you about the _____ activity, which can be a vital part of your patient assessment. This data is provided in the form of recognizable patterns, called arrhythmias. Arrhythmias are graphic representations of the heart's _____ activity.

electrical

electrical

11. To understand and interpret arrhythmias, it is necessary to understand the electrical activity that is occurring within the heart. This is because all arrhythmias are actually graphic displays of electrical activity. The term "electrocardiography" is given to the study of arrhythmias because arrhythmias are manifestations of _____ activity within the heart.

electrical

12. To help you understand and eventually be able to interpret individual arrhythmia patterns, you might want to know a little bit about the electrical processes that take place in the heart to produce the arrhythmia. To do this we'll consider the electrical component independent of the mechanical component. For now, we are only discussing the _____ activity in the heart.

electrical

13. In a cardiac cell the electrical charges are provided primarily by two chemicals: sodium (Na^+) and potassium (K^+). In a resting cell the potassium is mostly on the inside while the sodium is mostly on the outside. The sodium has a stronger charge than the potassium, making the outside of the cell more positive than the inside. In a manner of speaking, the inside of the cell is relatively negative to the outside (Fig. 1-A). Although both sodium and potassium carry _____ electrical charges, they are not equally positive. This means that the resting cell will carry a _____ charge on the outside and a relatively _____ charge on the inside.

positive
positive;
negative

14. This concept is really just background information for you. The important point is that the positive and negative charges are balanced in the resting state. In order for an electrical current to form, there must be a difference between the electrical charges. In the resting cell the charges are balanced, hence no electricity flows. This is called the "polarized" state; the cell charges are _____

balanced;

and ready for action. Polarization refers to a ready state where the electrical charges are _____ and no _____ current flows.

balanced;
electrical

15.   When the cell is in its resting state it is said to be _____ because all of the charges are _____ and there is no electrical _____.

polarized;
balanced;
flow

16.   The electrical cells in the heart are unique in that they have a property called automaticity. This means that they can discharge an electrical current without an external stimulus. These cells are able to modify their membrane and pull sodium into the cell while potassium exits. This causes a difference in the electrical charges resulting in initiation of an electrical flow. This phenomenon is commonly referred to as the "Sodium Pump" (Fig. 1). When the charges exchange places in the cell the result is formation of an _____ current. Once the pacemaker cells provide the stimulus, the flow is passed from cell to cell along the conduction pathway until the _____ cells are stimulated to contract.

electrical

muscle

17.   The polarized state is considered a "ready for action" phase. When the two chemical charges trade places, the electricity flows in a wave-like motion throughout the heart. This wave of electrical flow is called "depolarization" and is how the electrical stimulus travels through the heart. Polarization refers to the "ready" state, and _____ refers to the process of electrical discharge and flow of electrical activity.

depolarization

18.   After the cell depolarizes, the positive and negative electrical charges will again return to their original positions around the cell, and the cell will prepare itself for another discharge (Fig. 1C). The process which follows depolarization, when the cell charges are returning to their original state, is called "repolarization." Repolarization refers to the return of the electrical charges to their _____ position. Repolarization occurs _____ depolarization.

original
after

19.   If each of the positive charges on the outside of the cell is balanced by a negative charge on the inside of the cell, the electrical charges will be balanced, and there will be no movement of electricity. This state is called _____, and can be considered a "ready" state.

polarization

20.   The wave of electrical activity that takes place when the electrical charges surrounding the cell trade places is called _____, and the return of the electrical charges to their original state is called _____.

depolarization;

repolarization

21.   If polarization is considered the "ready" state, and _____ is considered the "discharge" state, then _____ would be considered the "recovery" state.

depolarization;
repolarization

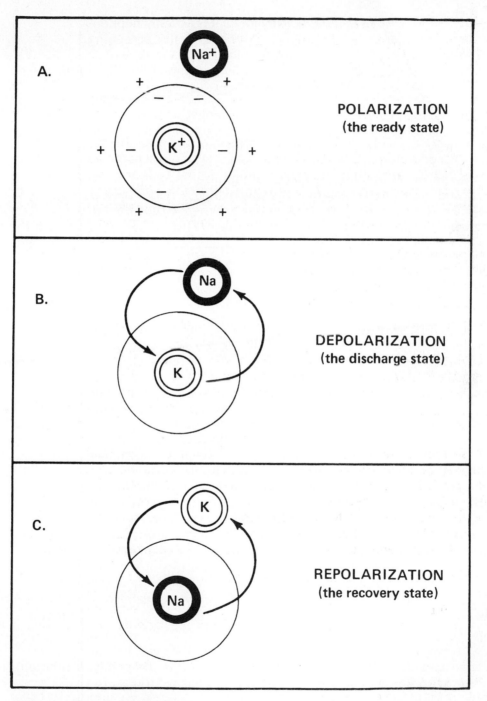

Figure 1. Chemical Basis for Impulse Formation

22.   Now let's relate this cellular activity to what is actually happening in the heart. All of the sequences described in the preceding frames are happening to single cells within the heart, but they do it in a _____-like movement, resulting in the entire heart responding electrically to the same activity.

wave

23.   The electrical cells in the heart are all arranged in a system of pathways called the conduction system. The physical layout of the conduction system is shown in Figure 2. This information is an essential part of arrhythmia interpretation, and should therefore be memorized now. Normally, the electrical impulse originates in the SA node and travels to the ventricles by way of the AV node. Look at Figure 2 and trace a normal electrical impulse. Where would the impulse go after it left the AV node and the Bundle of His? _____
_____

Down the left and right bundle branches and then to the Purkinje fibers

24.   In the normal heart, the first impulse which starts the flow of electrical current through the heart comes from the SA node. As it leaves the SA node, where does the current go? _____
_____

Down the internodal and intraatrial pathways

25.   The next area of conductive tissue along the conduction pathway is at the site of the AV node. The AV node is unique in that it does have conductive tissue, but it does not have any pacemaker cells like other areas of the conduction system. The pacemaking cells are actually located at the junction between the AV node and the atria, in an area called the AV junction. Thus, the term *AV Node* can be used when talking about conduction, but the term *AV Junction* is more accurate if you are specifically discussing formation of impulses. Don't let this confuse you. It is simply an explanation of what might otherwise appear to be indiscriminate use of the two phrases. We will use the term AV node if we're talking only about _____, but if we're specifically discussing pacemaking capabilities we will call it the AV _____.

conduction; junction

26.   After leaving the area of the AV node, the impulses go through the _____ to reach the right and left bundle branches. These branches are located within the right and left ventricles, respectively.

Bundle of His

27.   At the terminal ends of the bundle branches, smaller fibers distribute the electrical impulses to the muscle cells to stimulate contraction. These terminal fibers are called _____ fibers.

Purkinje

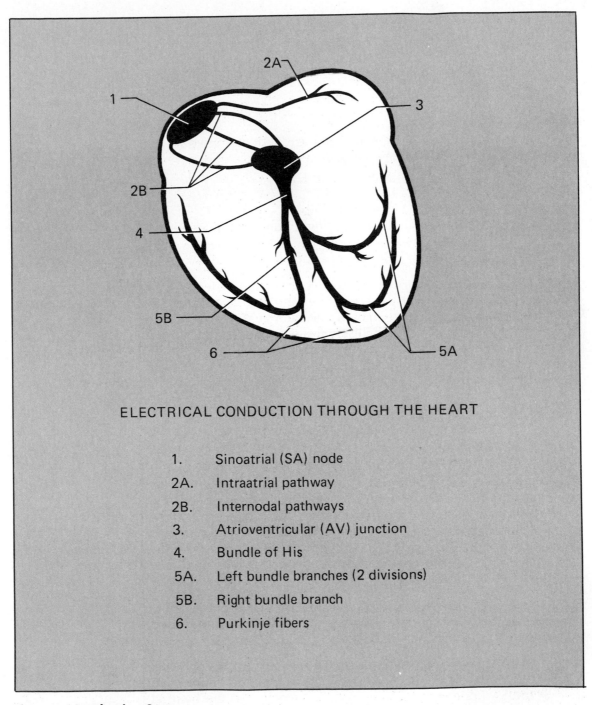

ELECTRICAL CONDUCTION THROUGH THE HEART

1.   Sinoatrial (SA) node
2A.   Intraatrial pathway
2B.   Internodal pathways
3.   Atrioventricular (AV) junction
4.   Bundle of His
5A.   Left bundle branches (2 divisions)
5B.   Right bundle branch
6.   Purkinje fibers

Figure 2. Conduction System

28. Are the muscle cells themselves part of the electrical conduction system? _____

No, they are made up of mechanical cells, not electrical cells.

29. Rearrange the following parts of the conduction system to place them in the actual order of conduction:

1) _____	a) Bundle of His	1. b
2) _____	b) SA node	2. f
3) _____	c) Purkinje fibers	3. e
4) _____	d) left and right bundle branches	4. a
5) _____	e) AV node	5. d
6) _____	f) intraatrial pathways	6. c

30. Each of the three major areas of the conduction system has its own built-in rate, called an *inherent* rate, at which it initiates impulses. An inherent rate simply means that each site has a rate range at which it usually produces impulses. A site can exceed or fall below its inherent rate, indicating that these rates are not concrete rules. But generally speaking, the sites will produce impulses at a rate within their own _____ rate ranges.

inherent

31. The inherent rate ranges of the major sites are outlined below:

SA Node   60–100 beats per minute
AV Junction   40–60 beats per minute
Ventricle   20–40 beats per minute

This information would give you a clue that if an EKG rate was between 20 and 40 beats per minute, the electrical impulse that stimulated the rhythm probably originated in the _____. If the rate was between 40 and 60 beats per minute, the impulse probably came from the _____, and it most likely came from the _____ if the rate was between 60 and 100 beats per minute.

ventricle

AV junction;
SA node

32. These rates are often helpful clues to be used in interpreting arrhythmias, but they can be misleading unless they are understood to be mere guidelines and not concrete _____.

rules

33. Generally speaking, the fastest inherent rate will become the pacemaker of the heart and override all other stimuli. The inherent rate of the SA node is the fastest, and therefore keeps the heart at a rate between _____ and _____ beats per minute. Thus the normal EKG is "sinus" in origin. The SA node is the normal pacemaker for the heart because the rate of the SA node is _____ than the other conduction sites.

60; 100

faster

34.   If, however, a site becomes irritable and begins to discharge impulses at a faster-than-normal rate, it can override the SA node and take over the pacemaking function for the heart. If the SA node is discharging at a rate of 72 and the AV junction begins to fire at a rate of 95, the _____ will become the pacemaker.

AV junction

35.   This mechanism of an irritable site speeding up and taking over as pacemaker is called "irritability." It is usually an undesirable occurrence, since it overrides the normal pacemaker and causes the heart to beat faster than it otherwise would. Irritability occurs when a site below the SA node _____ and takes over the pacemaking role.

speeds up

36.   Something very different happens if the normal pacemaker slows down for some reason. If the SA node drops below its inherent rate, or if it fails entirely, the site with the next highest inherent rate will usually take over the pacemaking role. The next highest site is within the _____, so that site would become the pacemaker if the SA node should fail. This mechanism is called "escape," and is a safety feature that is built into the heart to protect it in case the normal _____ fails.

AV junction

pacemaker

37.   Escape mechanism, unlike irritability, is a safety feature to protect the heart. Would you expect an irritable rhythm to be faster or slower than an escape rhythm? _____

faster

38.   The inherent rate of different areas of the conduction system refers to the rate at which that site _____ _____.

initiates impulses

39.   The SA node has an inherent rate of _____ to _____ beats per minute. This means that the normal rate of the heart will usually be within that range.

60;
100

40.   If the rate of an EKG is between 40 and 60, the impulse for that rhythm is probably coming from the _____.

AV junction

41.   What is the inherent rate of the ventricular conductive tissues? _____

20–40 beats/minute

42.   Because these rates cannot be relied upon as firm rules, they should be viewed only as _____. If they are used as clues the rates will be helpful in interpreting arrhythmias, but if they are considered inflexible they will simply confuse the learner.

guidelines

43.   A rule regarding the pacemaker function of the heart states that the site which initiates impulses at the _____ rate will usually become the pacemaker.

fastest

44.   In the normal heart the _____ initiates impulses at the fastest rate and therefore becomes the _____.

SA node
pacemaker

45.   If the AV junction or the ventricle became irritable, it could become the pacemaker if it were able to accelerate until it _____ _____.

became faster than the SA node

46.   The process described in the preceding frame is called _____.

irritability

47.   If the SA node failed as pacemaker, or if its rate dropped below the normal range, the _____ would probably take over as pacemaker.

AV junction

48.   The safety mechanism described in the preceding frame is called _____.

escape

49.   In addition to the inherent rates, the heart can be influenced by the autonomic nervous system. The two branches of this nervous system oppose each other, and thus keep the heart in a relative state of balance. The sympathetic branch influences both the atria (i.e., the SA node, the intraatrial and internodal pathways, and the AV junction) and the ventricles. If the sympathetic branch is stimulated it will cause both the atria and ventricles to react in these ways:

- increased rate
- increased conduction through the AV node
- increased irritability

The parasympathetic branch has the opposite effects, but it influences only the atria; it has little or no effect on the ventricles. While stimulation of the parasympathetic branch causes the atria to slow down as well as decreasing irritability and slowing conduction through the AV node, stimulation of the sympathetic branch would cause what three effects on the atria and ventricles?

_____

_____

_____

increased
   heart rate
increased AV
   conduction
increased
   irritability

These nervous influences are outlined in Figure 3.

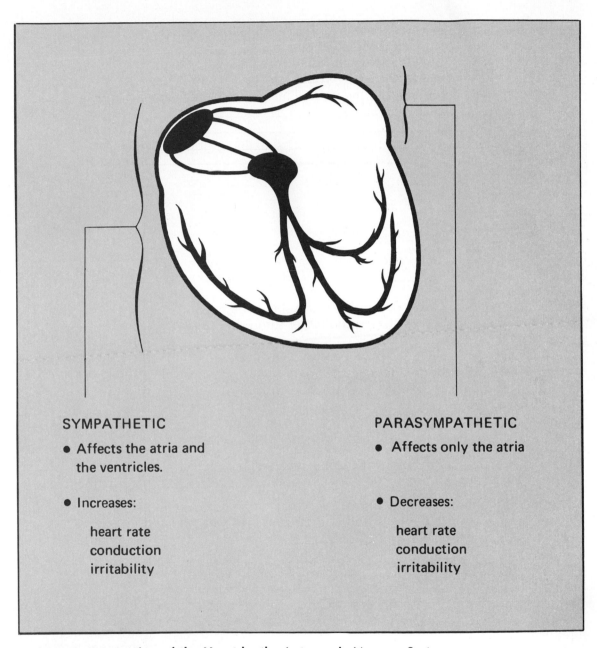

SYMPATHETIC

- Affects the atria and the ventricles.

- Increases:

    heart rate
    conduction
    irritability

PARASYMPATHETIC

- Affects only the atria

- Decreases:

    heart rate
    conduction
    irritability

Figure 3. Innervation of the Heart by the Autonomic Nervous System

50. If the vagus nerve (which is part of the parasympathetic branch) is stimulated, you would expect the heart rate to _____. On the other hand, if both the sympathetic and the parasympathetic branches are balanced, the heart rate would remain normal. Wh: would you expect if you blocked the normal influence of the vagus nerve? _____ _____ _____ _____

decrease

You would get a response similar to stimulation of the sympathetic branch; heart rate would increase as well as irritability and AV conduction.

51. If a patient had a heart rate that was too slow, you might try to speed it up by giving a drug that would either stimulate the sympathetic branch or _____.

block the parasympathetic branch

52. The two branches of the autonomic nervous system that influence heart rate are the _____ branch and the _____ branch.

sympathetic parasympathetic

53. Which of these branches, when stimulated, will produce an increase in heart rate, AV conduction, and irritability? _____

sympathetic

54. One of the branches has control over the atria and the ventricles, while the other influences only the atria. Which one affects both the atria and the ventricles? _____

sympathetic

55. If both branches are exerting equal influence over the heart, what will happen to the rates? _____ _____

They will stay within the ranges of the normal inherent rates.

56. What will happen if one of the branches of the autonomic nervous system is blocked? _____ _____

The heart would respond to the influence of the opposing branch.

57.   Using the reasoning described in the preceding frame, explain what would happen to the heart rate if the parasympathetic branch were blocked. _____

It would increase.

58.   The vagus nerve is part of the _____ branch of the autonomic nervous system. Therefore, stimulation of the vagus nerve would cause the heart rate to _____, and blocking of the vagus nerve would cause the heart rate to _____.

parasympa-thetic
decrease
increase

59.   All of this discussion is about _____ activity, and does not yet connect with mechanical activity. In order to discuss the heart contracting and producing a pulse, we must connect the electrical activity with _____ activity.

electrical

mechanical

60.   If the muscle cells receive an electrical stimulus they will respond to it by contracting. Sometimes, however, the muscle itself can't contract because it is injured or chemically imbalanced. In these cases the electrical component is all right, but the _____ component needs attention. In such a patient you would expect to find the EKG essentially normal, but the _____ would be absent or diminished.

mechanical

pulse

61.   The opposite situation is more common, and is the reason you are reading this book. This is when the heart muscle is able to respond but the electrical activity is erratic. Sometimes the electrical stimuli will make the ventricles contract before the atria do, or maybe there will just be too many electrical stimuli, so that the heart is not able to respond effectively to any of them. And sometimes the electrical impulse will discharge before the ventricles have time to fill with blood, thereby causing the ventricles to contract and eject insufficient blood for an adequate pulse. In all of these conditions, the erratic electrical activity will be seen on the EKG as an _____.

arrhythmia

Key Points – Electrophysiology

- The heart has two types of cells:
    - Electrical cells initiate and conduct impulses.
    - Mechanical cells contract in response to stimulation.

- Arrhythmias are graphic representations of electrical activity.

- Electrical activity precedes mechanical activity.

- Electrical activity can occur without mechanical response (pulse).

- If the electrical impulse stimulates the mechanical cells to contract, the heart is expected to contract and pump blood, thus producing a pulse.

- Polarization is when the electrical charges are balanced and ready for discharge.

- Depolarization is the discharge of energy that accompanies the transfer of electrical charges across the cell membrane.

- Repolarization is the return of electrical charges to their original state of readiness.

- Depolarization differs from contraction in that depolarization is an electrical phenomenon, while contraction is mechanical and is expected to follow depolarization.

- As shown in Figure 2, electrical flow in the heart originates in the SA node, travels via the intraatrial and internodal pathways to the AV node, then through the Bundle of His to the Left and Right Bundle Branches, and finally to the Purkinje Fibers, where the mechanical cells are stimulated.

- The inherent rates of the conduction system are:
    - SA Node   60–100 beats per minute
    - AV Junction   40–60 beats per minute
    - Ventricles   20–40 beats per minute.

- The site with the fastest rate will be the pacemaker.

- The SA node is the normal pacemaker of the heart.

- "Irritability" is when a site speeds up and takes over as pacemaker.

- "Escape" is when the normal pacemaker slows down or fails and a lower site assumes pacemaking responsibility.

- The influence of the autonomic nervous system can also affect the heart:
    - SYMPATHETIC stimulation causes:
    increased heart rate
    increased AV conduction
    increased irritability
    - PARASYMPATHETIC stimulation causes:
    decreased heart rate
    decreased AV conduction
    decreased irritability.

- The sympathetic branch influences both the atria (i.e., the SA node, the intraatrial and internodal pathways, and the AV junction) and the ventricles; the parasympathetic branch influences only the atria.

- If one branch of the autonomic nervous system is blocked, the effects of the opposing branch will prevail.

Self-Test: Electrophysiology

Directions:

Complete this self-evaluation of the information you have learned from this chapter. If your answers are all correct and you feel comfortable with your understanding of the material, proceed to the next chapter. However, if you missed any of the questions you should review the referenced frames before proceeding. If you feel uncomfortable with any of your understanding, invest the time now to go back over the entire chapter. DO NOT PROCEED WITH THE NEXT CHAPTER UNTIL YOU ARE VERY COMFORTABLE WITH THE MATERIAL IN THIS CHAPTER.

Question	Referenced Frames	
1. Name the two types of cardiac cells and tell what type of activity each is responsible for.	1, 2, 3, 4	electrical: conduction; mechanical: contraction
2. How do these two types of cells work together to produce cardiac activity?	1, 2, 3, 4	electrical cells stimulate muscle cells to contract
3. What physical signs are used to reflect the mechanical function of the heart?	5, 6, 7, 8, 9a	pulses, blood pressure, other perfusion parameters
4. How do you assess electrical activity in the heart?	5, 6, 7, 8, 10	analyze the EKG
5. Arrhythmias are manifestations of which type of cardiac activity?	9, 10, 11, 12	electrical
6. What happens when the positive and negative electrical charges exchange places across the cell membrane of a cardiac cell?	13, 14, 15, 16, 17	it initiates the flow of electrical current
7. Explain the polarized state.	14, 15, 16, 17, 19, 21	when electrical charges are balanced and in a state of readiness for discharge

Question	Referenced Frames	
8. Explain depolarization.	16, 17, 20, 22	the discharge of electrical energy that accompanies the transfer of electrical charges across the cell membrane
9. Is depolarization the same as contraction?	17	No, depolarization is an electrical phenomenon; contraction is mechanical and is expected to follow depolarization.
10. What is repolarization?	18, 20, 21	the return of the electrical charges to their original state of readiness
11. List the areas of the conduction system in the order in which the impulses travel through the heart.	23, 24, 25, 26, 27, 29	1. SA node; 2. intraatrial and internodal pathways; 3. AV node; 4. Bundle of His; 5. Bundle Branches 6. Purkinje Fibers
12. Which site is normally the pacemaker of the heart and why?	24, 33, 34, 43, 44	SA node, because it has the fastest inherent rate

Question	Referenced Frames	
13. Give the inherent rates for each of the following sites: Sinus Node _____ AV Junction _____ Ventricles _____	30, 31, 32, 38, 39, 40, 41, 42	60–100 times per minute 40–60 times per minute 20–40 times per minute
14. What process is responsible for a site speeding up and overriding a higher site, thus taking over as pacemaker?	33, 34, 35, 45, 46	irritability
15. What mechanism is in play if a lower site takes over responsibility for the pacemaking function following failure of a higher site?	33, 36, 37, 47, 48	escape
16. Which nervous system has two branches that control the activities of the heart?	49	autonomic
17. Name the two branches of the nervous system identified in the preceding question.	49, 52	sympathetic; parasympathetic
18. List three things that will happen to the heart if the sympathetic branch is stimulated.	49, 50, 51, 53	increased rate, increased AV conduction, increased irritability
19. List three things that will happen to the heart if the parasympathetic branch is stimulated.	49, 50, 51, 58	decreased rate, decreased AV conduction, decreased irritability
20. What part of the heart does the sympathetic branch innervate?	49, 54	the atria and ventricles
21. What part of the heart does the parasympathetic branch innervate?	49, 54	only the atria
22. What happens if one branch is blocked?	50, 51, 55, 56, 57, 58	the influence of the opposing branch will control the heart

2

Waves
and Measurements

...e last chapter you learned that arrhythmias are manifesta-
...s of the heart's _____ activity. And you learned that
the study of arrhythmias is called _____. In order to
study arrhythmias, we have to transform the electrical activity into
a format that can be seen.

electrical;
electrocardi-
ography

2. The electrical patterns of the heart can be picked up from the
surface of the skin by attaching an electrode to the skin and con-
necting it to a machine which will display the electrical activity on
graph paper. An electrode is a small item attached to the patient's
_____ and then connected by wire to a machine capable
of inscribing the patterns on graph _____.

skin;
paper

3. The electrical activity is displayed best if you can assure good
contact between the electrode and the skin. This can be done in
several ways:
  * abrade the skin slightly
  * remove any obstacles such as dirt or hair
  * use a contact medium such as saline or commercial gel
All of these measures are intended to improve _____
between the electrode and the skin.

contact

4. An _____ placed on the skin can pick up electrical
activity from within the heart and display it on graph paper using an
EKG machine. To ensure a good tracing you must provide good contact between the _____ and the _____.

electrode

skin; electrode

5. Contact between the skin and the electrode can be improved by
lightly _____ the skin, by wiping off excess _____,
or possibly even _____ excess hair. An important way to
ensure good contact is to use some type of contact medium, such as
_____ or commercial _____.

abrading; dirt;
shaving

saline; gel

6. When an EKG machine is turned on but isn't yet connected to
the patient's electrodes, the writing point (stylus) of the machine will
simply produce a straight line on the paper. This line is called the
"isoelectric line" because all of the electrical forces are equal; no current is flowing. Once the machine is connected to the patient's electrodes the needle will move up or down on the paper (above or below the isoelectric line) in response to the electrical forces it receives.
If no current is flowing, or if the forces balance each other out, the
graph paper will show a _____ _____. If the ma-
chine receives a flow of electricity, the needle will move _____
or _____ in response to the current.

straight line;
up;
down

7. A very basic rule of electrocardiography refers to the flow of
electricity through the heart and out to the electrodes. This rule
states that: If the electricity flows *toward* the *positive* electrode, the
patterns produced on the graph paper will be *upright*.

The converse of this rule is also true: if the electricity flows *away* from the positive electrode (or toward the negative electrode) the pattern will be a downward deflection. If the flow of electricity is toward the positive electrode the machine will produce an _____ | upright deflection on the graph paper (Fig. 4).

8.   Look at Fig. 4. If the electrical flow is toward the negative electrode, would you expect the graph paper to show a positive or a negative deflection? _____ | negative

9.   If the graph paper shows a positive deflection, you would assume the electrical activity is flowing primarily toward the _____ | positive electrode.

10.   If the deflection on the graph paper is negative, you can assume that the electrical flow is toward the _____ electrode and | negative away from the _____ electrode. | positive

11.   Thus we can determine the direction of electrical flow by the type of deflection made on the EKG paper. But to draw any conclusions based on this information, we must be sure that the electrodes are always in the same place on the patient so that the information is not misleading. The placement of the electrodes on patients is always _____ to avoid confusion or misinterpretation of | the same information. | (standardized)

12.   The positioning of electrodes for monitoring the EKG allows you to see a single view of the heart's electrical pattern. By rearranging electrodes, many such views are possible. (This concept can be compared to a camera which can photograph the heart from many angles, each one giving additional depth to the overall visualization of the heart itself.) Each view of the heart is called a "lead." Leads can be changed by a knob on the machine that diverts the flow of electricity through different electrodes. For sophisticated EKG interpretation, many leads are inspected to visualize the entire heart. However, for basic arrhythmia interpretation, it is only necessary to monitor a single lead. A monitoring lead shows only one _____ of | view the heart's electrical activity.

13.   When monitoring a patient for patterns of electrical activity such as arrhythmias, a lead is selected which gives the clearest picture of the basic waves. For simplicity, all of the information in this book will refer to a single lead, Lead II, since it is probably the most common monitoring lead. Another very common monitoring lead is the modified chest lead, or MCL_1. MCL_1 is becoming more widely used and may well be used in the area you work. When making simple arrhythmia interpretations, however, we do not need to get into a distinction between MCL_1 and Lead II. We will only be looking at how the various waves relate to each other within a single lead; we won't be

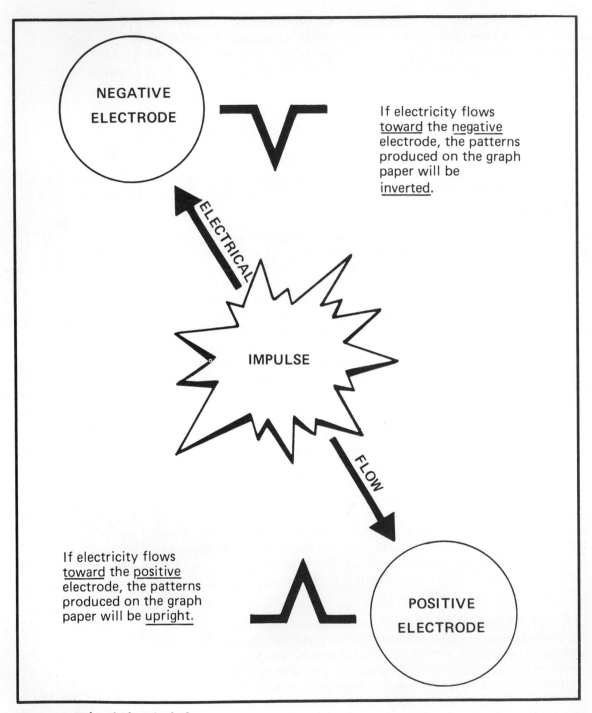

Figure 4. Rule of Electrical Flow

discussing how the leads compare to each other. Therefore, this book will refer only to Lead II, because it is a very common monitoring lead and shows clear views of the basic _____. All information in this book should be assumed to apply to _____ unless otherwise specified.

waves; Lead II

14.   Figure 5 shows the placement of electrodes to monitor Lead II. Note that the positive electrode is at the apex of the heart and the negative electrode is below the right clavicle. The third electrode is a ground electrode, and does not measure electrical flow in this lead. Since the pacemaker is normally in the _____ and the electrical current flows toward the ventricles, the primary thrust of electrical flow in the heart will be toward the positive electrode in Lead II. Thus the primary deflections in Lead II will be _____.

SA node

upright

15.   All EKG interpretation relies on the use of standardized, uniform graph paper. The size of the graph on the paper and the speed at which the paper travels through the EKG machine are both kept constant; all EKG paper is the same and all EKG machines operate at the same speed. By keeping the paper and the speed standardized, we can look at the patterns created by an individual's heart activity and compare them to what has been established as "normal" activity. If the graph paper were not _____, we would not be able to compare one person's EKG to any other EKG, nor would we be able to compare several EKGs taken on one person at different times. Similarly, if all EKG machines ran at different _____, we would not have a constant "norm" for comparing individual EKGs.

standardized

speeds

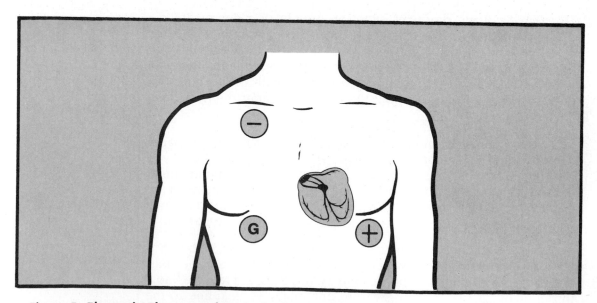

Figure 5. Electrode Placement for Monitoring Lead II

16. Since all graph paper has _____ markings we must | standardized
learn what these markings mean so that we will be able to interpret
the EKG tracings that are superimposed on the graph paper. Look at
the sample graph paper shown in Figure 6. You will notice that there
are lines going up and down (vertical) and lines going across (horizontal). Also, notice that every fifth line is heavier than the other
lighter lines. How many light lines are there between two heavy
ones? _____ | 4

17. The lines on the graph paper can help determine both the direction and the magnitude of deflections. When all electrical forces
are equal there is neither an upright nor a downward deflection; an
isoelectric line is created. If the electrical force is toward the positive
electrode, the stylus will draw an _____ wave. If the | upright
force travels primarily toward the negative electrode the wave will
be _____. If no current is present, or if positive and neg- | downward
ative forces are equal, the graph paper will show a _____ | (inverted)
line, called an isoelectric line. | straight

18. It is the strength of the current, or its voltage, that will determine
the magnitude of the deflection. If it is a very strong positive wave, it
will create a high spike above the isoelectric line. If it is a very weak
positive charge the deflection will go only slightly above the isoelectric line in response to the amplitude of the charge. Therefore, the
height of the deflection will indicate the _____ of the | voltage (or
electrical charge which produced that deflection. The same principle | amplitude)
holds for negative deflections. The stronger the charge, the deeper
the wave will go below the isoelectric line.

19. Since voltage produces either an upright or a downward deflection on the EKG, the magnitude of the current can be measured
by comparing the height of the spike against the horizontal lines on
the graph paper (Fig. 7). Voltage can be measured quantitatively (in
millivolts) but you need not concern yourself with these figures for
basic arrhythmia interpretation. On the graph paper the horizontal
lines measure _____. | voltage

20. The second, and more important, thing that the graph paper
can provide is a determination of time. The vertical lines can tell you
just how much time it took for the electrical current within the heart
to travel from one area to another. The vertical lines are the most important marking for simple arrhythmia identification because they
can tell you about the _____ it takes for the current to | time
travel about within the heart.

21. The standard rate at which the EKG machine runs paper past
the stylus is 25 millimeters per second. At this standard rate we know
that it takes .20 seconds to get from one *heavy* vertical line to the
next heavy vertical line. Therefore, if a deflection began on one

heavy line and ended on the next heavy line we would know that the electrical current within the heart that caused the deflection lasted _____ seconds. This is an essential figure to remember because it is the basis for many of the rates, rules, and normal values you will learn in later sections. The distance (in time) between two heavy vertical lines on the EKG graph paper is _____ seconds.

.20

.20

Figure 6: Sample EKG Graph Paper. The three vertical lines in the upper margin are measures of time standard to all EKG graph paper. The distance between two "tic" marks is 3 seconds, thus this strip measures 6 seconds in duration.

22.   If the time frame between two heavy vertical lines is .20 seconds and there are five small squares within this same area, it would follow that each of these small squares is equivalent to 1/5 of .20 seconds, or .04 seconds each. The distance (in time) between two light vertical lines, or across one small square, is _____ seconds.

.04

23.   You can see now that graph paper can be used to measure _____ and _____.

voltage; time

24.   As you know, the heart has four chambers. The upper two are the atria and the lower two are the ventricles. In most cases the atria function as a team and contract together, and the ventricles also operate as a single unit. So for nearly all of our discussions we will consider the atria as a single unit and the ventricles as a single unit, even though we realize they are actually the _____ separate chambers which make up the heart.

four

25.   The upper chambers of the heart are called the _____, and they will be considered a single _____. Likewise, the _____ are the lower chambers and will be considered a _____ unit.

atria;
unit;
ventricles;
single

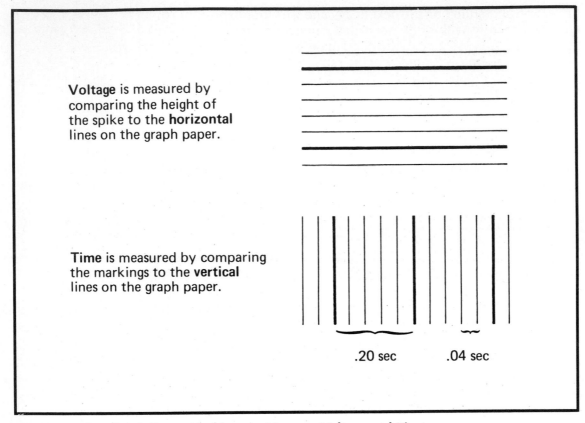

Voltage is measured by comparing the height of the spike to the **horizontal** lines on the graph paper.

Time is measured by comparing the markings to the **vertical** lines on the graph paper.

.20 sec   .04 sec

Figure 7. Using Graph Paper Markings to Measure Voltage and Time

26.   In the normal heart, blood enters both atria simultaneously and then is forced into both ventricles simultaneously as the atria contract. All of this is coordinated so that the atria fill while the ventricles contract, and when the ventricles are filling the atria contract. In considering a cardiac cycle we would expect the _____ to contract first.

atria

27.   Before the atria can contract, they must first receive an electrical stimulus to initiate the muscle cell response. In fact, for any myocardial cell to contract it must first receive an _____ stimulus. We know that the _____ cells have the ability to initiate an impulse. And we know that the same electrical impulses that eventually produce contraction of the heart can also produce deflections on the EKG graph paper. It is by careful scrutiny of these wave patterns that we are able to determine the _____ activity that is present in the heart, and sometimes we can even speculate on the type of _____ activity that could be expected. But to make these determinations we must first investigate the _____ patterns produced by the heart's electrical activity.

electrical;
electrical

electrical;

mechanical

wave

28. During each phase of the cardiac electrical cycle a distinct pattern is produced on the EKG _____ paper. By learning to recognize these wave patterns and the cardiac activity each represents, we can study the relationships between the different areas of the heart and begin to understand what is taking place within the heart at any given time. For each pacemaker impulse, the electrical flow travels down the _____ pathways, depolarizing the atria and then the ventricles as it goes. Following this, the pattern begins again with another impulse from the pacemaker. Each cardiac cycle includes all of the electrical activity that would normally be expected to produce a single heart beat. The cardiac cycle begins with the initiating impulse from the pacemaker and encompasses all phases until the ventricles are repolarized. On the EKG graph paper the cardiac cycle includes all of the wave patterns produced by electrical activity beginning with the _____ impulse and including ventricular _____ .

graph

conduction

pacemaker; repolarization

29. On the EKG, each of these phases is displayed by a specific wave pattern. Figure 8 shows a series of cardiac electrical cycles which makes up a typical EKG rhythm strip. In Figure 9 a single cardiac cycle has been enlarged so that we can see each of the individual patterns more closely. A single cardiac cycle is expected to produce one _____ beat. An EKG rhythm strip is composed of more than one _____ cycle.

heart; cardiac

30. In labeling the activity on the graph paper, the deflections above or below the isoelectric line are called waves. In a single car-

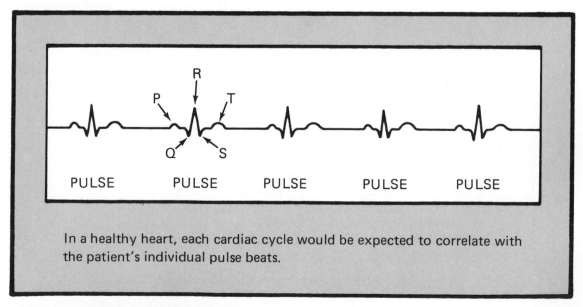

In a healthy heart, each cardiac cycle would be expected to correlate with the patient's individual pulse beats.

Figure 8. A Typical EKG Rhythm Strip

diac cycle there are five prominent waves, and each is labeled with a letter. Look at Figure 9 and find the P, Q, R, S, and T waves. An "interval" refers to the area between (and possibly including) waves, and a "segment" identifies a straight line or area of electrical inactivity between waves. Find the PR segment and the PR interval (PRI) on Figure 9. Does the PR segment include any waves? _____ What about the PR interval, does it include any waves? _____

No;
Yes—the PRI includes the P wave and the PR segment

31. The first wave you see on the cardiac cycle is the P wave. Locate it in Figure 9. The P wave starts with the first deflection from the isoelectric line. The _____ wave is indicative of atrial depolarization.

P

32. When you see a P wave on the EKG, does that mean that the atria contracted? _____

No, not necessarily. It means the atria were depolarized, but it is possible that the muscle cells did not contract in response. It is impossible to tell whether or not the atria contracted simply by looking at the EKG.

33. As the impulse leaves the atria and travels to the AV node it encounters a slight delay. The tissues of the node do not conduct impulses as fast as other cardiac electrical tissues. This means that the wave of depolarization will take a longer time to get through the AV node than it would in other parts of the heart. On the EKG this is translated into a short period of electrical inactivity called the PR segment. This is the straight line between the P wave and the next wave. Locate the PR segment on Figure 9. The PR segment is indicative of the delay in the _____.

AV node

34. The AV node is the area of the heart with the slowest conduction speed. That is, the conductive tissues of the sinus node, the atria, and the ventricles all conduct impulses faster than the AV node

does. This is necessary to allow time for atrial contraction and complete filling of the ventricles. On the EKG tracing this delay at the AV _____ is seen as a short isoelectric segment between the _____ wave and the next wave. This segment is called the _____ segment.

node;
P;
PR

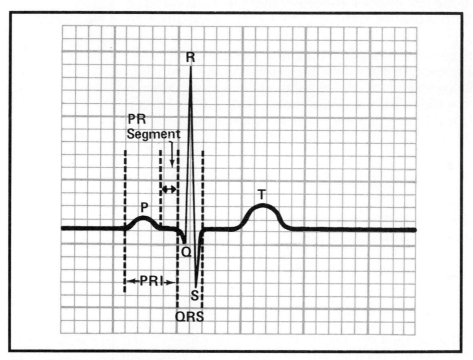

Figure 9. The EKG Complex

35.   If you wished to refer to all of the electrical activity in the heart before the impulse reached the ventricles you would look at the PR interval. This includes both the P wave and the PR segment. The P wave displays _____ depolarization and the PR segment is caused by the _____ in the AV node. Therefore, the PR _____ includes all atrial and nodal activity.

atrial;
delay;
interval

36.   By definition, the PR interval begins at the first sign of the P wave and ends at the first deflection of the next wave, called the QRS complex. The PR interval includes all _____ activity and all _____ activity, but does not include ventricular activity.

atrial;
nodal

37.   The ventricular depolarization is shown on the EKG by a large complex of three waves: the Q, the R, and the S. Collectively, these are called the QRS complex. This complex is significantly larger than the P wave because ventricular depolarization involves a greater muscle mass than atrial depolarization. The QRS complex starts with

the Q wave. The Q wave is defined as the first negative deflection following the P wave, but before the R wave. Locate the Q wave on Figure 9. The Q wave flows immediately into the R wave, which is the first positive deflection following the P wave. Next comes the S wave, which is defined as the second negative deflection following the P wave, or the first negative deflection after the R wave. Collectively, the QRS complex signifies _____ depolarization.   ventricular

38.   The QRS complex is larger and more complicated than the P wave, primarily because it involves a larger part of the heart. Very often, the QRS complex looks different from the complex shown in Figure 9, but it is still called the QRS complex. Several different configurations of the QRS complex are shown in Figure 10. Regardless of appearance, these still indicate depolarization of the _____.   ventricles

39.   After the ventricles depolarize they begin their repolarization phase, which results in another wave on the EKG. The T wave is indicative of ventricular repolarization. The atria also repolarize, but their repolarization usually occurs at the same time as ventricular depolarization, so the atrial repolarization wave is usually hidden in the _____ complex. Ventricular repolarization is much   QRS
more prominent, and is seen on the EKG as the _____   T
wave.

40.   Now that you have learned the definitions of all of the waves   Practice
on the EKG and what each one means, turn to Practice Sheet 1 and   Sheet 1
label each wave on each practice strip. Be sure to recall what each wave means as you mark them on the EKG. When you finish marking the waves, go back and identify the PR interval, the PR segment, and the QRS complex for each strip.

41.   To interpret arrhythmias you must be able to measure the PR interval and the duration of the QRS complex. The grid markings on the graph paper are used to determine just how many seconds it took for the impulse to create those intervals. In order for you to make these measurements you will use EKG calipers. Let's measure the PRI first. You can use Figure 9 for practice. Place one point of the calipers on the very first deflection that marks the beginning of the P wave. Then place the other point of the calipers on the final point of the PR interval, which you will recall is actually the very beginning of the _____ complex. Make sure you don't have any part   QRS
of the QRS complex included in your measurement. Now, count the number of small boxes within your caliper points, and multiply that number by _____ seconds, which is the amount of time   .04
allotted to each small box. What is your measurement? _____   .16
seconds

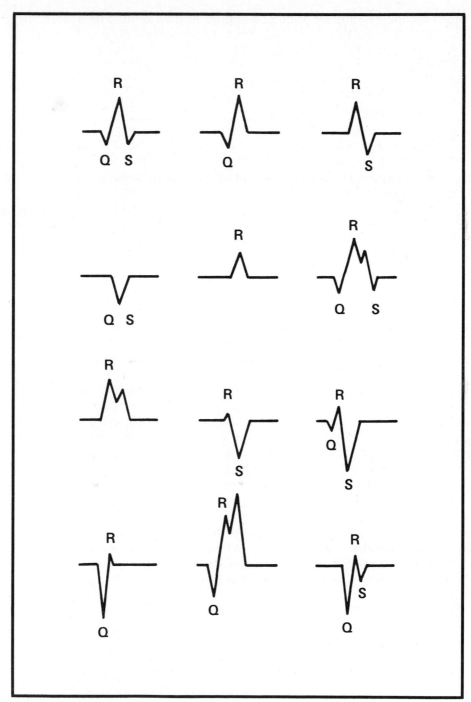

Figure 10. Various QRS Configurations

42. In order for the PR interval to be considered normal it must be between .12 and .20 seconds. If it is less than .12 seconds it is considered a short PRI, and if it is greater than .20 seconds it is said to be prolonged. The P wave itself does not contribute to a long PRI; it is actually the delay in the AV node, or the PR _____, that varies according to how long the node held the impulse before transmitting it. The normal PRI should be _____–_____ seconds; a long PRI would suggest _____ in the _____ _____.

segment

.12–.20; delay; AV node

43. Is the PRI measurement you determined for the complex shown in Figure 9 considered to be normal? _____.

Yes—it is .16 seconds, which is within the normal range of .12–.20 seconds.

44. You measure the QRS complex in the same way as the PR interval. Just make sure your caliper points are exactly where the definitions tell you they should be. The Q wave should be measured where the deflection first begins to go below the isoelectric line. This part usually isn't so hard. The S wave is more difficult. Between the S wave and the T wave is a section called the ST segment. Although segments are supposed to be straight lines, the ST segment often gets caught up in the transition between the QRS complex and the T wave, and is very rarely a cut-and-dried configuration. So you must look for some clue that indicates to you where the S wave stops and the _____ wave begins. If such an indication is present, it will usually be a very small notch or other movement suggesting an alteration of electrical flow. At any rate, this should be the outside measurement of the QRS complex. Include in your measurement the entire S wave, but don't let it overlap into the ST segment or the T wave. The QRS complex measurement should include the beginning of the _____ wave and the end of the _____ wave.

T

Q; S

45. For practice, measure the QRS complex shown in Figure 9. What is your measurement? _____ seconds.

.08

46. People very rarely agree on what a normal time range is for the QRS measurement. It is usually considered to be between .06 and .11 seconds. For simplicity, we'll define the normal QRS complex measurement as anything less than .12 seconds. This means that the ventricles took a normal amount of time to depolarize if they did it in less than _____ seconds.

.12

47.   Is the QRS measurement shown in Figure 9 considered to be normal? _____

Yes – it measures .08 seconds, which is less than .12 seconds.

48.   Now that you know how to measure PRIs and QRSs, the rest is up to you. All it takes is practice, practice, and more practice. It is particularly helpful if you can get someone to check your measurements in the beginning so you don't develop bad habits. You can start by measuring the PRI and QRS on each of the practice strips on Practice Sheet 2. The answer key shows you where the calipers were placed to obtain the answers, so if your measurements differ from those given, look to see where the complex was measured to arrive at the answer shown.

Practice Sheet 2

49.   The complexes on an EKG tracing are created by electrical activity within the heart. But it is possible for things other than cardiac activity to interfere with the tracing you are trying to analyze. Some common causes of interference, or artifact, are:
   • muscle tremors, shivering
   • patient movement
   • loose electrodes
   • the effect of other electrical equipment in the room (called 60–cycle interference)
Each of these situations can cause _____ on the EKG tracing that may interfere with your interpretation of the arrhythmia. When such external factors cause deflections on an EKG strip, those deflections are considered to be artifact, and are important to recognize because they can _____ with your interpretation of the arrhythmia.

artifact

interfere

50.   Figure 11 shows you what each of these types of interference can look like on an EKG tracing. As you can see, _____ can often confuse you and lead you to believe that the deflection was caused by cardiac activity when it was not. As you practice identifying the P waves and QRS complexes you will become more and more familiar with the normal configurations of these wave forms, and will be more apt to distinguish them from artifact. When trying to determine whether or not a deflection was caused by artifact, you should try to identify the _____ waves and _____ complexes of the underlying rhythm and compare these configurations with the questionable deflections.

artifact

P; QRS

51.   Let's go back to electrophysiology to make one final point. Since depolarization takes place when the electrical charges begin

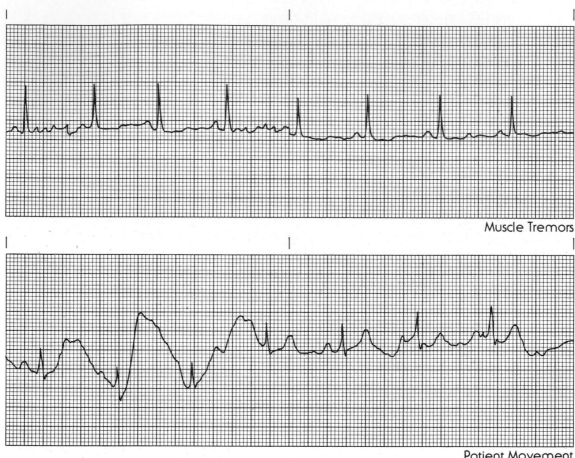

Muscle Tremors

Patient Movement

Figure 11. Types of Interference

their wave of movement by exchanging places across the cell membrane, it would follow that this process can not take place unless the charges are in their original position. This means that the cell cannot depolarize until the _____ process is complete. In order for depolarization to take place, repolarization must be _____.

repolarization
complete

52.   When the charges are depolarized and have not yet returned to their polarized state, the cell is said to be electrically "refractory" because it cannot accept another impulse yet. If a cell is _____ it cannot accept an impulse because it isn't yet _____.

refractory;
repolarized

53.   On the EKG the refractory period of the ventricles is when they are depolarizing or repolarizing. Thus the QRS and the T wave on the EKG would be considered the _____ period of the cardiac cycle, since it signifies a period when the heart would be unable to respond to an impulse.

refractory

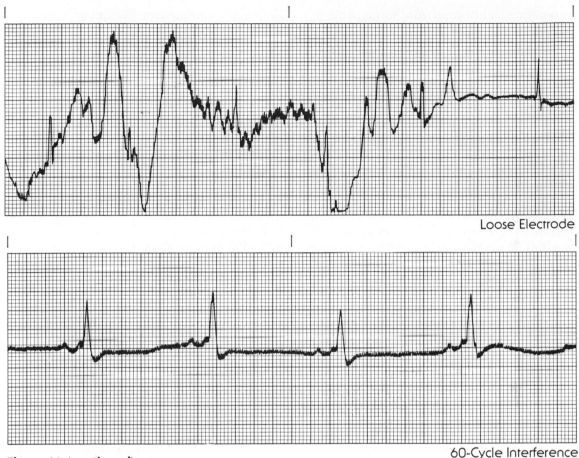

Loose Electrode

60-Cycle Interference

Figure 11 (continued)

54.   Sometimes an electrical impulse will try to discharge the cell before repolarization is fully complete. In most cases nothing will happen because the cells aren't back to their original position and therefore can't _____. But once in a while, if the stimulus is strong enough, an impulse might find several of the charges in the right position and thus discharge them before the rest of the cell is ready. This results in abnormal depolarization, and hence is an undesirable occurrence. This premature depolarization can occur only if most of the cell charges are back to the _____ position. Thus there is a small part of the refractory period that is not absolutely refractory. This small section is called the "relative" refractory period because some of the charges are polarized and thus can be _____ if the impulse is strong enough.

depolarize

original

depolarized

55.   So, there are actually two refractory periods: an absolute refractory period, when no impulse could cause depolarization, and a relative refractory period, when a strong impulse could cause a

premature, abnormal discharge. The _____ refractory | relative
period would allow depolarization if the impulse were strong enough,
while the _____ refractory period would not allow any | absolute
response at all.

56.   Figure 12 shows you where these refractory periods are located
on the EKG. Notice that while all of the T wave is considered a
refractory period, the downslope of the T wave is only relatively refractory. This means that if a strong impulse fell on the downslope of
the T wave it could result in ventricular _____. This fact | depolarization
will become more important to you when we begin to look at specific arrhythmias.

57.   You now have all of the information you need to begin analyzing EKG rhythm strips. You can identify all of the different waves that
make up a cardiac cycle, and you can measure the PRI and the QRS
complex. You are now ready to turn to Chapter 3 and learn how to
apply this knowledge as you develop a technique for analyzing EKG
rhythm strips.

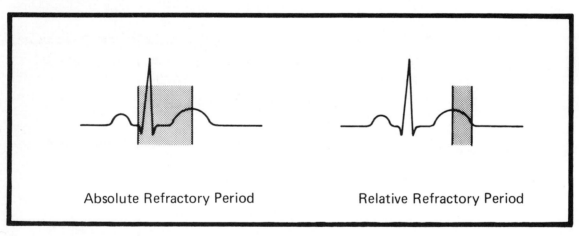

Absolute Refractory Period   Relative Refractory Period

Figure 12. Refractory Periods

Key Points — Waves and Measurements

- Electrodes are devices which are applied to the skin to detect electrical activity and convey it to a machine for display.

- Electrode contact can be improved by:
    - abrading the skin
    - cleaning or drying the skin
    - using contact medium.

- If electricity flows toward the positive electrode the patterns produced on the graph paper will be upright; if the electrical flow is toward the negative electrode the patterns will be inverted.

- Electrode placement is standardized to avoid confusion in EKG interpretation (Fig. 5).

- A lead is a single view of the heart, often produced by a combination of information from several electrodes.

- A monitoring lead is one that shows clear wave configuration, very frequently Lead II.

- Graph paper is standardized to allow comparative analysis of EKG wave patterns.

- The isoelectric line is the straight line made on the EKG when no electrical current is flowing.

- Vertical lines on the graph paper measure time; horizontal lines measure voltage (Fig. 7).

- A small square on the graph paper (the distance between two light vertical lines) is .04 seconds.

- A large square on the graph paper (the distance between two heavy vertical lines) is .20 seconds.

- The atria normally contract before the ventricles.

- A single cardiac cycle on the EKG includes everything from depolarization of the atria up to and including repolarization of the ventricles.

- A single cardiac cycle is expected to produce a single heart beat (a pulse).

- The P wave represents atrial depolarization.

- The PR segment represents delay in the AV node.

- The PR interval includes the P wave and the PR segment, and represents both atrial depolarization and delay in the AV node.

- The PRI is measured from the beginning of the P wave to the beginning of the QRS complex.

- The PRI is normally between .12 and .20 seconds.

- The QRS complex represents ventricular depolarization.

- The QRS interval is measured from the beginning of the Q wave to the end of the S wave.

- The Q wave is the first negative deflection following the P wave, but before the R wave.

- The R wave is the first positive wave following the P wave, or the first positive wave of the QRS complex.

- The S wave is the second negative deflection following the P wave, or the first negative deflection following the R wave.

- The QRS interval is usually less than .12 seconds.

- External factors capable of producing artifact on the EKG tracing include: muscle tremors, shivering, patient movement, loose electrodes, and 60–cycle electrical current.

- A cell is electrically refractory when it has not yet repolarized and thus cannot accept and respond to another stimulus.

- The absolute refractory period occurs when the cells cannot respond to any stimulus at all.

- The relative refractory period occurs when some of the cells are capable of responding if the stimulus is strong enough.

- If an impulse falls during the relative refractory period the heart might be depolarized, but in an abnormal way.

- The absolute refractory period encompasses the QRS and the first part of the T wave.

- The relative refractory period is the downslope of the T wave.

Self-Test: Waves and Measurements

Directions:

Complete this self-evaluation of the information you have learned from this chapter. If your answers are all correct and you feel comfortable with your understanding of the material, proceed to the next chapter. However, if you missed any of the questions you should review the referenced frames before proceeding. If you feel uncomfortable with any of your understanding, invest the time now to go back over the entire chapter. DO NOT PROCEED WITH THE NEXT CHAPTER UNTIL YOU ARE VERY COMFORTABLE WITH THE MATERIAL IN THIS CHAPTER.

Question	Referenced Frames	
1. What is an electrode used for?	1, 2, 4	To pick up electrical activity from the skin surface.
2. List three ways to improve contact between the electrode and the skin.	2, 3, 4, 5	abrade skin; clean skin; use contact medium
3. If the electrical current flows toward the positive electrode, will the deflection on the graph paper be upright or downward?	6, 7, 8, 9, 10, 17	upright
4. Why is it important to standardize electrode placement?	11, 12	To avoid confusion when interpreting EKG patterns.
5. What is a lead, and how does it differ from an electrode?	12, 13	A lead is a single view of the heart, often produced by a combination of information from several electrodes.
6. How many leads do you need to know to interpret arrhythmias?	12, 13	one; only a monitoring lead

Question	**Referenced Frames**	
7. Which lead will be discussed throughout this book?	13	Lead II
8. What are the electrode positions for the lead identified in the preceding question?	14	negative electrode below right clavicle; positive electrode at the apex; ground electrode below the right nipple
9. What features are important for a good monitoring lead?	12, 13	clear visualization of the basic waves
10. In Lead II, will the primary deflections be upright or downward on the EKG?	14	Upright, because the current is flowing toward the positive electrode.
11. Why is it important to use standardized EKG graph paper?	15, 16	Standardized markings enable you to measure the EKG and compare it to "normal."
12. What is an isoelectric line?	17	The straight line on the EKG made when no electrical current is flowing.
13. What do the vertical lines on the graph paper tell you?	16, 17, 20, 21, 22, 23	time

Question	**Referenced Frames**	
14. What do the horizontal lines on the graph paper tell you?	16, 17, 18, 19, 23	voltage
15. How much time is involved between two heavy lines on the graph paper?	16, 21, 22	.20 seconds
16. How much time is involved in one small square on the graph paper?	16, 21, 22	.04 seconds
17. Which chambers contract first in a single cardiac cycle?	24, 25, 26	the atria
18. What must occur in order for the heart to contract?	27	The muscle cells must receive an electrical stimulus.
19. What cardiac activity is included in a single cardiac cycle on the EKG?	28	Everything from depolarization of the atria up to and including repolarization of the ventricles.
20. How many heart beats would you expect a single cardiac cycle to produce?	28, 29	one
21. What are the five waves found in a single cardiac cycle on the EKG?	30, 40	P, Q, R, S, and T
22. Differentiate between waves, segments, and intervals.	30	waves are deflections, segments are straight lines, and intervals include both waves and segments
23. What does the P wave represent and how is it found on the EKG?	31	atrial depolarization; it is measured from the first

Question	**Referenced Frames**	
		deflection on the cardiac cycle until the deflection returns to the isoelectric line
24. What does the PR segment represent?	33, 34	delay in the AV node
25. What is the PR interval, how is it measured, and what is its normal duration?	35, 36, 41, 42, 43, 48	The PRI includes the P wave and the PR segment; it is measured from the beginning of the P wave to the very beginning of the QRS complex; it is normally .12–.20 seconds.
26. What does the QRS represent; how is it measured and what is its normal duration?	37, 38, 44, 45, 46, 47, 48	ventricular depolarization; measure from the beginning of the Q wave to the end of the S wave; normally less than .12 seconds
27. What does the T wave represent?	39	ventricular repolarization
28. List four external factors capable of producing artifact on the EKG tracing.	49, 50	muscle tremors, shivering; patient movement;

Question	**Referenced Frames**	
		loose electrodes; 60–cycle electrical current
29. What is meant by electrical refractoriness?	51, 52, 53	The cells are not yet repolarized and thus cannot accept and respond to another stimulus.
30. Differentiate between absolute refractory period and relative refractory period.	54, 55, 56	Absolute refractory period means the heart cannot accept any stimulus at all; relative refractory period means that some of the cells are capable of responding to a strong stimulus.
31. What is so important about the relative refractory period?	54, 55, 56	If an impulse hits on the relative refractory period the heart can be discharged in an abnormal way.
32. What part of the EKG complex signifies the relative refractory period?	56	The down-slope of the T wave.

Practice Sheet 1: Labeling Waves

Directions

For each of the rhythm strips below, label the P, Q, R, S, and T waves of a single cardiac cycle. (Some of the tracings may not have all of these waves.) As you finish each strip, check your answers with the key on p. 368.

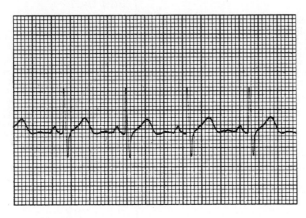

1.1

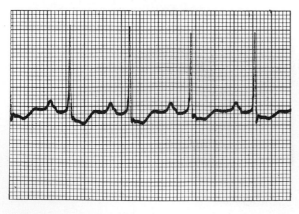

1.2

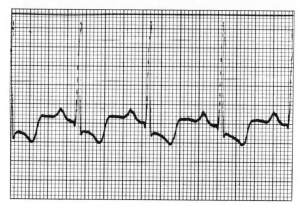

1.3

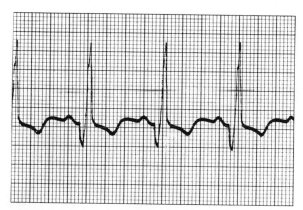

1.4

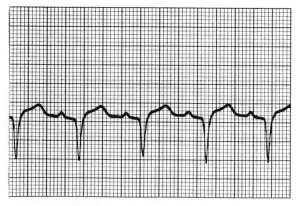

1.5

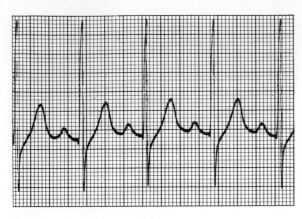

1.6

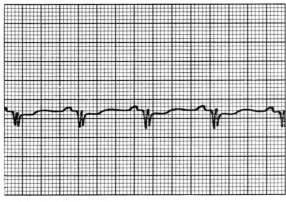

1.7

When you have completed this exercise, check your answers with the key on page 368; then return to Frame 41 in Chapter 2 (page 30).

Practice Sheet 2:
Measuring Intervals

Directions

For each of the rhythm strips below, measure the PR interval and the QRS complex. As you do each strip, check with the answer key on page 371.

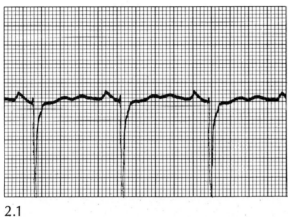

2.1

PRI: _____ seconds
QRS: _____ seconds

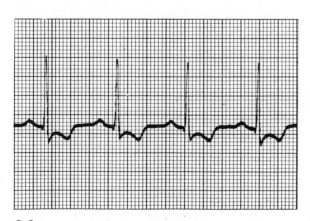

2.2

PRI: _____ seconds
QRS: _____ seconds

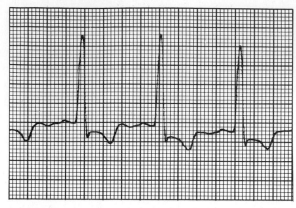

2.3

PRI: _____ seconds
QRS: _____ seconds

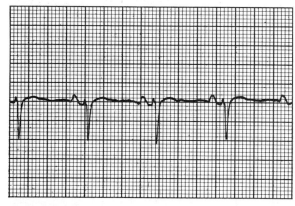

2.4

PRI: _____ seconds
QRS: _____ seconds

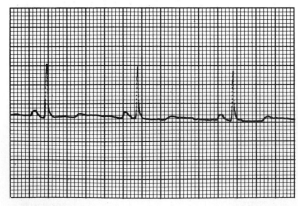

2.5

PRI: _____ seconds
QRS: _____ seconds

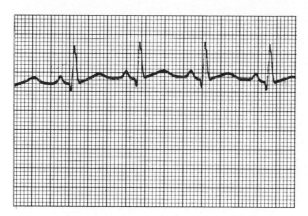

2.6

PRI: _____ **seconds**
QRS: _____ **seconds**

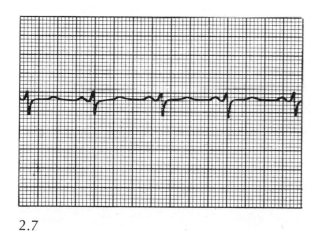

2.7

PRI: _____ **seconds**
QRS: _____ **seconds**

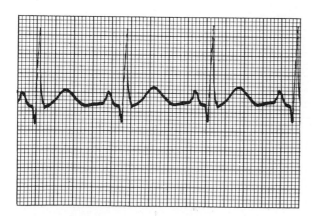

2.8

PRI: _____ **seconds**
QRS: _____ **seconds**

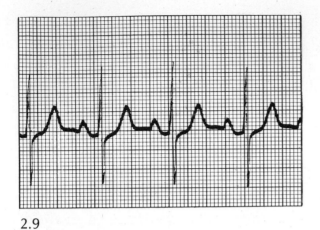

2.9

PRI: _____ seconds
QRS: _____ seconds

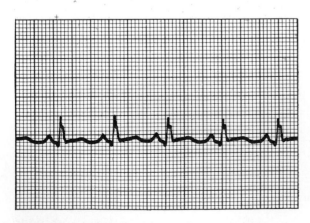

2.10

PRI: _____ seconds
QRS: _____ seconds

2.11

PRI: _____ seconds
QRS: _____ seconds

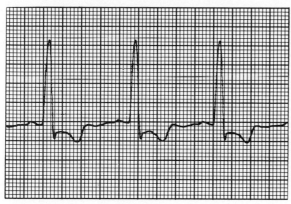

2.12

PRI: _____ **seconds**
QRS: _____ **seconds**

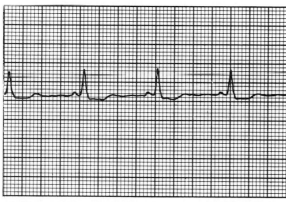

2.13

PRI: _____ **seconds**
QRS: _____ **seconds**

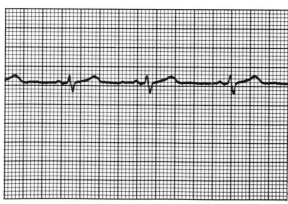

2.14

PRI: _____ **seconds**
QRS: _____ **seconds**

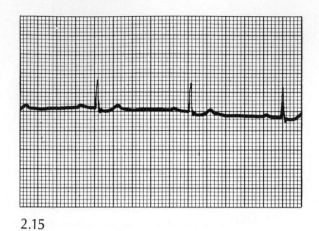

2.15

PRI: _____ **seconds**
QRS: _____ **seconds**

When you complete this exercise, return to Frame 49 in Chapter 2 (page 33).

3

Analyzing
EKG Rhythm Strips

1.   In the last chapter you learned that there are five distinct wave patterns which make up a single _____ _____ on the EKG. You also learned that a beating heart will produce a series of these _____ _____, which together become an EKG rhythm strip.

cardiac cycle;

cardiac cycles

2.   EKGs are even more complex than fingerprints. Not only does every person on earth have his or her own individual EKG, distinct from all others, but one person's EKG can look very different from one moment to the next. This is why it is inadequate to simply memorize 8 or 10 of the most common EKG patterns and hope you can recognize one next time you see it. This type of EKG analysis is called "pattern recognition" and is a common but haphazard way to approach arrhythmias. A much more reliable way to approach an EKG tracing is to take it apart, wave by wave, and interpret exactly what's happening within the heart. This method of EKG interpretation is more sophisticated than _____ _____, and will be far more valuable to you because it's more reliable.

pattern recognition

3.   Arrhythmias can be categorized into groups according to which pacemaker site initiates the rhythm. The most common sites, and thus the major categories of arrhythmias, are:
- sinus
- atrial
- junctional
- ventricular

Arrhythmias are categorized this way because the _____ impulse for that rhythm came from one of these sites.

pacemaker

4.   The most common cardiac rhythm is sinus in origin, because the _____ node is the usual pacemaker of the heart. Therefore, a normal, healthy heart would be in "Normal Sinus Rhythm," or "NSR" because it originated in the _____ node.

SA

sinus (SA)

5.   To get an idea of the variety of EKG patterns possible, look at Practice Sheet 3. All of the EKG tracings shown are sinus rhythm. You can see why it is necessary to have an organized format for approaching arrhythmia interpretation. Without a format for deciphering EKGs, you could easily be intimidated even by a group of "normal" tracings. To develop competency and confidence in interpreting EKGs, you must have an organized _____ for approaching arrhythmias.

format

6.   Each EKG tracing provides a multitude of clues as to what is happening in that heart. These clues include wave configurations, rates, measurements, and wave relationships. Experts have compiled this data and found that each cardiac arrhythmia has its own set of clues. That is, each specific arrhythmia will repeatedly give off the same set of clues. By looking at the clues available from the strip, you can tell

what the rhythm is, but only if you know in advance the kinds of clues that any specific arrhythmia is known to produce. We call these clues the "rules" for a specific arrhythmia. For example, NSR has a set of rules, including a specific relationship between P waves and QRS complexes, and a range for both rate and wave measurements. If you memorize these rules in advance and then come across a rhythm that meets these rules, you have reason to believe that this rhythm is NSR. Therefore, it is necessary to memorize the rules for each rhythm strip, and then look for the _____ available   clues
from each strip you approach.

7.   EKG interpretation is a true "gray" area; there is no black and white to any of the information you will learn here. When it comes right down to naming a rhythm, you'll find that this isn't always possible, particularly in the more complex tracings. However, the clues you get from the strip should collectively eliminate most of the possibilities and point to one or two specific patterns. From there, it is a matter of which possibility has the most clues in its favor. Even though you can't always identify the rhythm exactly, the _____   clues
you get from the strip should fit the rules of one or two arrhythmias, thus suggesting the category of arrhythmia you are trying to identify.

8.   Let's repeat the point we just made in the preceding frame, because it will be important as we go over the analysis process. As you approach an arrhythmia, look at the _____ and compare   clues
them to the rules for arrhythmias. If there are two possibilities, or two people who disagree on the interpretation, it will be decided by who has the most clues in his/her favor. Therefore, it is critical to pick up the clues from the strip and compare them to the _____   rule
for each arrhythmia. Now you can see why it will be essential to memorize the rules for each arrhythmia and have them comfortably available for recall as you begin arrhythmia interpretation.

9.   Although EKG interpretation is acknowledged to be a very negotiable field, and everyone is entitled to a personal opinion of each arrhythmia's true identity, we have been able to agree on a fairly standard format for approaching arrhythmias. This format is outlined in Figure 13, and will be discussed point by point in the next several frames. Look at Figure 13 and determine which item we will look at first, when starting to analyze an EKG. _____   regularity

10.   The regularity, or _____, of an EKG pattern is deter-   rhythm
mined by looking at the R–to–R interval (RRI). This interval is measured by placing one point of the calipers on one R wave (or any other fixed, prominent point on the QRS complex) and placing the other point on the same spot of the next QRS complex. The R wave is indicative of ventricular _____, and thus *should* corre-   depolarization;
spond to the patient's _____.   pulse

king to see if the rhythm is regular or irregular, mea- | R–R intervals
_____ _____ *across the entire strip.* If the pat-
the RRI should remain constant throughout. A con-
...RRI would mean that the rhythm is _____. | regular

12. A key point in determining regularity is to measure *all* the
RRIs across the rhythm strip. If you skip around and don't measure
_____ the RRIs, you will frequently miss a pattern of | all
irregularity.

REGULARITY (also called Rhythm)

- is it regular?
- is it irregular?
- are there any patterns to the irregularity?
- are there any ectopic beats; if so, are they early or late?

RATE

- what is the exact rate?
- is the atrial rate the same as the ventricular rate?

P WAVES

- are the P waves regular?
- is there one P wave for every QRS?
- is the P wave in front of the QRS or behind it?
- is the P wave normal and upright in Lead II?
- are there more P waves than QRS complexes?
- do all the P waves look alike?
- are the irregular P waves associated with ectopic beats?

PR INTERVAL

- are all the PRIs constant?
- is the PRI measurement within normal range?
- if the PRI varies, is there a pattern to the changing measurements?

QRS COMPLEX

- are all the QRS complexes of equal duration?
- what is the measurement of the QRS complex?
- is the QRS measurement within normal limits?
- do all the QRS complexes look alike?
- are the unusual QRS complexes associated with ectopic beats?

Figure 13. Systematic Approach to Arrhythmia Interpretation

13.   If the pattern is not regular, you must determine whether it is:

- *regularly irregular*
  (it has a pattern of irregularity)
- *basically regular*
  (it is a regular rhythm which has a beat or two that interrupts it)
- *totally irregular*
  (it has no patterns at all)

If the rhythm has a pattern to the irregularity, it is said to be _____ regularly;
irregular; if it has a beat or two that interrupts the regular pattern, it
would be basically _____; if it is totally irregular, it would   regular;
have _____ patterns.   no

14.   If the rhythm is regular across the entire strip, you can consider
it a _____ rhythm. Sometimes a rhythm will be very   regular
nearly regular, but will be "off" by one or even two small squares.
This can be especially disconcerting to the student, who is usually
still looking for everything to fit exactly. However, as you now
know, EKG interpretation isn't always exact, and regularity determination is no exception. It is not uncommon for a rhythm, especially
a slow one, to be "off" by a small square and still be considered regular. A general guideline is that faster rates should be more exactly
_____, while slower rates can sometimes have a little   regular
more leeway. The key issue is to make sure that there are no other
areas of irregularity. If there are other areas of irregularity, or if there
are patterns of irregularity, you really can't consider the rhythm to
be _____.   regular

15.   If the rhythm is not regular, measure all combinations of RRIs to
see if there is a pattern to the irregularity. Possible patterns include:

- a regular rhythm with one or more disrupting (ectopic) beats
- a combination of normal beats and ectopic beats that produces a pattern of "grouped" beats

If these possibilities are eliminated, you should consider the rhythm
totally irregular. An irregular EKG strip will be considered totally irregular if it has no _____ of irregularity.   patterns

16.   The next major step in the analysis process as shown in Figure 13
is rate. There are several common ways to calculate heart rate, and
the method you choose depends primarily on the regularity of the
rhythm. In order to select the method of calculating rates, you must
first determine whether or not the rhythm is _____.   regular

17.   If the rhythm is regular, the most accurate way to calculate heart
rate is to count the number of small squares between two R waves
and divide it into 1500. A faster way is to count the number of large
squares between two R waves and divide it into 300. If you count

small squares, you would divide it into _____ but if you | 1500
count large squares, you divide it into _____, since there | 300
are five small squares in each large square.

18.   There is an even simpler (but less accurate) way to calculate
rate of regular rhythm. It is based on the system of dividing the
number of large squares into 300, but it requires that you memorize
the simple rate scale shown in Figure 14. This rate scale is well worth
memorizing, since it will probably be the method you use most often.
It is a quick and fairly accurate way to calculate rate, but the rhythm
must be _____ in order to use this method. | regular

METHOD	DIRECTIONS	FEATURES
A	Count the number of R waves in a 6-second strip and multiply by 10.	• not very accurate • used only with very quick estimate
B	Count the number of large squares between 2 consecutive R waves and divide into 300. —OR— *Memorize this Scale:* 1 large square = 300 bpm 2 ″ ″ = 150 ″ 3 ″ ″ = 100 ″ 4 ″ ″ = 75 ″ 5 ″ ″ = 60 ″ 6 ″ ″ = 50 ″	• very quick • not very accurate with fast rates • only used with regular rhythms
C	Count the number of small squares between 2 consecutive R waves and divide into 1500.	• most accurate • used only with regular rhythms • time consuming

Figure 14: Calculating Heart Rates

19.   If the rhythm is irregular, it's very easy to estimate the rate. Look
at the sample rhythm strip in Figure 15. On each strip, you will notice little vertical notches in the upper margin of the paper. Each of
these notches is 3 seconds away from the next. So, if you count the
number of QRS complexes in a 6-second span, you can multiply that
by 10 to get the heart rate for 1 minute. This method of estimating
rate for irregular rhythms requires that you count the number of QRS

complexes in a 6 second span and multiply by _____ to | 10
get the heart rate in beats per minute.

20.   The method described in the preceding frame is the quickest
and easiest way to estimate rate, but it is not very accurate, and
shouldn't be used unless the rhythm is irregular and can't be calculated any other way. For regular rhythms, you should count the
number of small squares between two R waves and divide it into
_____, or count the number of large squares between | 1500;
two R waves and divide it into _____. Again, the most | 300
convenient way to estimate rate for a regular rhythm will be to memorize the chart shown in Figure 14.

21.   By now, you would have looked at the rhythm strip and de- | Practice
cided whether or not it was regular, and then would have deter- | Sheet 3
mined the heart rate. Turn to Practice Sheet 3 and make both of
these determinations for each strip shown.

22.   Now that you have determined regularity and rate for the strip
you are analyzing, your next step is to begin figuring out the wave
patterns. This is a very basic step that you should always follow when
approaching arrhythmias. Before you can interpret the arrhythmia,
you must first locate and identify each _____ so that you | wave
can understand what's happening in the heart.

23.   To begin marking waves, first identify the P wave. The QRS
complex is tempting because it is usually the largest and most con-
spicuous, but you will soon learn that the P wave can be your best
friend because it's more reliable than the other waves. To begin
identifying the waves, look first for the _____ waves. | P

24.   The P wave has a characteristic shape that will often stick out
even among a lot of unidentifiable waves. The morphology (shape)
of the P wave is usually rounded and uniform. Sometimes, P wave
morphology can change if the pacemaker begins moving out of the
sinus node. But if the sinus node is the pacemaker, and it isn't dis-
eased or hypertrophied (enlarged), the P wave will have a smooth,
rounded, uniform _____. | morphology
| (shape)

25.   Another characteristic of the _____ P wave is that | sinus
it is upright and uniform. If you look back at Figure 5 in Chapter II,
you will see that the electrical flow is toward the positive electrode
in Lead II, which explains why the P wave will be upright as long as
the impulse begins in the sinus node and travels toward the ventricles. As you get more sophisticated in your understanding of arrhythmias, you will learn that a P wave can sometimes be negative. But
for now, you need to remember that a normal sinus P wave will al-
ways be upright. If the P wave originates in the _____ | SA;
node, it will be a smooth, rounded, _____ wave. | upright

26.   Now, you know that P waves usually come before _____ complexes, so begin looking at the rhythm strips on Practice Sheet 3 and label each P wave. It might help you keep things straight if you mark the P above the wave directly on the strip. NOTE: this is a helpful way to learn arrhythmias, but be careful not to mark up an EKG if it's the patient's one-and-only original.

27.   Were you able to locate each P wave all across each strip? If you ever have trouble finding a P wave, or if you can't decide whether or not a wave is a P wave, there are several tips you can remember. First, you know that the normal PRI is _____ seconds. So set your calipers at .20 seconds and measure that distance in front of the QRS complex. If there is a wave there, it's likely to be a _____ wave. To determine whether or not a P wave precedes the QRS, look for the P wave between _____ and _____ seconds in front of the QRS complex, since that is the normal PRI measurement.

28.   P waves are the most reliable of the waves, so map out the Ps across the strip. If most of them are regular but a space is missing near the T wave, it is probable that a P is hidden in another wave. Because P waves are reliably _____, you can often assume a P wave is present just by noting the patterns of the visible P waves.

29.   Let's take a minute here to talk about "losing" waves. This is a phenomenon that occurs when two electrical activities take place at

QRS
Practice
Sheet 3

.12–.20

P

.12; .20

regular

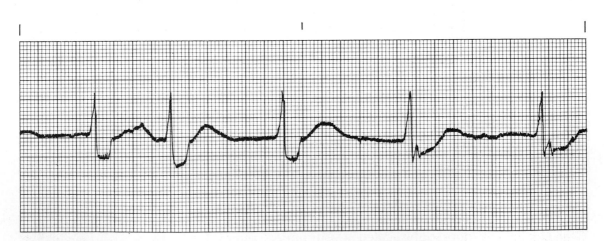

Figure 15. Figuring Rates Based on the Number of QRS Complexes in a 6-Second Strip. This sample strip has five R waves within the 6-second period defined by the notches in the margin. To figure the heart rate, multiply the R waves by 10 for a rate of 50 beats in 60 seconds.

the same time. For instance, if the atria depolarize at the same time the ventricles repolarize, then the P wave will be in the same spot on the EKG as the _____. When this happens, the largest wave will usually obscure all or most of the smaller wave. In this situation, the P wave would be said to be "lost" or "hidden" in the T wave. If the P wave is _____ in the T wave, you may be able to tell it's there by mapping out the other P waves, or by looking for a suspicious notch on the T wave where you expect the P wave to be.

| | T wave |
| | lost (hidden) |

30.   Once all the P waves are marked, it's usually not as difficult to identify the other waves. Go back to Practice Sheet 3 and mark the Q, R, S, and T waves. As you're doing this, make a mental note of the relationships between the waves. That is, does a P wave precede every QRS complex? Is there only one P wave for every QRS, or are there more P waves than QRS complexes?

See Practice Sheet 3

31.   Now that all the waves are identified, go through the rhythm strips and measure the PRIs and QRS complexes to determine whether or not they are within the normal ranges. If you've forgotten the normal measurements, review the Key Points for Chapter 2.

32.   You now have all the data you need from these arrhythmias in order to identify them. The reason you can't name them now is that you have not yet learned the rules, and thus do not know into which category each tracing falls. To identify an arrhythmia, you must first collect the data from the strip and then compare it to the _____ for each arrhythmia.

rules

33.   In the next chapter, you will begin learning the rules for each of the arrhythmias. Before you go on to that, there are one or two more points that must be covered for you to be able to interpret arrhythmias, rather than just recognizing them. For example, the measurements you have just learned are actually measurements of time. As we go on to the next chapters, it will become increasingly important for you to think of measurements such as PRI and QRS as actual activity within the heart, and not just normal or abnormal figures. That is, a PRI is considered abnormal if an impulse took too long to get from the sinus node through the _____ and the _____ _____; similarly, a QRS is considered abnormal if the impulse took too long to travel through the _____. The actual figure is not as critical as being able to understand what occurred within the heart to produce that figure.

atria; AV node ventricles

34.   Let's carry this point a bit further. We know from information gathered during research that it takes .12–.20 seconds for an impulse to get from the sinus node through the atria and AV node of a normal heart. On the EKG, this time frame is depicted as the _____

PR

interval. If this time is extended, and the PRI is elongated, we can deduce that there was some delay somewhere in the atria or the node.

35.   The _____ includes the P wave and the PR segment. The P wave itself indicates the amount of time it took the impulse to travel through the _____ and depolarize them. The isoelectric component of the PRI, or the PR segment, shows the delay in the AV node. Together, these two parts of the cardiac cycle show us what happened to the impulse *before* it reached the _____. Therefore, the PRI represents the cardiac activity that takes place above the ventricles in the atria and AV node; this category of activity is referred to as "supraventricular" activity. Supraventricular refers to the part of the heart _____ the ventricles.

PRI

atria

ventricles

above

36.   In Chapter 2 you learned that the _____ _____ is the area of the heart with the slowest conduction speed. That is, the conductive tissues of the sinus node, the atria, and the ventricles all conduct impulses _____ than the node. There is one more thing you should know about the AV node. Because it is the doorway between the atria and the ventricles, the node has the responsibility of "holding" impulses until the ventricles are able to receive them. This is why there is a slight delay at the node before each impulse passes through to the ventricles. In the normal heart, this is not a particularly critical feature, but occasionally the atria will become irritable and begin firing impulses very rapidly. The ventricles cannot respond effectively to all these impulses, so the AV node "screens" some of them, allowing only a few to get through. This vital function of the node is called the heart's "fail safe" mechanism, and you will learn much more about it later as you learn about the more complex arrhythmias. The AV node is a vital structure within the heart, because it protects the _____ from having to respond to too many impulses.

AV node

faster

ventricles

37.   When a rhythm originates in the sinus node, the atria, or the AV junction, it is considered to be in the general category of supraventricular arrhythmias because it originated above the ventricles. _____ rhythms include all those that originate above the ventricles; in fact, the only rhythms *not* included in the supraventricular category are those that originate in the ventricles. This basic categorization separates rhythms that originate in the ventricles from those that originate _____ the ventricles.

Supraventricular

above

38.   The major EKG finding that can help you distinguish between supraventricular and ventricular rhythms is the width of the QRS complex. This is because research data shows us that the only way an impulse can get all the way through the ventricles in less than .12 seconds is if it follows normal conduction pathways; all other means of depolarizing the ventricles will take a longer time. Therefore, if a rhythm has a normal QRS measurement of less than .12 seconds, it

must have been conducted normally, and thus would have to be _____ in origin. This tells us that a rhythm is known to be supraventricular, meaning it originated *above* the ventricles, if it has a QRS measurement of less than _____ seconds.

supraventricular

.12

39.   Unfortunately, this rule does not apply in the reverse. That is, just because the QRS is wide does not mean that the rhythm is ventricular. A wide QRS complex can be caused by:

- a supraventricular impulse that reaches an obstruction in the bundle branches
- a supraventricular impulse that cannot be conducted normally through the ventricles because they are still refractory from the preceding beat
- an irritable focus in the ventricles that assumes pacemaking responsibility

Of these possibilities, the third is by far the most common, telling us that a _____ _____ very frequently is caused by a ventricular impulse. However, it can get you into trouble if you assume that all wide QRSs are ventricular in origin. So, a normal QRS complex *must* be supraventricular, while a wide QRS complex can be ventricular, but it can also be supraventricular with a conduction defect. A wide QRS can be either ventricular or supraventricular, but a QRS of less than .12 seconds must be _____ in origin.

wide QRS

supraventricular

40.   By definition, supraventricular arrhythmias must have a normal QRS measurement of less than _____ seconds. However, as was shown in the preceding frame, they can frequently have prolonged ventricular _____. When this happens, you must note it along with your interpretation of the rhythm. For example, a Normal Sinus Rhythm should have a QRS of _____ than .12 seconds, but if it had a _____ disturbance in the ventricles, it would fit all the rules of NSR except that the QRS would be too _____. It should then be called Sinus Rhythm *with a wide QRS complex.* It is not necessary for you to be more specific in identifying which type of disturbance is present; if you choose to learn more about EKGs at a later time, you will most likely also learn to distinguish between these conduction irregularities. For now, you will simply call attention to an abnormal QRS complex by calling it a _____ _____ _____. Regardless of whether or not ventricular conduction is normal, you must give primary attention to identifying the basic arrhythmia.

.12

conduction

less
conduction

wide

wide QRS complex

41.   You now have the necessary knowledge to begin learning specific arrhythmias. The secret to arrhythmia interpretation is practice. So if you have time now, turn to Practice Sheet 4 and practice gathering data from those tracings.

Practice Sheet 4

Key Points — Analyzing EKG Rhythm Strips

- The beating heart produces a series of cardiac cycles, which together become an EKG rhythm strip.

- Arrhythmias are categorized according to which pacemaker site initiates the rhythm.

- The normal heart rhythm originates in the sinus node, and thus is called Normal Sinus Rhythm.

- It is necessary to memorize the rules for each arrhythmia in order to interpret it in the future.

- EKG interpretation is based on how closely the clues gathered from the rhythm strip comply with the rules for a given arrhythmia.

- Because EKG interpretation can be so complex, it is essential to develop a routine format for analyzing rhythm strips, and then use it consistently when identifying arrhythmias. An example of such a format is shown here:

  Rhythm (also called regularity)
  Rate
  P Wave
  PR Interval (PRI)
  QRS Complex (QRS)

- Rhythm, or regularity, is determined by measuring the R–R intervals, or possibly the P–P intervals, across the entire strip. If the pattern is not regular, note whether it is regularly irregular, basically regular, or totally irregular. Look for patterns to the irregularity which could indicate ectopics or grouped beating.

- Rate can refer to either the ventricular rate (most common) or the atrial rate if they differ. Rate can be calculated in one of three ways:

  1. Count the number of small squares between two R waves and divide it into 1500.
  2. Count the number of large squares between two R waves and divide it into 300. Standard tables giving this information are available, and can be memorized for quick reference.
  3. Count the number of R waves in a 6-second strip and multiply by 10. This last method should only be used on irregular arrhythmias because it is the least accurate.

- The P wave should be found preceding the QRS complex. It should be upright and uniform. The P waves should be regular across the entire strip, and there should be only one P wave for each QRS complex. It is possible for the P wave to be hidden in the T wave of the preceding complex.

- The PR interval is an indication of the electrical activity taking place within the atria and the AV node. It encompasses all electrical activity above the ventricles. The PRI consists of the P wave and the PR segment. The PR segment is caused by the delay of the impulse at the AV node. The PRI should be constant across the strip, and should measure between .12 and .20 seconds.

- The QRS complex can help you determine whether the rhythm originated from a supraventricular focus or from the ventricles. A supraventricular focus normally produces a QRS less than .12 seconds. However, it is possible for a supraventricular rhythm to have a wider QRS complex if there was a conduction disturbance within the ventricles. If the rhythm originated in the ventricles, the QRS complex will be .12 seconds or greater. A narrow QRS complex indicates that the impulse is supraventricular, while a wide QRS complex can be either supraventricular with a conduction disturbance, or it can be ventricular.

Self-Test: Analyzing EKG Rhythm Strips

Directions:

Complete this self-evaluation of the information you have learned in this chapter. If your answers are all correct and you feel comfortable with your understanding of the material, proceed to the next chapter. However, if you missed any of the questions you should review the referenced frames before proceeding. If you feel uncomfortable with any of your understanding, invest the time now to go back over the entire chapter. DO NOT PROCEED WITH THE NEXT CHAPTER UNTIL YOU ARE VERY COMFORTABLE WITH THE MATERIAL IN THIS CHAPTER.

Question	Referenced Frames	
1. What is a cardiac cycle on the EKG?	1	The electrical impulses associated with a single heart beat; the P, Q, R, S, and T waves.
2. What is the name of the normal cardiac rhythm associated with a healthy heart?	4	Normal Sinus Rhythm
3. Why is it necessary to have an organized format for approaching arrhythmia interpretation?	2; 5; 9	There are so many possible configurations of EKGs that you would never be able to memorize all of them. You must be able to systematically gather all of the available information and then compare it to the rules for the rhythms.

Question	Referenced Frames	
		Without a routine format, you would overlook important clues.
4. Why do you have to memorize the rules for each of the arrhythmias?	2; 6; 7; 8; 9	So that you can compare them to the findings on an EKG strip, and thus determine the identity of the arrhythmia.
5. What are the five parts of the analysis format you learned in this Chapter?	9	Regularity (rhythm) Rate P Wave PR Interval QRS Complex
6. How can you tell whether or not an arrhythmia is regular?	10; 11; 12; 14	Measure the R–R interval, or the P–P interval.
7. What does the phrase "regularly irregular" mean?	13; 15	There is a pattern to the irregularity.
8. What does the phrase "basically regular" mean?	13; 15	The underlying rhythm is regular but it is interrupted by ectopics.
9. What does it mean when you call an arrhythmia "totally irregular?"	13; 15	There is no pattern to the irregularity.
10. If you wanted to calculate accurately the rate of a regular rhythm, you could count the number of *small* squares between two R waves and divide it into what number?	16; 17; 18; 20	1500

Question	**Referenced Frames**	
11. If you counted the number of *large* squares between two R waves, what number would you divide that into to determine the heart rate?	16; 17; 18; 20	300
12. When an arrhythmia is irregular, you should determine the heart rate by counting the number of R waves in 6 seconds and multiplying that by what number?	19; 20	10
13. What is the first wave you should try to locate and map out when analyzing a rhythm strip?	22; 23	the P wave
14. What does a normal sinus P wave look like?	23; 24; 25	It has a smooth rounded shape; it is upright and uniform.
15. Where can you normally find the P wave?	26	It is usually located immediately in front of the QRS complex.
16. Are P–P intervals usually regular or irregular?	23; 28	They are usually very regular.
17. What is meant when a P wave is said to be "lost" in the T wave?	29	It means that the P wave occurred on or near the T wave, and is thus obscured beyond clear identification.
18. In your analysis of a rhythm strip, what waves should you look for next after you have located the P waves?	30; 31	the QRS and the T waves

Question	**Referenced Frames**	
19. Why is it important for you to know all these waves and measurements?	32; 33	because they reflect cardiac activity
20. What is a "supraventricular" arrhythmia?	33; 34; 35; 36; 37; 38; 39; 40	An arrhythmia which originates above the ventricles.
21. If a QRS complex measures less than .12 seconds, where can you assume it originated?	38; 39; 40	from a supraventricular focus
22. If a QRS complex measures .12 seconds or greater, it could possibly be a supraventricular rhythm with a ventricular conduction disturbance. What is the other possible explanation for a wide QRS complex?	38; 39; 40	A rhythm that originates in the ventricles will have a QRS measurement of .12 seconds or more.

Practice Sheet 3:
Analyzing EKG Strips

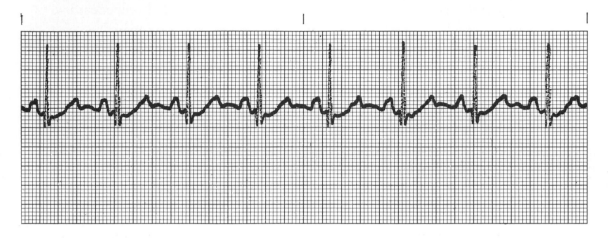

3.1   Regularity: _____
           Rate: _____
           P Waves: _____
           PRI: _____
           QRS: _____

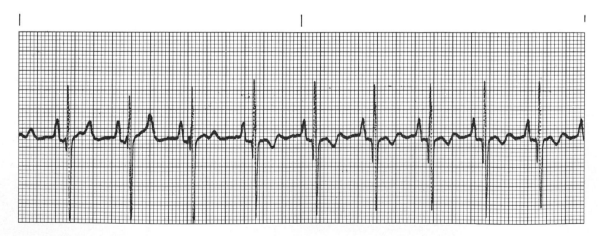

3.2   Regularity: _____
           Rate: _____
           P Waves: _____
           PRI: _____
           QRS: _____

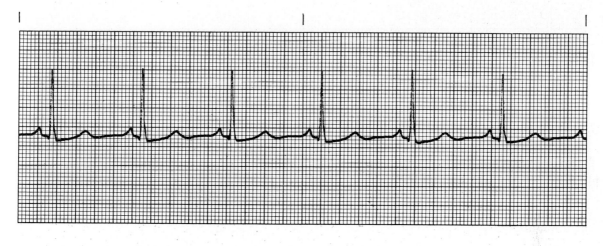

3.3   Regularity: _____
           Rate: _____
           P Waves: _____
           PRI: _____
           QRS: _____

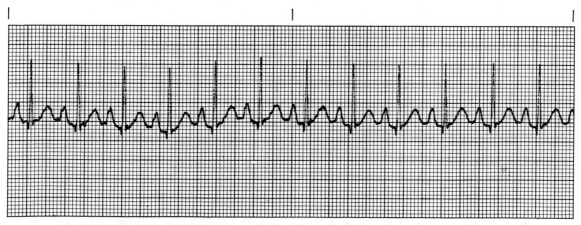

3.4   Regularity: _____
           Rate: _____
           P Waves: _____
           PRI: _____
           QRS: _____

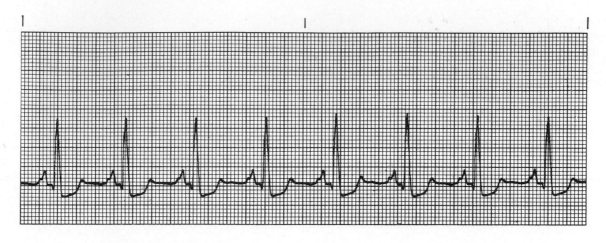

3.5   Regularity: _____

             Rate: _____

             P Waves: _____

             PRI: _____

             QRS: _____

Practice Sheet 4:
Gathering Information from Strips

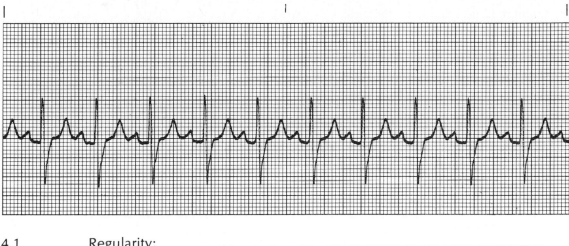

4.1   Regularity: _____
          Rate: _____
          P Waves: _____
          PRI: _____
          QRS: _____

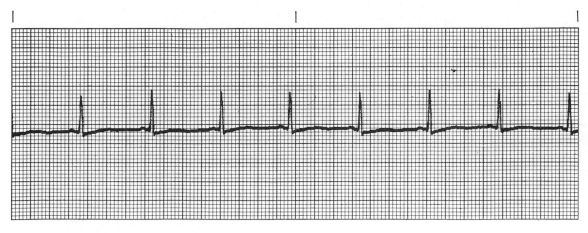

4.2   Regularity: _____
          Rate: _____
          P Waves: _____
          PRI: _____
          QRS: _____

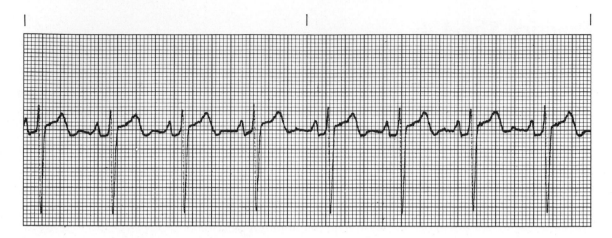

4.3   Regularity: _____

        Rate: _____

        P Waves: _____

        PRI: _____

        QRS: _____

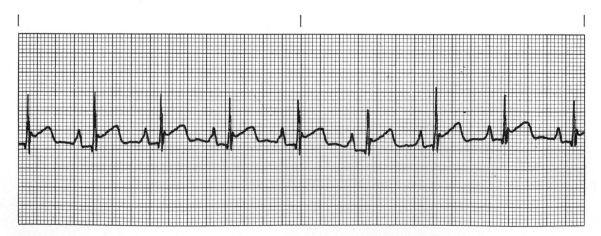

4.4   Regularity: _____

        Rate: _____

        P Waves: _____

        PRI: _____

        QRS: _____

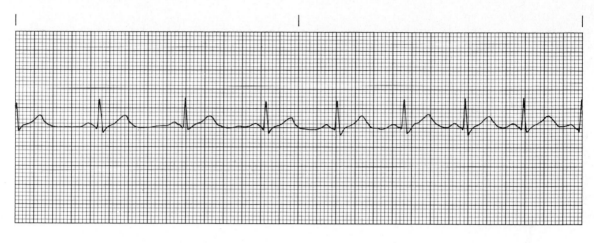

4.5   Regularity: _____
          Rate: _____
          P Waves: _____
          PRI: _____
          QRS: _____

4

Sinus Rhythms

1. The first category of arrhythmias you will learn is the category of rhythms that originate in the sinus node. This group includes:

> Normal Sinus Rhythm (NSR)
> Sinus Bradycardia
> Sinus Tachycardia
> Sinus Arrhythmia

Each of these arrhythmias will be discussed individually. You will need to memorize the information provided, because it will provide the rules necessary for you to later be able to identify that arrhythmia again. You will eventually need to memorize the _____ for all of the arrhythmias, but we will begin just with those originating in the _____ node.

rules;

sinus

2. First, we will discuss normal sinus rhythm. We will look at what a normal rhythm is, and what defines it as normal, and then we will begin looking at arrhythmias and how they differ from _____. Technically speaking, NSR is not an arrhythmia because it is a normal, rhythmic pattern. However, you will often hear phrases like arrhythmia, dysrhythmia, or rhythm being loosely used to describe both normal and abnormal EKG patterns. Although NSR is not actually an _____ because it has a normal, rhythmic pattern, we will include it in general discussions of all arrhythmias.

normal

arrhythmia

3. In normal sinus rhythm, the pacemaker impulse originates in the sinus node and travels through the normal conduction pathways within normal time frames. Because the pacemaker originates in the _____ node, the P waves will be uniform, and since conduction is normal, one P wave will be in front of every QRS complex. In NSR, there will be _____ P waves, one in front of every _____ complex.

sinus

uniform;
QRS

4. In NSR, the atria are stimulated by the sinus impulse and contract before the ventricles do. Because the major thrust of the electrical current is traveling *toward* the positive electrode in Lead II, there will be an upright _____ wave.

P

5. Since the SA node inherently fires at a rate of 60–100 times per minute, a normal sinus rhythm must, by definition, fall within this rate range. If an EKG rhythm is slower than _____ beats per minute or faster than _____ beats per minute, it is not _____ _____ _____.

60;
100;
normal sinus
rhythm

6. NSR is defined as being a regular rhythm. That is, the _____ interval must be regular across the entire strip. Even if a normal sinus rhythm is interrupted by an ectopic beat, the underlying pattern must have a regular R–R measurement in order to be called _____ _____ _____.

R–R

normal
sinus rhythm

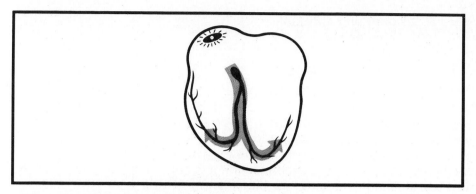

Figure 16. Normal Sinus Rhythm

Sinus node is the pacemaker, firing at a regular rate of 60–100 times per minute. Each beat is conducted normally through to the ventricles.

7.   You now know that a normal sinus rhythm must be a regular pattern, at a rate between _____ and _____, with an upright P wave in front of every QRS complex. When you measure the PR interval, it must fall between .12 and .20 seconds, and it must be of the same duration across the entire strip. That is, if it is less than _____ seconds or greater than _____ seconds, it is outside the normal range and not defined as _____. Further, if the PRI is, for instance, .16 seconds, then each PRI on the strip must be .16 seconds, if the PRI changes from one complex to the next, even if it stays within the normal range, it would not be considered a normal sinus rhythm. In NSR, the PRI must be between _____ and _____ seconds, and must be constant across the _____ strip.

60; 100
.12; .20; NSR
.12; .20; entire

8.   Finally, the QRS measurement for a true NSR must be within the normal range, i.e., _____ than .12 seconds. This can be a little tricky, because a sinus rhythm might fit all the other rules, but still have a wide QRS complex. When this happens, the rhythm must be qualified by calling it a "sinus rhythm with a wide _____ _____." Notice that the pattern is no longer called "normal" sinus rhythm, but simply sinus rhythm. If you go on to study EKGs to greater depth, you will learn the reasons behind this phenomenon of the wide QRS complex, and will learn the proper terminology for identifying it, but for now, just remember that unless the QRS is less than _____ seconds, the rhythm is not a _____ sinus rhythm.

less
QRS complex
.12; normal

9.   To summarize the rules for the EKG findings in NSR:
    Regularity: regular
        Rate: 60–100 beats minute
      P Wave: uniform shape: one P wave in front of every QRS complex

PRI: .12–.20 seconds and constant
QRS: less than .12 seconds

For a rhythm to be called NSR, it must have _____ P waves, one in front of every QRS complex; the rate must be _____ to _____ beats per minute, with a _____ R–R interval across the entire strip. It must have a PRI that measures between _____ and _____ seconds, and the PRI must be _____ across the entire strip. Finally, the QRS measurement must be less than _____ seconds, or if it is not, the interpretation must be qualified by calling it a sinus rhythm with a wide QRS complex.

uniform
60;
100; regular;

.12; .20;
constant;
.12

10.   Now go back to Practice Sheets 3 and 4. Look at all the data available from each strip. Each of these strips has been identified as Sinus Rhythm. Compare your findings with the rules for NSR to see which patterns comply with the rules for NSR.

All are NSR
except 3.4,
4.1, 4.5.

11.   If a rhythm originates in the sinus node, but doesn't follow one or more of the rules for NSR, it might fall into one of the other categories of sinus rhythms. If the rate is slower than 60 beats per minute, it is called a bradycardia, meaning *slow heart*. When a rhythm originating in the sinus node has a normal, upright P wave in front of every QRS complex, a normal PRI and QRS, and it is regular, it is called Sinus Bradycardia, if the only reason it doesn't fit into NSR is because the rate is too slow. A rhythm can be identified as Sinus Bradycardia when it fits all of the rules for NSR except that the rate is less than _____ beats per minute.

60

12.   Here are the rules for the EKG findings in Sinus Bradycardia:

Regularity: regular
Rate: less than 60 beats per minute
P Wave: uniform shape; one P wave in front of every QRS complex
PRI: .12–.20 seconds and constant
QRS: less than .12 seconds

13.   The same thing is true for a rhythm that fits all of the rules for NSR except that the rate is too fast. When the heart beats too fast, it is called tachycardia, meaning *fast heart*. So, a rhythm that originates in the sinus node and fits all rules for NSR except that the rate is too _____ would be called a Sinus Tachycardia. When a rhythm is regular, has a uniform P wave in front of every QRS complex, has a normal and constant PRI and QRS, but the rate is greater than 100 beats per minute, it is called _____ _____.

fast

Sinus
Tachycardia

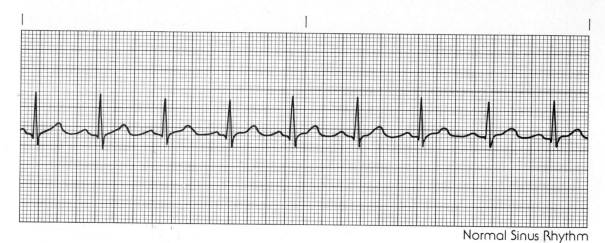

Normal Sinus Rhythm

Figure 17. Rules for NSR

REGULARITY: **The R–R intervals are constant; the rhythm is regular.**
RATE: **The atrial and ventricular rates are equal; heart rate is between 60 and 100 beats per minute.**
P WAVE: **The P waves are uniform. There is one P wave in front of every QRS complex.**
PRI: **The PR interval measures between .12 and .20 seconds; the PRI measurement is constant across the strip.**
QRS: **The QRS complex measures less than .12 seconds.**

14. The rules for Sinus Tachycardia are:

Regularity: regular
Rate: greater than 100 beats per minute (usually does not exceed 160 beats per minute)
P Wave: uniform shape; one P wave in front of every QRS complex
PRI: .12–.20 seconds and constant
QRS: less than .12 seconds

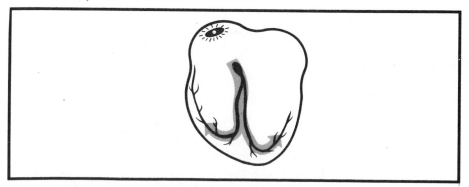

Figure 18. Sinus Bradycardia

Sinus node is the pacemaker, firing regularly at a rate of less than 60 times per minute. Each impulse is conducted normally through to the ventricles.

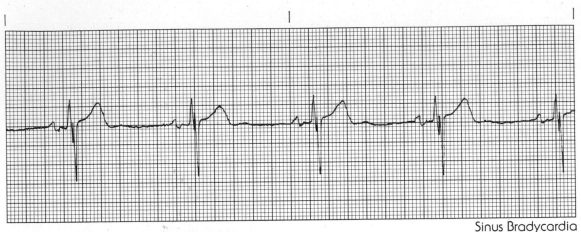

Sinus Bradycardia

Figure 19. Rules for Sinus Bradycardia

REGULARITY: **The R–R intervals are constant; the rhythm is regular.**

RATE: **The atrial and ventricular rates are equal; heart rate is less than 60 beats per minute.**

P WAVE: **There is a uniform P wave in front of every QRS complex.**

PRI: **The PR interval measures between .12 and .20 seconds; the PRI measurement is constant across the strip.**

QRS: **The QRS complex measures less than .12 seconds.**

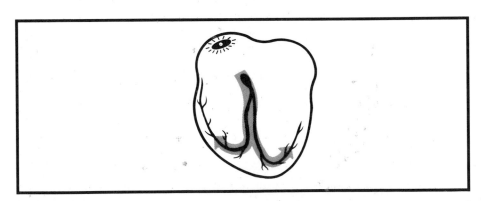

Figure 20. Sinus Tachycardia

Sinus node is the pacemaker, firing regularly at a rate of greater than 100 times per minute. Each impulse is conducted normally through to the ventricles.

15.   The last of the sinus rhythms we will learn is Sinus Arrhythmia. This rhythm is characterized by a pattern that would normally be considered NSR, except that the rate changes with the patient's respirations. When the patient breathes in the rate increases, and when he/she breathes out the rate slows. This causes the _____ _____ to be irregular across the strip. The result is a pattern with an upright P wave in front of every QRS complex, a normal

R–R interval

and constant PRI, a normal QRS complex, but an _____ | irregular
R–R interval. The difference between NSR and Sinus Arrhythmia is
that NSR is regular and Sinus Arrhythmia is _____. | irregular

16. Here are the rules for the EKG findings in Sinus Arrhythmia:

Regularity: irregular
     Rate: 60–100 beats per minute (usually)
  P Wave: uniform shape; one P wave in front of every QRS
        complex
      PRI: .12–.20 seconds and constant
    QRS: less than .12 seconds

17. You now know the rules for the first four arrhythmias. Normal
Sinus Rhythm originates in the _____ node and has nor- | sinus
mal conduction within normal time frames. This means that the
_____ wave will be uniform in front of every QRS complex, | P
and that the PRI and QRS measurements will be within _____ | normal;
limits, and that the _____ will be constant. For NSR, the rate | PRI
must fall between _____ and _____ beats per minute. | 60; 100
If the rate drops below 60 beats per minute but all the other rules

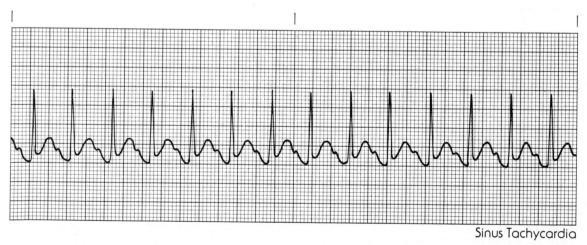

Sinus Tachycardia

Figure 21. Rules for Tachycardia

REGULARITY: The R–R intervals are constant; the rhythm is regular.
       RATE: The atrial and ventricular rates are equal; heart rate is
           greater than 100 beats per minute (usually between 100
           and 160 beats per minute).
   P WAVE: There is a uniform P wave in front of every QRS complex.
        PRI: The PR interval measures between .12 and .20 seconds;
           the PRI measurement is constant across the strip.
     QRS: The QRS complex measures less than .12 seconds.

apply to NSR, the rhythm is called _____ _____; if the rate is faster than 100 beats per minute, the rhythm is called _____ _____. If the rhythm fits all the rules of NSR except that it is irregular, the rhythm is called _____ _____.

Sinus Bradycardia; Sinus Tachycardia; Sinus Arrhythmia

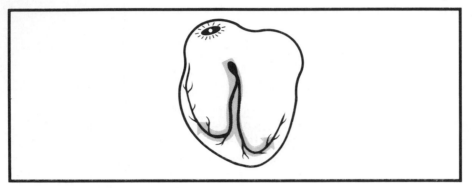

Figure 22. Sinus Arrhythmia

Sinus node is the pacemaker, but impulses are initiated in an irregular pattern. The rate increases as the patient breathes in and decreases as the patient breathes out. Each beat is conducted normally through to the ventricles.

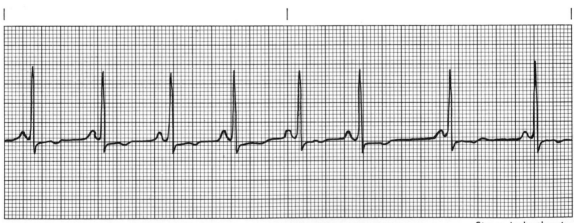

Sinus Arrhythmia

Figure 23. Rules for Sinus Arrhythmia

REGULARITY: The R–R intervals vary; the rate changes with the patient's respirations.

RATE: The atrial and ventricular rates are equal; heart rate is usually in a normal range (60–100 beats per minute), but can be slower.

P WAVE: There is a uniform P wave in front of every QRS complex.

PRI: The PR interval measures between .12 and .20 seconds; the PRI measurement is constant across the strip.

QRS: The QRS complex measures less than .12 seconds.

18.   If a rhythm originates in the sinus node, it will have uniform, upright _____ waves because the electrical impulses are traveling from the atria downward through the ventricles, and thus are heading toward the _____ electrode in Lead II.

P

positive

19.   With NSR, Sinus Tachycardia, Sinus Bradycardia, and Sinus Arrhythmia, the PRI will always be between _____ and _____ seconds and constant.

.12;
.20

20.   Of the four sinus rhythms you have learned, the only one that does not have a regular R–R interval is _____ _____ .

Sinus
Arrhythmia

21.   With all rhythms that originate in the sinus node, the QRS measurement should be _____. If it is greater than .12 seconds, it cannot be considered _____, and this should be noted along with your interpretation of the underlying pattern. For the time being, you can qualify your interpretation by naming the rhythm and including "_____." If you continue to study EKGs you will learn the proper terminology for this phenomenon.

less than .12
seconds;
normal

with a
wide QRS

22.   Now you must memorize all of the rules for each of the sinus arrhythmias. Then you can begin gathering data from the strips shown in Practice Sheet 5 and compare them to the rules for each pattern. You should be able to identify each of the strips. If you have any trouble, or are unsure about the process, you should seek help before going on to the next section. If you would like more practice after you finish Practice Sheet 5, go back to Practice Sheets 3 & 4. With the information you now know, you should be able to identify each of these rhythm strips. Check your results with the answer keys (beginning on page 365). If you missed any of these arrhythmias, spend the time *now* to review this section. Do not go on until you are very comfortable with the information in this chapter.

Practice
Sheet 5

Practice
Sheets 3 & 4

Key Points – Sinus Rhythms

- Rhythms that originate in the sinus node include:

    Normal Sinus Rhythm
    Sinus Bradycardia
    Sinus Tachycardia
    Sinus Arrhythmia.

- All rhythms that originate in the sinus node will have upright P waves. This is because the electrical current flows from the atria toward the ventricles, which is toward positive electrode in Lead II.

- Here are the rules for *NSR*:

    Regularity: regular
         Rate: 60–100 beats per minute
       P Wave: normal and upright; one P wave in front of every QRS complex
          PRI: .12–.20 seconds and constant
          QRS: less than .12 seconds.

- Here are the rules for *Sinus Bradycardia*:

    Regularity: regular
         Rate: less than 60 beats per minute
       P Wave: normal and upright; one P wave in front of every QRS complex
          PRI: .12–.20 seconds and constant
          QRS: less than .12 seconds.

- Here are the rules for *Sinus Tachycardia*:

    Regularity: regular
         Rate: greater than 100 beats per minute (usually 100–160 beats
               per minute)
       P Wave: normal and upright; one P wave in front of every QRS complex
          PRI: .12–.20 seconds and constant
          QRS: less than .12 seconds.

- Here are the rules for *Sinus Arrhythmia*:

    Regularity: regular
         Rate: 60–100 beats per minute (usually)
       P Wave: normal and upright; one P wave in front of every QRS complex
          PRI: .12–.20 seconds and constant
          QRS: less than .12 seconds.

- When a rhythm is determined to have originated in the sinus node, but has a QRS measurement greater than .12 seconds, this should be noted in the interpretation by calling it a sinus rhythm with a wide QRS complex.

Self-Test: Sinus Rhythms

Directions:

Complete this self-evaluation of the information you have learned from this chapter. If your answers are all correct and you feel comfortable with your understanding of the material, proceed to the next chapter. However, if you missed any of the questions you should review the referenced frames before proceeding. If you feel uncomfortable with any of your understanding, invest the time now to go back over the entire chapter. DO NOT PROCEED WITH THE NEXT CHAPTER UNTIL YOU ARE VERY COMFORTABLE WITH THE MATERIAL IN THIS CHAPTER.

Question	Referenced Frames	
1. Why do sinus rhythms have upright P waves?	3; 4; 7; 17; 18	Because an impulse that originates in the sinus node will travel downward through the atria to the ventricles; in Lead II, the positive electrode is placed below the apex, thus the major electrical flow is toward the positive electrode in Lead II.
2. In a Normal Sinus Rhythm, what will the rate range be?	5; 7; 9; 17	60–100 beats per minute
3. What is the defined PRI for a NSR?	3; 7; 9; 17; 19	.12–.20 and constant
4. Is NSR defined as being regular or irregular?	6; 7; 9; 17; 20	regular
5. What should the QRS measurement be in order to be called a Normal Sinus Rhythm?	8; 9; 17; 21	less than .12 seconds

Question	Referenced Frames	
6. What would you call a rhythm that originated in the sinus node and fit all the rules for NSR except that the QRS was too wide?	8; 9; 21	sinus rhythm with a wide QRS
7. What will the P wave be like for Sinus Bradycardia?	3; 11; 17; 18	normal and upright; one P wave in front of every QRS complex
8. In Sinus Bradycardia, what is the rate range?	11; 12	less than 60 beats per minute
9. Is Sinus Bradycardia regular or irregular?	11; 12; 20	regular
10. What will the PRI measurement be in a Sinus Bradycardia?	11; 12; 19	.12–.20 seconds and constant
11. What is the normal QRS measurement in a Sinus Bradycardia?	11; 12; 21	less than .12 seconds
12. How does Sinus Bradycardia differ from Normal Sinus Rhythm?	11; 12	the rate in Sinus Bradycardia is slower than NSR
13. Is Sinus Tachycardia regular or irregular?	13; 14; 20	regular
14. What is the rate range for Sinus Tachycardia?	13; 14	greater than 100 beats per minute (usually does not exceed 160 beats per minute)
15. What is the PRI for Sinus Tachycardia?	13; 14; 19	.12–.20 seconds and constant
16. What is the normal QRS measurement for Sinus Tachycardia?	13; 14; 21	less than .12 seconds

Question	Referenced Frames	
17. What do the P waves look like in Sinus Tachycardia?	13; 14; 18	normal and upright; one P wave in front of every QRS complex
18. How does Sinus Tachycardia differ from NSR?	13; 14	the rate in Sinus Tachycardia is faster than NSR
19. Describe the rhythm (regularity) of Sinus Arrhythmia.	15; 16; 20	it is irregular; the rate increases with each respiratory inspiration and decreases with each expiration
20. What is the rate range for Sinus Arrhythmia?	15; 16	usually 60–100 beats per minute
21. What is the PRI measurement in a Sinus Arrhythmia?	15; 16; 19	.12–.20 seconds and constant
22. What is the normal QRS measurement in a Sinus Arrhythmia?	15; 16; 21	less than .12 seconds
23. How does Sinus Arrhythmia differ from NSR?	15; 16; 20	Sinus Arrhythmia is irregular while NSR is regular

Practice Sheet 5:
Sinus Rhythms

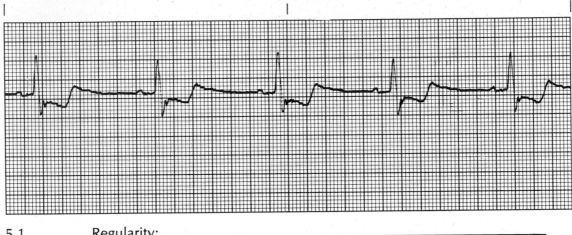

5.1

Regularity: _____

Rate: _____

P Waves: _____

PRI: _____

QRS: _____

Interp: _____

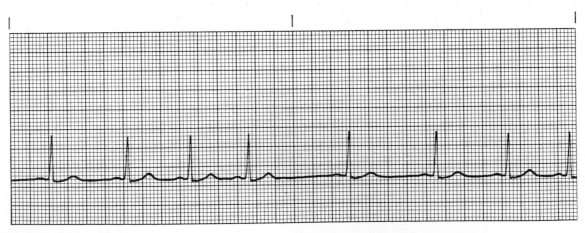

5.2

Regularity: _____

Rate: _____

P Waves: _____

PRI: _____

QRS: _____

Interp: _____

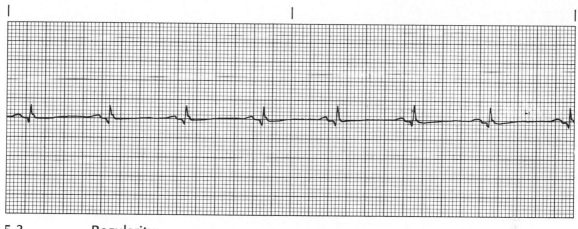

5.3   Regularity: _____
       Rate: _____
       P Waves: _____
       PRI: _____
       QRS: _____
       Interp: _____

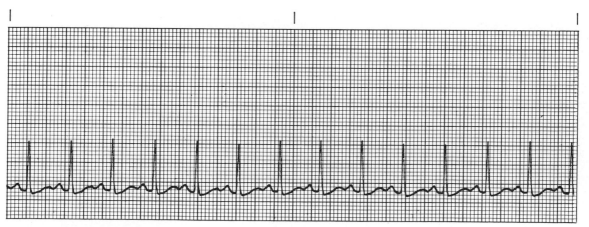

5.4   Regularity: _____
       Rate: _____
       P Waves: _____
       PRI: _____
       QRS: _____
       Interp: _____

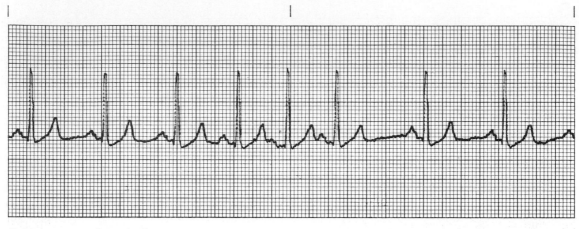

5.5

Regularity: _____

Rate: _____

P Waves: _____

PRI: _____

QRS: _____

Interp: _____

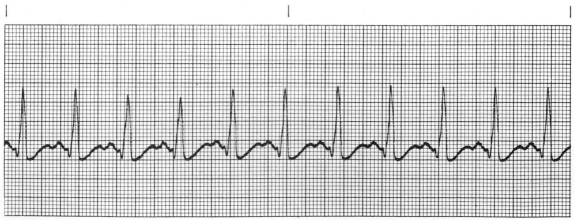

5.6

Regularity: _____

Rate: _____

P Waves: _____

PRI: _____

QRS: _____

Interp: _____

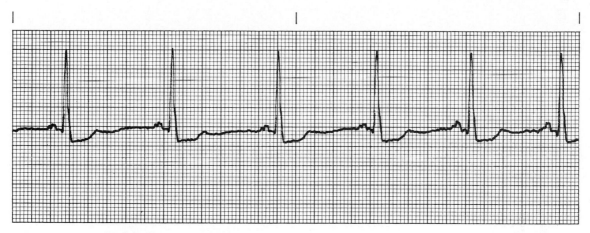

5.7   Regularity: _____
           Rate: _____
           P Waves: _____
           PRI: _____
           QRS: _____
           Interp: _____

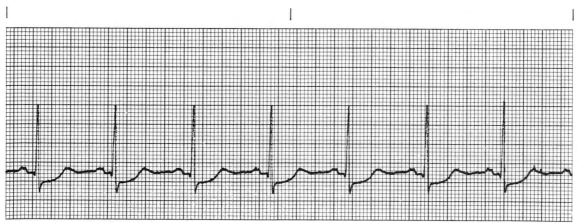

5.8   Regularity: _____
           Rate: _____
           P Waves: _____
           PRI: _____
           QRS: _____
           Interp: _____

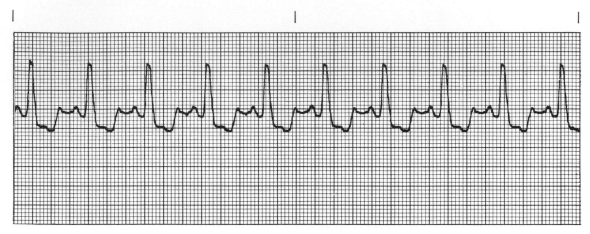

5.9

Regularity: _____

Rate: _____

P Waves: _____

PRI: _____

QRS: _____

Interp: _____

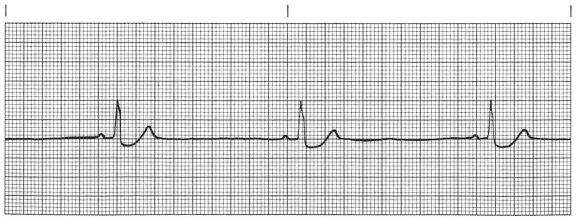

5.10

Regularity: _____

Rate: _____

P Waves: _____

PRI: _____

QRS: _____

Interp: _____

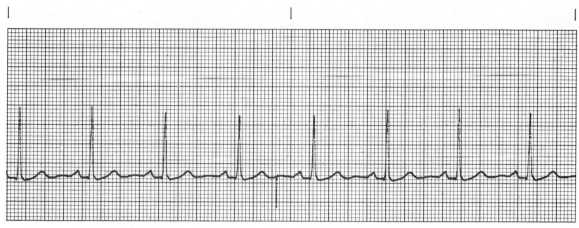

5.11   Regularity: _____
        Rate: _____
        P Waves: _____
        PRI: _____
        QRS: _____
        Interp: _____

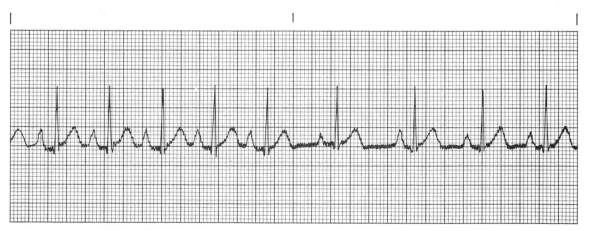

5.12   Regularity: _____
        Rate: _____
        P Waves: _____
        PRI: _____
        QRS: _____
        Interp: _____

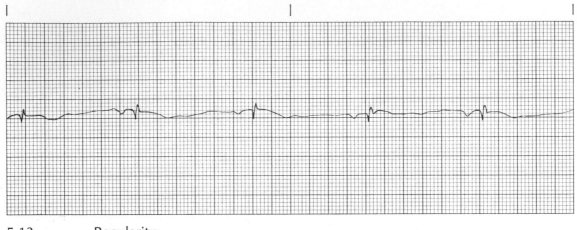

5.13   Regularity: _____
            Rate: _____
            P Waves: _____
            PRI: _____
            QRS: _____
            Interp: _____

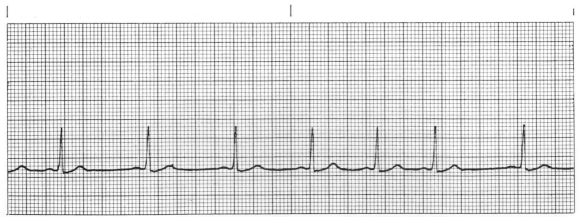

5.14   Regularity: _____
            Rate: _____
            P Waves: _____
            PRI: _____
            QRS: _____
            Interp: _____

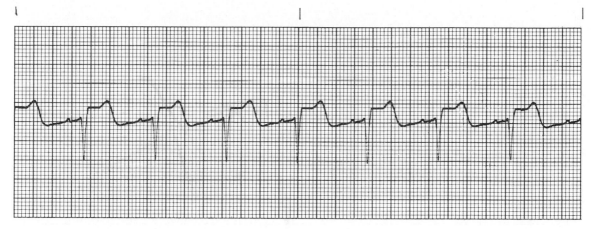

5.15   Regularity: _____
            Rate: _____
            P Waves: _____
            PRI: _____
            QRS: _____
            Interp: _____

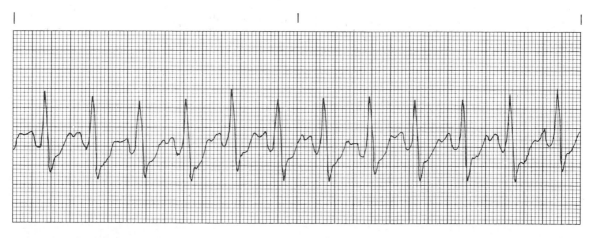

5.16   Regularity: _____
            Rate: _____
            P Waves: _____
            PRI: _____
            QRS: _____
            Interp: _____

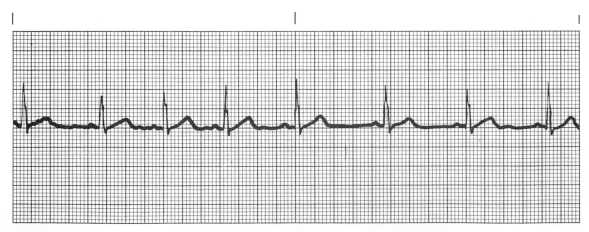

5.17   Regularity: _____
            Rate: _____
            P Waves: _____
            PRI: _____
            QRS: _____
            Interp: _____

5.18   Regularity: _____
            Rate: _____
            P Waves: _____
            PRI: _____
            QRS: _____
            Interp: _____

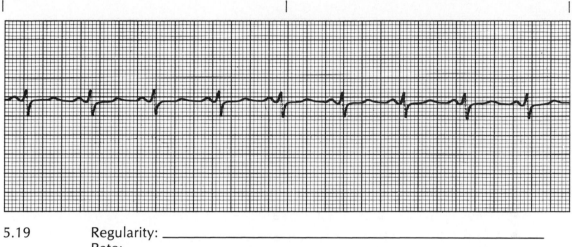

5.19   Regularity: _____

            Rate: _____

            P Waves: _____

            PRI: _____

            QRS: _____

            Interp: _____

5

Atrial Rhythms

1. In the last section you learned that NSR, Sinus Bradycardia, Sinus Tachycardia, and Sinus Arrhythmia all originate in the _____ node. These are all rhythms that originate in the normal pacemaker of the heart. Sometimes, for one reason or another, the _____ node loses its pacemaking role and this function is taken over by another site along the conduction system. The site with the fastest inherent rate usually controls the _____ function. Since the atria have the next highest rate after the SA node, it is common for the atria to take over from the SA node. Rhythms that originate in the atria are called atrial arrhythmias.

sinus

sinus

pacemaking

2. Atrial _____ are caused when the atrial rate becomes faster than the sinus rate, either by irritability or by escape, and an impulse from somewhere along the atrial _____ pathways is able to override the SA node and stimulate _____. When an atrial impulse is able to take over the pacemaking function from the SA node and initiate depolarization, the resulting pattern is termed an _____ arrhythmia.

arrhythmias

conduction; depolarization

atrial

3. As with a sinus rhythm, an impulse that originates in the atria will travel through the atria to the AV junction, and then through the _____ conduction pathways to the Purkinje fibers. The only difference is in the atria, where the conduction will be a little slower and rougher than it is with sinus rhythms. Since atrial depolarization is seen on the EKG as a P wave, you would expect the unusual atrial depolarization seen with _____ arrhythmias to show up in unusual or atypical _____ waves.

ventricular

atrial;
P

4. The normal sinus P wave is described as having a nice, rounded, uniform wave shape which precedes the _____ _____. An atrial P wave will have a different morphology than the _____ P wave. It can be flattened, notched, peaked, sawtoothed, or even diphasic (meaning that it goes first above the isoelectric line and then dips below it). A P wave that is uniformly rounded would most likely be coming from the _____ node, but a P wave that is notched, flattened, or diphasic would be called an _____ P wave.

QRS complex;
sinus

sinus;
atrial

5. Atrial arrhythmias have several features in common. They originate above the ventricles, and would therefore have a _____ QRS complex. The impulse has a little trouble getting through the atria, since it originated outside the SA node, and would thus produce an atrial P wave rather than a typical _____ P wave. We will be discussing five atrial arrhythmias, each of which will have a _____ QRS complex and a _____ wave that has a different shape from the _____ P wave.

narrow

sinus;

normal
(narrow); P;
sinus

6.   The first atrial arrhythmia we'll learn is called Wandering Pace-maker. Wandering Pacemaker is caused when the pacemaker role switches from beat to beat from the SA node to the atria and back again. The result is a rhythm made up of interspersed sinus and atrial beats. The sinus beats are preceded by nice rounded P waves, but the P wave changes as the pacemaker drops to the atria. The P waves of the atrial beats are not consistent, and can be any variety of atrial configuration, e.g., flattened, notched, or diphasic. Sometimes the pacemaker site will drop even lower, into the AV junction, resulting in inverted or even absent P waves. This concept is dealt with in greater detail in Chapter 6. Wandering Pacemaker is categorized as an atrial arrhythmia characterized by _____ in the _____ waves from one beat to the next.

changes; P

7.   Because the pacemaker site is changing between beats, each of the impulses will vary in the time it takes to reach the ventricles. Therefore, the PRI may be slightly different from one beat to the next. This can also cause a slightly irregular R–R interval. In Wandering Pacemaker, the rhythm is usually slightly _____, and the _____ can vary somewhat from one beat to the next, but will always be less than .20 seconds. Both the R–R interval and the PR interval are usually slightly _____.

irregular; PRI

irregular

8.   The rules for Wandering Pacemaker are:
      Regularity: slightly irregular
          Rate: usually normal, 60–100 beats/minute
      P wave: morphology changes from one complex to the
                  next
           PRI: less than .20 seconds; may vary
          QRS: less than .12 seconds

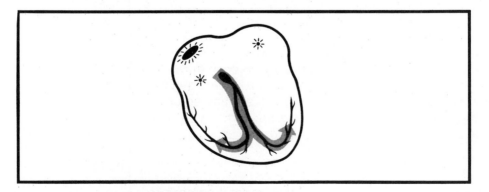

Figure 24. Wandering Pacemaker

The pacemaker site wanders between the sinus node, the atria, and the AV junction. Although each beat originates from a different focus, the rate usually remains within a normal range, but can be slower. Conduction through to the ventricles is normal.

9.   The next atrial arrhythmia is not really a rhythm at all, but is actually a single beat. When a single beat arises from an ectopic focus (a site outside of the SA node) within the conduction system, that beat is called an ectopic beat. An _____ beat is a single beat that arises from a focus outside of the _____ _____.

ectopic
SA node

10.   When an ectopic beat originates in the atria, it is called an atrial ectopic. An ectopic beat arises when a site somewhere along the _____ system becomes irritable and overrides the SA node for a single beat. By definition, an ectopic can also be caused when an ectopic focus initiates an impulse as an escape mechanism, but the most common usage of the term suggests that the site became _____ and overrode the _____ node.

conduction

irritable; sinus

11.   When you see a single ectopic beat interrupting a rhythm, you can easily tell whether it is caused by irritability or escape. An irritable beat will come earlier than you expected it to, while an escape beat will be delayed because it only fires after the expected beat is skipped. An early, or premature, beat would be an indication of _____, while an _____ beat would be preceded by a prolonged R–R cycle.

irritability;
escape

12.   An atrial ectopic that is caused by irritability is called a Premature Atrial Contraction, or PAC. This is really a misnomer, since the ectopic indicates depolarization, rather than contraction. We can't assume that contraction followed the depolarization. However, this term is very widely used and seems resistant to more accurate titles. So, a PAC is an ectopic beat that comes _____ in the cardiac cycle and originates in the _____.

early;
atria

13.   When you look for a PAC on an EKG tracing, keep in mind that it is a single beat, and not an entire rhythm. So you really have two jobs: to identify the underlying rhythm, and to locate any ectopics. When interpreting an arrhythmia that has ectopics in it, you must identify both the _____ _____ and the _____.

underlying
rhythm;
ectopics

14.   The first thing you will notice about a PAC is that it comes prematurely; that is, it comes _____ you would expect the next beat. This causes a normally regular rhythm to be _____, since the ectopic(s) will interrupt the regular underlying rhythm. A rhythm with PACs will be _____ because the ectopics come prematurely and interrupt the _____ rhythm.

before
irregular

irregular;
underlying

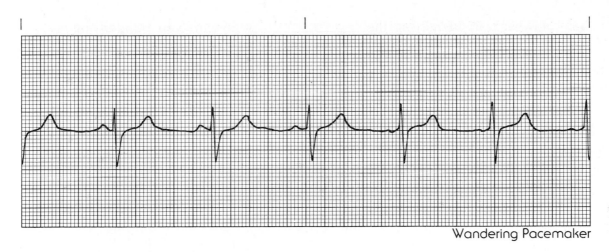

Wandering Pacemaker

Figure 25. Rules for Wandering Pacemaker

REGULARITY: The R–R intervals vary slightly as the pacemaker site changes; the rhythm can be slightly irregular.

RATE: The atrial and ventricular rates are equal; heart rate is usually within a normal range (60–100 beats per minute) but can be slower.

P WAVE: The morphology of the P wave changes as the pacemaker site changes. There is one P wave in front of every QRS complex, although some may be difficult to see depending on the pacemaker site.

PRI: The PRI measurement will vary slightly as the pacemaker site changes. All PRI measurements should be less than .20 seconds; some may be less than .12 seconds.

QRS: The QRS complex measures less than .12 seconds.

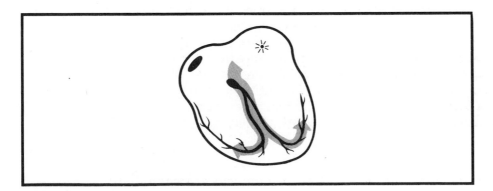

Figure 26. Premature Atrial Contraction

The pacemaker is an irritable focus within the atrium which fires prematurely and produces a single ectopic beat. Conduction through to the ventricles is normal.

15. However, in identifying the _____ rhythm, you should determine whether or not it is regular in places where there are no ectopics to interrupt it. It would be inaccurate to label a normally regular rhythm as irregular simply because it is interrupted by PACs. In order to determine whether or not the underlying rhythm is regular, you should measure the R–R intervals on a section of the strip where there are no _____.

underlying

ectopics (PACs)

16. Because PACs originate in the atria, they will have a characteristic atrial P wave that differs in morphology from the _____ P waves. An atrial P wave will usually be _____.

sinus; flattened, notched, or diphasic

17. As with Wandering Pacemaker, conduction through the AV node and the ventricles is usually _____ with a PAC; therefore, the PRI will usually be _____–_____ seconds, and the QRS will be less than _____ seconds. It is possible, though, for the PRI to be prolonged if the AV node is refractory.

normal
.12–.20
.12

18. Since a PAC comes _____ in the cardiac cycle, it will usually fall very close to the end of the preceding QRS complex. This often means that the atrial P wave which initiated the PAC will fall very near the T wave, and may be "lost" in it entirely. If visible, the PAC will have a typical atrial P wave, but it might not be visible, since it can be _____ in the preceding _____ _____.

early

lost; T wave

19. As with all other supraventricular rhythms, a PAC should have normal _____ through the AV node and ventricles, and therefore has a QRS complex of normal duration. It is possible, though, for any of these arrhythmias to have a conduction problem, thus causing a prolonged QRS complex. For all of our purposes, it is sufficient to simply call attention to this abnormality by calling it a PAC with a wide QRS complex. However, in order for an ectopic with a wide QRS complex to fit the rule of a PAC, it must have an atrial P wave in front of it. A PAC with a QRS complex greater than .12 seconds in duration should be called a PAC with a _____. _____ _____.

conduction

wide
QRS complex

20. When an atrial focus becomes irritable and fires a pacemaker impulse to override the sinus node, the premature ectopic beat is called a _____. This beat will be characterized by P waves with a morphology that is different from _____ P waves. However, the PRI and QRS measurements will be _____. PACs cause an _____ rhythm because they come earlier than expected and interrupt the regularity of the underlying rhythm.

PAC;
sinus;
normal;
irregular

21. The rules for PACs are:
  Regularity: depends on the underlying rhythm; will usually
      be regular except for the PAC
  Rate: usually normal; depends on underlying rhythm
  P Wave: P wave of early beat differs from sinus P waves;
      can be flattened or notched; may be lost in pre-
      ceding T wave
  PRI: .12–.20 seconds; can exceed .20 seconds
  QRS: less than .12 seconds

22. A PAC is caused when an irritable focus in the _____ | atria
takes over the pacemaking function for a single beat. It is also possible for a single focus in the atria to become so irritable that it begins
to fire very regularly and thus overrides the SA node for the entire
rhythm. This arrhythmia is called Atrial Tachycardia, or AT. AT is
caused by a single focus in the _____ that fires rapidly to | atria
override the SA node and thus assumes pacemaking responsibility
for the entire rhythm.

23. Atrial Tachycardia will have all of the characteristics of a PAC,
except that it is an entire _____ instead of a single beat. | rhythm
All of the P waves in AT will have an atrial configuration; they will be
peaked, flattened, notched, or diphasic. The PRI is usually normal,
and the QRS should be normal. As with PACs, Atrial Tachycardia will
have a normal _____ interval and a normal _____ | PR; QRS
duration. The P waves will be typically _____ in configura- | atrial
tion, and hence different from sinus P waves.

24. Atrial Tachycardia is characteristically a very regular arrhythmia. It is usually very rapid, with a rate range between 150 and 250
beats per minute. At this rate, it is very common for the P waves
to be hidden on the preceding T waves. The usual rate for AT is
_____–_____ beats per minute, and the rhythm is charac- | 150–250;
teristically very _____. | regular

25. When you see a very regular supraventricular rhythm which
has atrial P waves and a rate between 150 and 250 beats per minute,
you should suspect that it is _____ _____. | Atrial
Tachycardia

26. The rules for Atrial Tachycardia are:
  Regularity: regular
  Rate: 150–250 beats per minute
  P Wave: atrial P wave; differs from sinus P wave; can be
      lost in T wave
  PRI: .12–.20 seconds
  QRS: less than .12 seconds

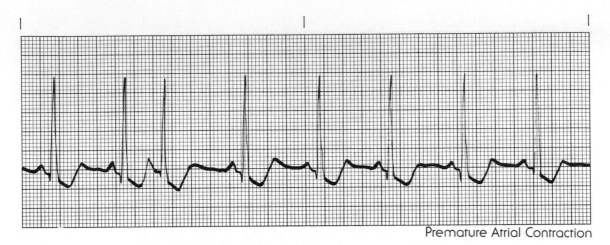

Premature Atrial Contraction

Figure 27. Rules for Premature Atrial Contraction

REGULARITY: Since this is a single premature ectopic beat, it will interrupt the regularity of the underlying rhythm.

RATE: The overall heart rate will depend on the rate of the underlying rhythm.

P WAVE: The P wave of the premature beat will have a different morphology than the P waves of the rest of the strip. The ectopic beat will have a P wave, but it can be flattened, notched, or otherwise unusual. It may be hidden within the T wave of the preceding complex.

PRI: The PRI should measure between .12 and .20 seconds, but can be prolonged; the PRI of the ectopic will probably be different from the PRI measurements of the other complexes.

QRS: The QRS complex measurement will be less than .12 seconds.

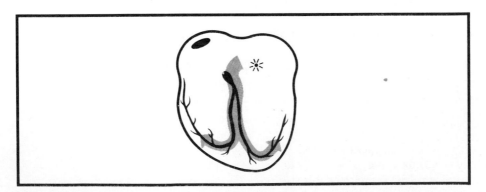

Figure 28. Atrial Tachycardia

The pacemaker is a single irritable site within the atrium which fires repetitively at a very rapid rate. Conduction through to the ventricles is normal.

27.   When the atria become so irritable that they fire faster than 250 beats per minute, they are said to be "fluttering." It is theorized that an area in the atrium initiates an impulse which is conducted in a repetitive, cyclic pattern, creating a series of atrial waves with a saw-tooth appearance (called Flutter or "F" waves). This rhythm is called Atrial Flutter. Atrial Flutter is an atrial arrhythmia that occurs when ectopic foci in the atria exceed a rate of _____ beats per minute; the atrial rate is usually in the range of 250–350 beats per minute.

250

28.   The problem with a heart rate this rapid is that the ventricles don't have enough time to fill with blood between each beat. The result is that the ventricles will continue to pump but they won't be ejecting adequate _____ volume to meet body needs. The heart has a built-in protective mechanism to prevent this from happening: the AV node. The AV _____ is responsible for preventing excess impulses from reaching the ventricles. So,

blood

node

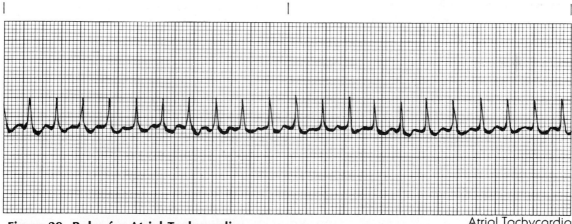

Figure 29. Rules for Atrial Tachycardia   Atrial Tachycardia

REGULARITY: The R–R intervals are constant; the rhythm is regular.
RATE: The atrial and ventricular rates are equal; the heart rate is usually 150–250 beats per minute.
P WAVE: There is one P wave in front of every QRS complex. The configuration of the P wave will be different than that of sinus P waves; they may be flattened or notched. Because of the rapid rate, the P waves can be hidden in the T waves of the preceding beats.
PRI: The PRI is between .12 and .20 seconds and constant across the strip. The PRI may be difficult to measure if the P wave is obscured by the T wave.
QRS: The QRS complex measures less than .12 seconds.

when the heart beats too fast, the _____ _____   AV node;
will prevent some of the impulses from reaching the _____.   ventricles
This blocking action allows the ventricles time to fill with blood before they have to contract.

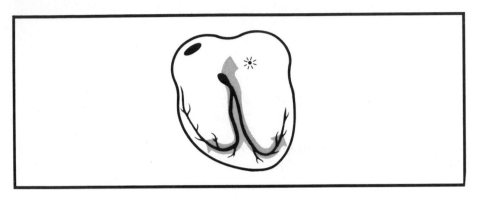

Figure 30. Atrial Flutter

**A single irritable focus within the atria issues an impulse that is conducted
in a rapid, repetitive fashion. To protect the ventricles from receiving too
many impulses, the AV node blocks some of the impulses from being conducted through to the ventricles.**

29. In Atrial Flutter, the atrial rate is between 250 and 350 beats per
minute. Therefore, the AV node seeks to block some of these impulses and slow the ventricular rate. This will be seen on the EKG as
a very rapid series of P waves (Flutter waves) with an atrial rate of
250–350, but not every one is followed by a QRS complex. The ventricular rate will thus be quite a bit slower than the atrial rate. In
Atrial Flutter the atrial rate will be between _____ and _____   250; 350
beats per minute, but the ventricular rate will be _____.   slower

30. The AV node usually allows only every second, third, or fourth
impulse to be conducted through to the ventricles. On the EKG this
will look like two, three, or four sawtooth F waves between each
QRS complex. If the node is consistent in how it lets the impulses
through, the ventricular rhythm will be regular. However, the node
can be very erratic about conducting impulses. When this happens
the ratio between F waves and QRS complexes can vary between
2:1, 3:1, and 4:1, thus creating an irregular R–R interval. This is
called variable block, and causes the R–R interval in Atrial Flutter to
be _____.   irregular

31. When the atria are fluttering, it is virtually impossible to accurately determine the PRI. So when you gather data from the strip, the
PRI is not measured. In an Atrial Flutter, the _____ is not   PRI
measured.

32.   The QRS complex is normal in Atrial Flutter. As with other supraventricular arrhythmias, if the rhythm is normal, the QRS complex will be less than .12 seconds. If the QRS is greater than .12 seconds, the arrhythmia should be considered abnormal and should be labeled Atrial Flutter with a _____ _____ _____.

wide QRS complex

33.   When you see an EKG tracing that has more than one P wave for every QRS complex, with an atrial rate of 250–350 beats per minute, particularly if the P waves have a sawtooth configuration, you would know that there is a lot of irritability in the atria, and that they are fluttering. This rhythm is called _____.

Atrial Flutter

34.   The rules for Atrial Flutter are:
      Regularity: atrial rhythm is regular; ventricular rhythm is usually regular but can be irregular if there is variable block
      Rate: atrial rate 250–350 beats per minute; ventricular rate varies
      P Wave: characteristic sawtooth pattern
      PRI: unable to determine
      QRS: less than .12 seconds

35.   The last atrial arrhythmia you will learn about is called Atrial Fibrillation. This rhythm results when the atria become so irritable that they are no longer beating, but are merely quivering ineffectively. This ineffective quivering is called fibrillation. On the EKG tracing it is seen as a series of indiscernible waves along the isoelectric line. In most arrhythmias the P wave is reliably present, and nearly always regular, thus providing a helpful clue for interpreting the rhythm. But in Atrial Fibrillation, there are no discernible P waves, and when you do see one or two here or there, they cannot be mapped out across the strip. Atrial Fibrillation characteristically has no discernible _____ waves. The fibrillatory waves characteristic of Atrial Fibrillation are called "f" waves.

P

36.   In Atrial Fibrillation, the atria are quivering at a rate in excess of 350 times per minute. But this is an academic point, since there are no _____ waves with which we can measure the atrial rate. We do know, though, that the atria are fibrillating so rapidly that the AV _____ must block some of the impulses in order to keep the ventricular rate reasonable. Unlike Atrial Flutter, where the sawtooth P waves are conducted through in a semi-regular fashion, the fibrillatory waves of Atrial Fibrillation are conducted in an extremely chaotic pattern, producing a grossly irregular _____ interval. The rhythm of Atrial Fibrillation is grossly _____ because the fibrillatory waves are conducted in a very chaotic way.

P

node

R–R; irregular

37.   The two most characteristic features of Atrial Fibrillation, and the reasons why this arrhythmia is so easily recognized, are that there are no discernible P waves and the rhythm is grossly irregular. As the ventricular rate becomes faster, the R waves get closer together on the EKG paper, which makes the rhythm appear more regular. But even with rapid rates, Atrial Fibrillation is grossly _____ and has no discernible _____ waves.

irregular;
P

38.   Because Atrial Fibrillation originates above the ventricles, conduction through to the ventricles will proceed within normal time frames (for those impulses that are conducted), thus resulting in a _____ QRS measurement. The QRS measurement in Atrial Fibrillation will normally be less than .12 seconds.

normal
(narrow)

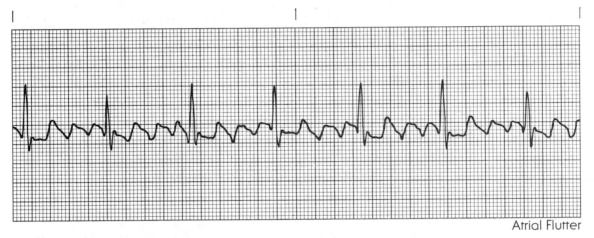

Atrial Flutter

Figure 31. Rules for Atrial Flutter

REGULARITY: **The atrial rhythm is regular. The ventricular rhythm will be regular if the AV node conducts impulses through in a consistent pattern. If the pattern varies, the ventricular rate will be irregular.**

RATE: **Atrial rate is between 250 and 350 beats per minute. Ventricular rate will depend on the ratio of impulses conducted through to the ventricles.**

P WAVE: **When the atria flutter they produce a series of well-defined P waves. When seen together, these "Flutter" waves have a sawtooth appearance.**

PRI: **Because of the unusual configuration of the P wave (Flutter wave) and the proximity of the wave to the QRS complex, it is often impossible to determine a PRI in this arrhythmia. Therefore, the PRI is not measured in Atrial Flutter.**

QRS: **The QRS complex measures less than .12 seconds; measurement can be difficult if one or more flutter waves is concealed within the QRS complex.**

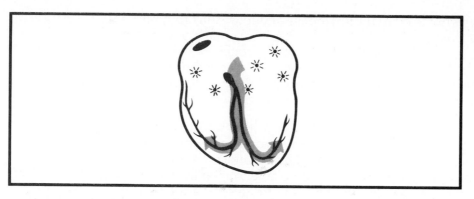

Figure 32. Atrial Fibrillation

The atria are so irritable that a multitude of foci initiate impulses, causing the atria to depolarize repeatedly in a fibrillatory manner. The AV node blocks most of the impulses, allowing only a limited number through to the ventricles.

39.   One other thing is important to note about Atrial Fibrillation. There is a big difference between an Atrial Fibrillation with a ventricular response within a normal rate range (less than 100 beats per minute), and an Atrial Fibrillation with an excessively rapid ventricular response. This is because the rapid rate will create symptoms in the patient, whereas the slower rate is less likely to cause problems. If the ventricular rate is less than 100 beats per minute, the rhythm is called Atrial Fibrillation with a controlled ventricular response. If the rate is greater than 100 beats per minute, the rhythm is called Atrial Fibrillation with a rapid ventricular response. A controlled ventricular response indicates that the ventricular rate is _____   less than 100 beats per minute, while a rapid ventricular response means that the ventricles are beating at _____ than 100 beats   more per minute.

40.   Since you can't identify legitimate P waves in an Atrial Fibrillation, it is impossible to determine a _____ interval. You   PR would note this on your data sheet as "not able to measure." In an Atrial Fibrillation, the PRI is not _____.   measurable

41.   The rules for Atrial Fibrillation are:
      Regularity: grossly irregular
          Rate: atrial rate greater than 350 beats per minute
                ventricular rate varies greatly
    P Wave: no discernible P waves, atrial activity is referred
                to as fibrillatory waves (f waves)
       PRI: unable to measure
      QRS: less than .12 seconds

42. You now know five atrial arrhythmias and four sinus rhythms. You know that rhythms originating in the sinus node have a characteristic, _____ P wave. The P wave associated with atrial arrhythmias can be flattened, peaked, notched, or even diphasic. But all of these patterns should have a normal QRS measurement since they originate _____ the ventricles.

uniform

above

43. As with the sinus rhythms, you must now memorize all of the rules for each of the atrial arrhythmias. Then you can begin gathering data from the strips shown in Practice Sheet 6 and compare them to the rules for each pattern. You should be able to identify each of the strips with relative ease. If you have any trouble, or are unsure about the process, you must seek help before going on to the next section.

Practice
Sheet 6

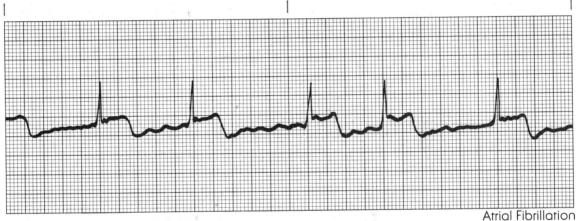

Atrial Fibrillation

Figure 33. Rules for Atrial Fibrillation

REGULARITY: The atrial rhythm is unmeasurable; all atrial activity is chaotic. The ventricular rhythm is grossly irregular, having no pattern to its irregularity.

RATE: The atrial rate cannot be measured because it is so chaotic; research indicates that it exceeds 350 beats per minute. The ventricular rate is significantly slower because the AV node blocks most of the impulses. If the ventricular rate is below 100 beats per minute the rhythm is said to be "controlled"; if it is over 100 beats per minute it is considered to have a "rapid ventricular response."

P WAVE: In this arrhythmia the atria are not depolarizing in an effective way; instead, they are fibrillating. Thus, no P wave is produced. All atrial activity is depicted as "fibrillatory" waves, or grossly chaotic undulations of the baseline.

PRI: Since no P waves are visible, no PRI can be measured.

QRS: The QRS complex measurement should be less than .12 seconds.

Key Points – Atrial Rhythms

- All supraventricular arrhythmias should have a normal QRS measurement; if they don't, it should be noted by naming the rhythm but saying it has "a wide QRS complex."

- Atrial arrhythmias occur when an ectopic focus in the atria assumes responsibility for pacing the heart, either by irritability or escape.

- An ectopic focus is one that originates outside of the SA node.

- Because an atrial focus is outside of the SA node, any impulse coming from it would cause an unusual depolarization wave, thus causing the P wave to have an unusual configuration; this atrial P wave can be either flattened, notched, peaked, or diphasic.

- In Wandering Pacemaker the pacemaker shifts between the SA node and the atria, causing each P wave to differ slightly from those around it.

- Here are the rules for *Wandering Pacemaker*:

    Rhythm: slightly irregular
      Rate: usually normal, 60–100 beats/minute
    P Wave: morphology changes from beat to beat
       PRI: less than .20 seconds; may vary
      QRS: less than .12 seconds.

- Premature Atrial Contractions (PACs) are single beats that originate in the atria and come early in the cardiac cycle.

- Ectopic beats that come early in the cardiac cycle are caused by irritability; ectopic beats that come later than expected in the cardiac cycle are caused by the escape mechanism.

- When confronted with ectopics, you must identify both the ectopic and the underlying rhythm.

- A rhythm with ectopics in it will be irregular, even if the underlying rhythm is characteristically regular; this is because the ectopic(s) interrupt the regularity of the underlying pattern.

- Here are the rules for *Premature Atrial Contractions*:

    Rhythm: depends on the underlying rhythm; will usually be regular
            except for the PAC
      Rate: usually normal; depends on underlying rhythm
    P Wave: P wave of early beat differs from sinus P waves;
            can be flattened or notched; may be lost in preceding
            T wave.
       PRI: .12–.20 seconds; can be greater than .20 seconds
      QRS: less than .12 seconds.

- Atrial Tachycardia is caused when a single focus in the atria fires very rapidly and overrides the SA node.

- Here are the rules for *Atrial Tachycardia*:

  Rhythm: regular
    Rate: 150–250 beats per minute
  P Wave: atrial P wave; differs from sinus P wave; can be
            lost in preceding T wave
    PRI: .12–.20 seconds
    QRS: less than .12 seconds.

- In Atrial Flutter and Atrial Fibrillation the atria are beating too rapidly for the ventricles to respond, so the AV node blocks some of the impulses.

- Here are the rules for *Atrial Flutter*:

  Rhythm: atrial rhythm is regular; ventricular rhythm is usually regular
            but can be irregular if there is variable block
    Rate: atrial rate 250–350 beats per minute;
            ventricular rate varies
  P Wave: characteristic sawtooth pattern (F waves)
    PRI: unable to determine
    QRS: less than .12 seconds.

- Here are the rules for *Atrial Fibrillation*:

  Rhythm: grossly irregular
    Rate: atrial rate greater than 350 beats per minute;
            ventricular rate varies greatly
  P Wave: no discernible P waves; atrial activity is referred to as
            fibrillatory waves (f waves)
    PRI: unable to measure
    QRS: less than .12 seconds.

Self-Test: Atrial Rhythms

Directions:

Complete this self-evaluation of the information you have learned from this chapter. If your answers are all correct and you feel comfortable with your understanding of the material, proceed to the next chapter. However, if you missed any of the questions you should review the referenced frames before proceeding. If you feel uncomfortable with any of your understanding, invest the time now to go back over the entire chapter. DO NOT PROCEED WITH THE NEXT CHAPTER UNTIL YOU ARE VERY COMFORTABLE WITH THE MATERIAL IN THIS CHAPTER.

Question	Referenced Frames	
1. How does an atrial P wave differ from a sinus P wave?	3; 4; 5; 42	Sinus P waves are upright and uniform. Atrial P waves can be flattened, notched, irregular, or even inverted.
2. What two basic mechanisms can cause an atrial focus to take over pacemaking responsibilities?	1; 2; 11	irritability or escape
3. What is an ectopic focus?	9; 10	a site of electrical activity *other than* the SA node
4. Which atrial arrhythmia is characterized by a pacemaker which shifts between the SA node and various foci in the atria, sometimes even dropping down to the AV junction?	6; 7; 8	Wandering Pacemaker
5. What is a PAC (Premature Atrial Contractions)?	9; 10; 11; 12; 13; 14; 20; 21; 22	a single beat that originates in the atrium and comes early in the cardiac cycle

Question	Referenced Frames	
6. Is a PAC an ectopic?	9; 10; 11; 12; 13; 22	Yes, because it originates outside of the SA node.
7. If an ectopic is caused by irritability, will it come earlier than expected, or later than expected?	11; 14; 18; 22	Earlier; if the ectopic comes later than expected it was caused by escape mechanism.
8. Is Wandering Pacemaker a single ectopic beat?	6; 9	No, it is an entire arrhythmia.
9. What is the most characteristic feature of Wandering Pacemaker?	6	the changing shapes of the P waves as the pacemaker site shifts locations
10. What should the QRS measurement be for a PAC?	5; 17; 19; 21; 42	less than .12 seconds
11. What will the P wave look like on a PAC?	5; 16; 19; 20; 21; 42	it would have the characteristic look of atrial P waves: it could be flattened, notched, diphasic, or peaked
12. If the P wave of a PAC was not clearly visible, where might you consider looking for it?	18	in the T wave of the preceding complex
13. Is Atrial Tachycardia caused by one irritable focus, or by many?	22	only one; this is why it is usually so regular

Question	**Referenced Frames**	
14. What is the usual rate range for Atrial Tachycardia?	24; 25; 26	150–250 beats per minute
15. Does Atrial Tachycardia have a P wave in front of every QRS complex?	26	Yes, although you may have some trouble seeing them if they are superimposed on the T waves of the preceding complexes.
16. What does the P wave look like in an Atrial Tachycardia?	5; 23; 26; 43	just like the P wave of a PAC; in fact, AT looks very much like a lot of PACs connected together
17. What happens if the atria begin beating too rapidly for the ventricles to respond to them?	28; 29; 30	The AV node may block some of the impulses so that they aren't conducted to the ventricles. This results in more P waves than QRS complexes.
18. Which two atrial arrhythmias do you know that involve the phenomenon described in the preceding question?	29; 36	Atrial Flutter and Atrial Fibrillation
19. What's the atrial rate in Atrial Flutter?	27; 29; 33; 34	250–350 beats per min

Question	Referenced Frames	
20. Is the ventricular rhythm regular or irregular in Atrial Flutter?	30; 34	This depends on how the AV node is blocking impulses. If atrial impulses are being conducted in a regular pattern, e.g., 2:1 or 4:1, the ventricular rhythm would be regular. But if the conduction ratio varied, e.g., 2:1, 3:1, 2:1, etc., the ventricular rhythm would be irregular.
21. In Atrial Flutter, would the ventricular rate be faster or slower than the atrial rate?	29; 30; 33; 34	The ventricular rate would always be slower, unless the conduction ratio was 1:1. This is because not all of the P waves are able to produce QRS complexes.
22. What does the atrial activity look like in an Atrial Flutter?	29; 30; 33; 34	The Flutter waves usually take on a characteristic sawtooth appearance, although not always.

Question	**Referenced Frames**	
23. How would you describe the atrial activity in Atrial Fibrillation?	35; 36; 41	The atria are not contracting; instead they are quivering chaotically. This causes the isoelectric line to undulate in a very irregular fashion. There are no visible P waves, only fibrillatory waves (f waves).
24. What is the atrial rate in Atrial Fibrillation?	36; 41	over 350 beats per min
25. Is there a relationship between atrial activity and ventricular activity in Atrial Fibrillation?	36; 38; 41	Yes, there is; some of the impulses are conducted through to the ventricles, but it is not possible to determine a PRI because there is no clear P wave.
26. What is the ventricular rate for Atrial Fibrillation?	36; 39; 41	That depends on how many of the impulses are conducted through to the ventricles. If the ventricular rate is less than 100 beats per minute, the rhythm is called Atrial

Question	**Referenced Frames**	
		Fibrillation with "controlled" ventricular response. If the rate is over 100 beats per minute, it is called a "rapid ventricular response."
27. What are the two most characteristic features of Atrial Fibrillation?	36; 37; 41	It has no discernible P waves, and the R–R interval is grossly irregular.

Practice Sheet 6:
Atrial Rhythms

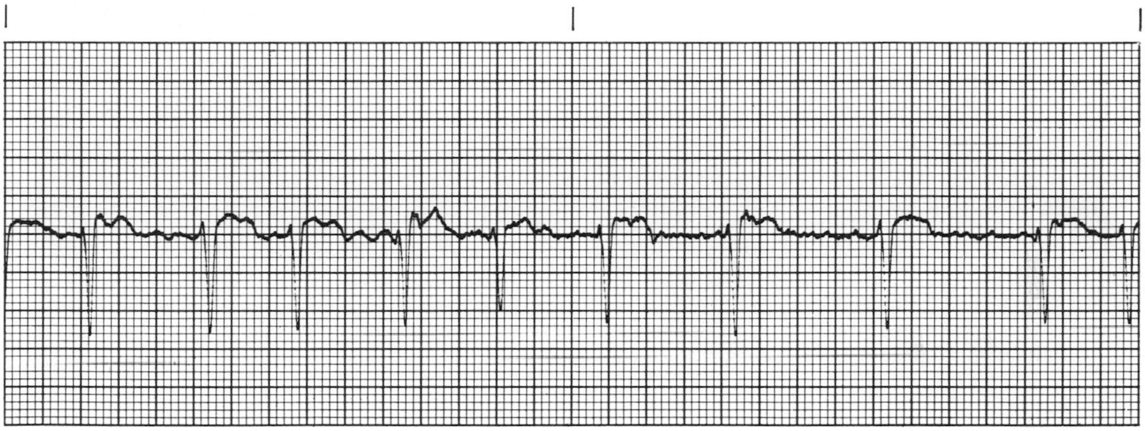

6.1   Regularity: _____
           Rate: _____
           P Waves: _____
           PRI: _____
           QRS: _____
           Interp: _____

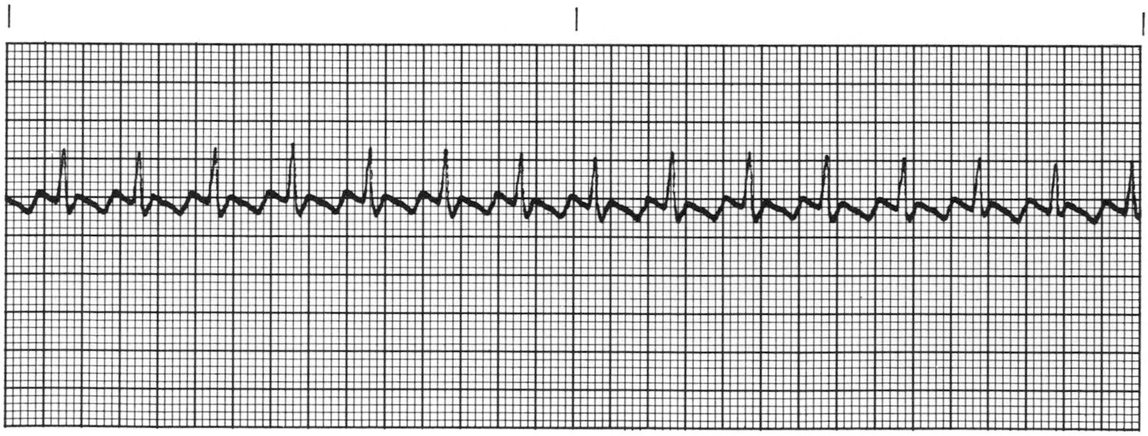

6.2   Regularity: _____
           Rate: _____
           P Waves: _____
           PRI: _____
           QRS: _____
           Interp: _____

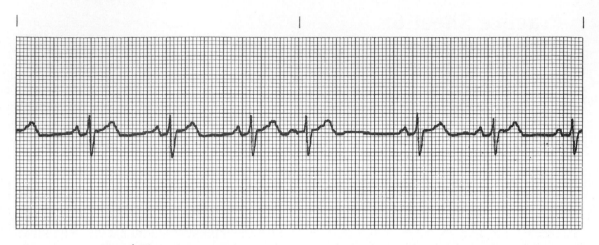

6.3   Regularity: _____
       Rate: _____
       P Waves: _____
       PRI: _____
       QRS: _____
       Interp: _____

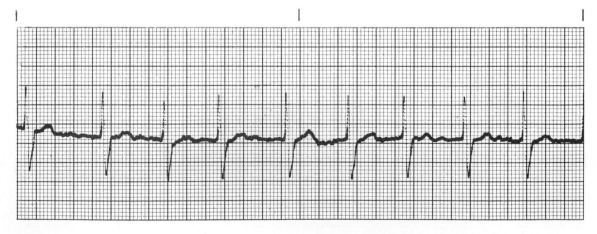

6.4   Regularity: _____
       Rate: _____
       P Waves: _____
       PRI: _____
       QRS: _____
       Interp: _____

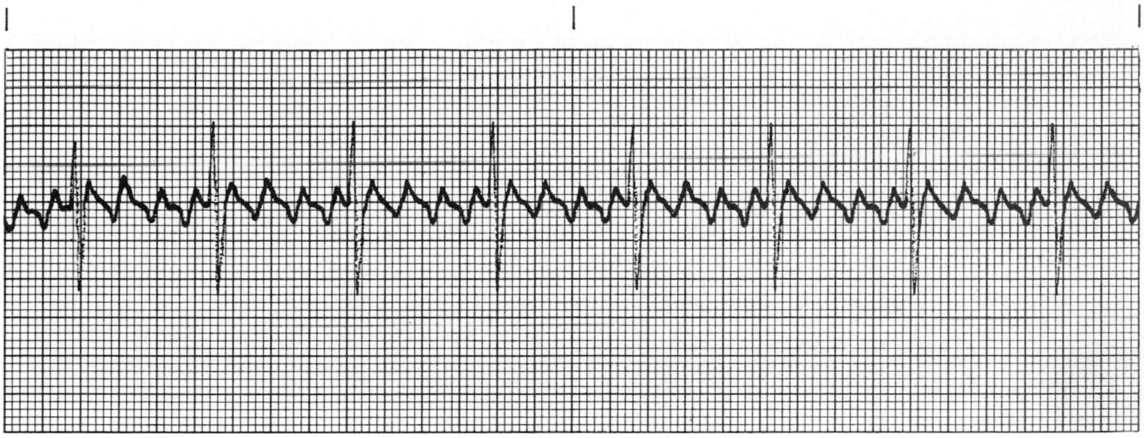

6.5   Regularity: _____
            Rate: _____
            P Waves: _____
            PRI: _____
            QRS: _____
            Interp: _____

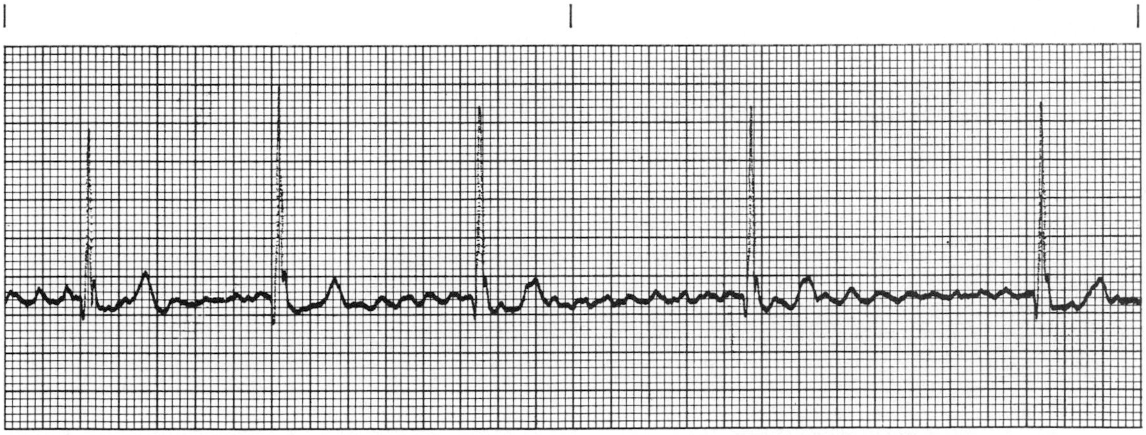

6.6   Regularity: _____
            Rate: _____
            P Waves: _____
            PRI: _____
            QRS: _____
            Interp: _____

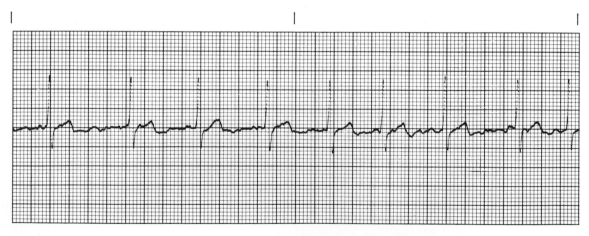

6.7   Regularity: _____
       Rate: _____
       P Waves: _____
       PRI: _____
       QRS: _____
       Interp: _____

6.8   Regularity: _____
       Rate: _____
       P Waves: _____
       PRI: _____
       QRS: _____
       Interp: _____

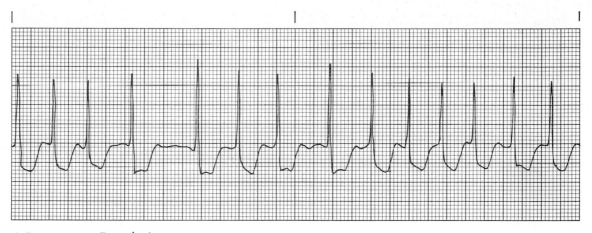

6.9   Regularity: _____
            Rate: _____
            P Waves: _____
            PRI: _____
            QRS: _____
            Interp: _____

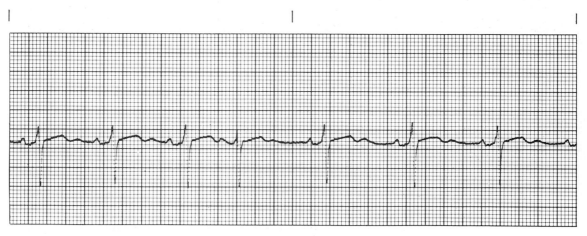

6.10   Regularity: _____
            Rate: _____
            P Waves: _____
            PRI: _____
            QRS: _____
            Interp: _____

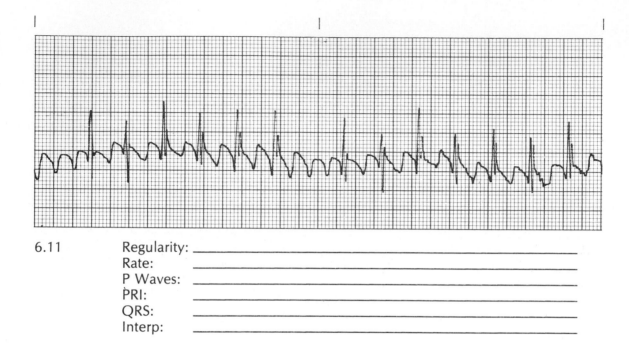

6.11   Regularity: _____

            Rate: _____

            P Waves: _____

            PRI: _____

            QRS: _____

            Interp: _____

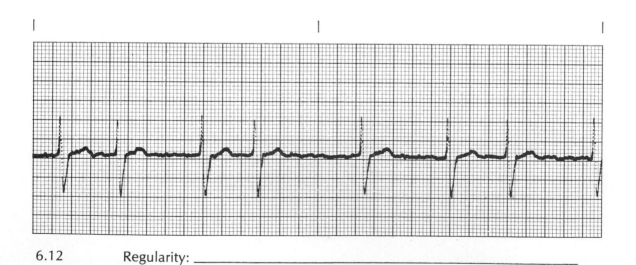

6.12   Regularity: _____

            Rate: _____

            P Waves: _____

            PRI: _____

            QRS: _____

            Interp: _____

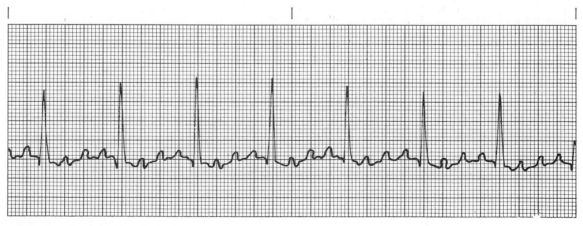

6.13   Regularity: _____
            Rate: _____
            P Waves: _____
            PRI: _____
            QRS: _____
            Interp: _____

6.14   Regularity: _____
            Rate: _____
            P Waves: _____
            PRI: _____
            QRS: _____
            Interp: _____

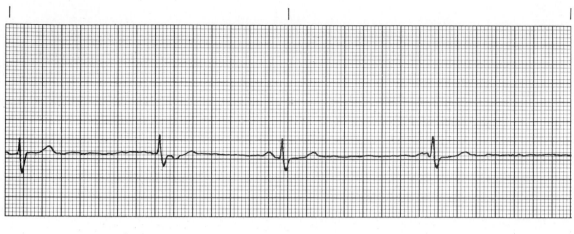

6.15   Regularity: _____
              Rate: _____
              P Waves: _____
              PRI: _____
              QRS: _____
              Interp: _____

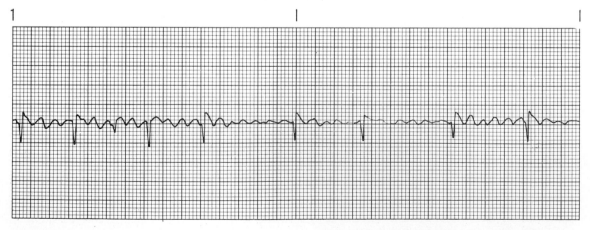

6.16   Regularity: _____
              Rate: _____
              P Waves: _____
              PRI: _____
              QRS: _____
              Interp: _____

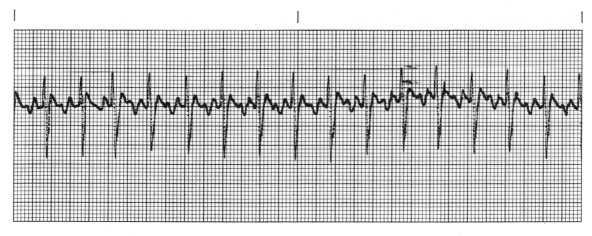

6.17   Regularity: _____
        Rate: _____
        P Waves: _____
        PRI: _____
        QRS: _____
        Interp: _____

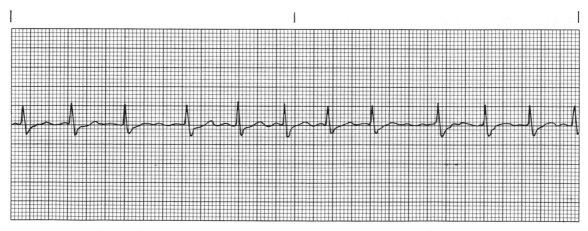

6.18   Regularity: _____
        Rate: _____
        P Waves: _____
        PRI: _____
        QRS: _____
        Interp: _____

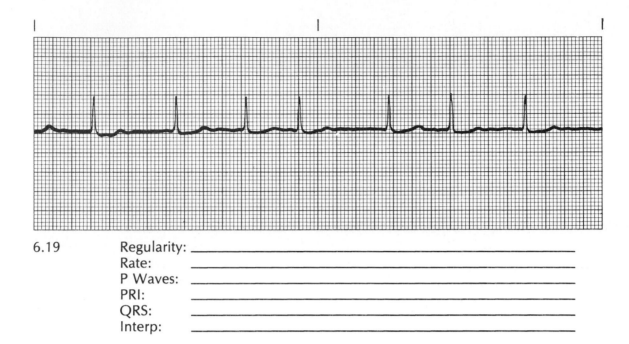

6.19   Regularity: _____
        Rate: _____
        P Waves: _____
        PRI: _____
        QRS: _____
        Interp: _____

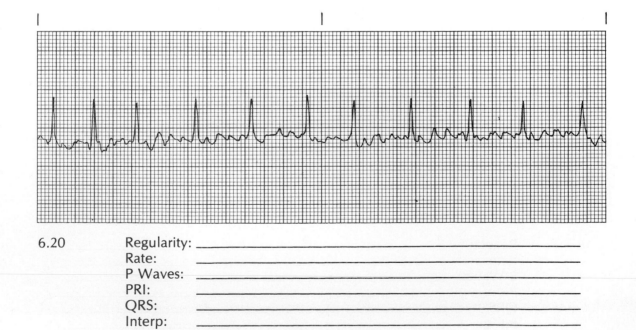

6.20   Regularity: _____
        Rate: _____
        P Waves: _____
        PRI: _____
        QRS: _____
        Interp: _____

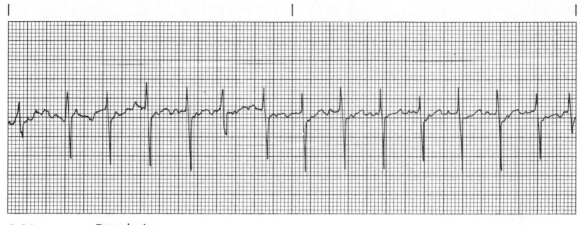

6.21   Regularity: _____
         Rate: _____
         P Waves: _____
         PRI: _____
         QRS: _____
         Interp: _____

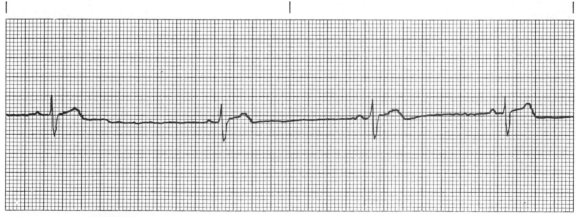

6.22   Regularity: _____
         Rate: _____
         P Waves: _____
         PRI: _____
         QRS: _____
         Interp: _____

6

Junctional Rhythms

1.   You learned in Chapter 1 that the AV node is responsible for conducting impulses from the _____ _____ and the _____ down the conduction pathways into the ventricles. And you learned that the node has the ability to hold impulses or even block them from getting through to the ventricles. The one property the node does not have is the ability to initiate impulses. It was once thought that the node could be a pacemaker, but research now suggests that the pacemaker cells are not in the node at all. They are in the tissues located at the junction between the atria and the node. This area is called the AV junction. Arrhythmias that originate in the area of the AV node really come from the junctional tissues; thus they are called AV _____ rhythms.

SA node;
atria

junctional

2.   Since the electrical impulses originate in the AV junction the heart is depolarized in a somewhat unusual fashion. With the pacemaker located in the middle of the heart, the electrical impulses spread in two directions simultaneously. This is unusual because the heart is normally depolarized by a single force spreading downward toward the _____. However, when the AV junction assumes _____ responsibility, the atria and the ventricles will be depolarized at very nearly the same time because the impulse spreads in _____ directions at one time. This concept is pictured in Figure 34.

ventricles;
pacemaking

two

3.   As you recall, electrode positions for Lead II place the _____ electrode above the right atria and the _____ electrode below the ventricle. (See Figure 35.) In the normal heart, the major thrust of electrical flow is toward the ventricles (and toward the positive electrode in Lead II), thus producing an upright P wave and an upright QRS complex. In a junctional rhythm, the ventricles are depolarized by an impulse traveling down the conduction system toward the positive electrode; thus the QRS complex is _____. But at the same time, the impulse spreads upward through the atria toward the _____ electrode. The method by which the atria are depolarized is called "retrograde conduction," because the electrical impulse is traveling in the opposite direction it usually takes. The mechanism which enables the AV junction to depolarize the atria with a backward flow of electricity is called _____ conduction.

negative;
positive

upright

negative

retrograde

4.   We know that the QRS complex is upright in junctional arrhythmias because the ventricles were depolarized by an impulse traveling toward the _____ electrode. We also know that the atria are depolarized by a _____ impulse which travels toward the negative electrode. We can thus deduce that the electrical pattern on the EKG which depicts atrial depolarization will be shown as an inverted P wave. In other words, the P wave of an AV junctional arrhythmia should be _____, since it was produced by an impulse traveling toward the negative electrode.

positive;
retrograde

inverted
(downward)

5. In AV junctional arrhythmias, the atria are depolarized via _____ conduction at approximately the same time as the ventricles are depolarized in the normal manner. The production of two simultaneous electrical force flows, one retrograde and the other normal, results in an inverted _____ wave and an upright _____ complex.

retrograde

P;
QRS

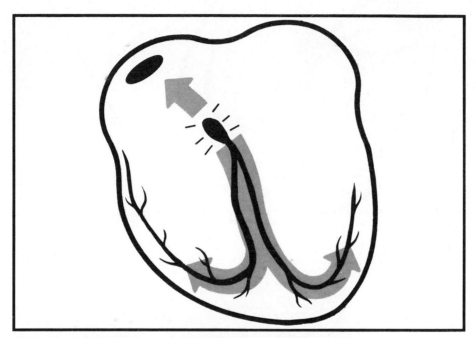

Figure 34. Electrical Flow in Junctional Arrhythmias

6. In junctional arrhythmias a single impulse originates in the AV junction and causes electricity to flow in two directions. One electrical force flows upward (retrograde) to depolarize the _____ while the other flows downward to depolarize the _____. Even though both electrical forces originate from a single impulse in the junction, the force that depolarizes the atria is not the same force that depolarizes the ventricles. For this reason, you will not always see a consistent relationship between the inverted P wave and the QRS complex. The P wave will not have a consistent relationship to the QRS complex because the force that depolarizes the atria is not the same force that depolarizes the _____.

atria
ventricles

ventricles

7. In junctional arrhythmias the P wave does not always have to precede the QRS complex, because it is possible for the ventricles to be depolarized before the atria, if the force reaches them first. The position of the P wave in relation to the QRS complex will depend on whether the atria or the ventricles were _____ first.

depolarized

NEGATIVE
ELECTRODE

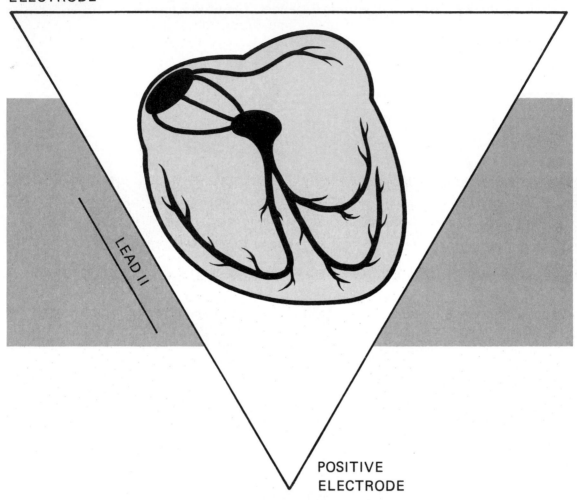

LEAD II

POSITIVE
ELECTRODE

Figure 35. Electrode Placement for Monitoring EKG

If the ventricles are depolarized before the atria, the QRS will come before the P wave. If the atria depolarize first, the P wave will precede the QRS complex. If they both depolarize simultaneously, the _____ wave will be hidden within the QRS complex. In junctional arrhythmias, the P wave is always _____, because the atria are depolarized via retrograde conduction. But the P wave can come before, during, or after the _____ complex, depending on which depolarized first, the atria or the ventricles (See Fig. 36).

P
inverted

QRS

8.   The biggest clue to a junctional rhythm is the inverted P wave. But this same phenomenon occurs with some atrial arrhythmias

when the impulse originates so low in the atria that it is very near the AV junction. In such cases the impulse will have to depolarize parts of the atria with retrograde conduction, thus producing an inverted P wave. Therefore, while all junctional rhythms must have inverted P waves, a rhythm with an inverted P wave can be either _____ or _____ in origin.

atrial;
junctional

9. When you see an arrhythmia with an inverted P wave following the QRS complex, you know that it had to have originated in the AV _____. But if the inverted P wave precedes the QRS complex, you need to determine whether it originated in the AV junction or in the _____. The important clue will come from the PR interval. If the impulse originated in the atria, the impulse would take the normal length of time getting through the node and into the ventricles. Thus, the PRI would be normal, or _____–_____ seconds. But if the impulse originated in the AV junction, it would take less time to get to the ventricles, and thus would have a PRI of less than .12 seconds. If the rhythm has an inverted P wave and a normal PRI measurement, you would know that it originated in the _____, whereas if the PRI was less than .12 seconds, it had to have originated in the _____.

junction

atria

.12–.20

atria;

AV junction

10. You now know quite a bit about junctional rhythms in general. You know that the QRS measurement is _____, and that the P wave will be _____. The P wave will be seen either before or after the QRS complex, but the rhythm might not have a visible P wave at all if it is hidden within the QRS complex. Finally, you know that the PRI must be less than .12 seconds; if it is greater than .12 seconds the arrhythmia would be _____ in origin. All of these rules pertain to all junctional arrhythmias, regardless of the mechanism displayed. For example, a junctional tachycardia could have an inverted P wave before, during, or after the QRS complex, and the same goes for other types of junctional arrhythmias. So for each of the individual arrhythmias you will now learn about, you know that all of the above rules apply; all _____ arrhythmias will comply with the above rules, regardless of the mechanism.

normal;
inverted

atrial

junctional

11. All junctional arrhythmias will have an inverted P wave because the atria are depolarized via _____ conduction.

retrograde

12. Atrial arrhythmias can also have _____ P waves since they can be produced by retrograde conduction.

inverted

13. Junctional arrhythmias will have a PRI of less than _____ seconds; atrial arrhythmias will have a PRI of _____–_____ seconds.

.12;
.12–.20

14. An inverted P wave which precedes the QRS complex and has a PRI of less than .12 seconds indicates that the pacemaker impulse

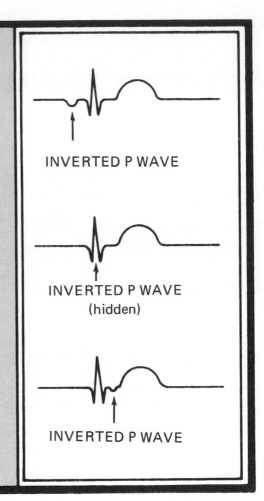

The P wave will precede the QRS complex if the atria are depolarized before the ventricles. In such a case, the PRI will be less than .12 seconds.

If the atria and the ventricles are depolarized simultaneously there will be no visible P wave, since it is hidden within the QRS complex.

The P wave will follow the QRS complex if the ventricles are depolarized before the atria.

Figure 36. P Wave Placement in Junctional Rhythms

originated in the _____ _____, and the atria depolarized _____ the ventricles.

AV junction; before

15. If the junctional impulse reached the ventricles first and depolarized the ventricles before the atria, it would produce an inverted P wave _____ the QRS complex.

following

16. You would not see a P wave if the impulse originated in the junction but reached the atria and the ventricles simultaneously, since this would cause the P wave to be _____ within the QRS complex.

hidden

17. If visible, a junctional P wave will be _____, but it can be hidden within the QRS complex if both the atria and the ventricles are _____ simultaneously.

inverted

depolarized

18.   The junctional pacemaker site can produce a variety of arrhythmias depending on the mechanism employed. We will discuss four basic mechanisms common to the AV junction:
- premature junctional contraction
- junctional escape rhythm
- accelerated junctional rhythm
- junctional tachycardia

Although these are four different mechanisms, each of these arrhythmias originates in the AV _____.

junction

19.   The first junctional arrhythmia we will learn about is called a Premature Junctional Contraction, or PJC. As with Premature Atrial Contractions (PAC), this is something of a misnomer, since it applies to depolarization, rather than actual _____. But the general implication is still the same: an irritable focus in the junction stimulates an early cardiac cycle, which interrupts the underlying rhythm for a single _____. When such a premature ectopic originates in the AV junction it is called a PJC, or _____ _____ _____.

contraction

beat
premature
junctional
contraction

20.   Since a PJC is a single beat, it will interrupt the rhythm of the underlying pattern. The R–R interval will be regular or irregular, depending on the regularity of the underlying rhythm, but the PJC will come earlier than expected, and thus will cause the overall rhythm to be irregular. Because a PJC is a single early beat, it will cause the overall rhythm to be _____.

irregular

21.   As with regularity, the rate will depend on the rate of the underlying arrhythmia. Being a single beat, a PJC does not have a rate of its own. To determine heart rate, you would have to look at the overall rate of the _____ rhythm.

underlying

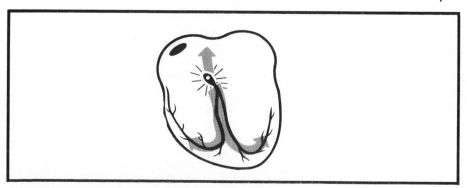

Figure 37. Premature Junctional Contraction

The pacemaker is an irritable focus within the AV junction which fires prematurely and produces a single ectopic beat. The atria are depolarized via retrograde conduction. Conduction through the ventricles is normal.

22. The P wave of a PJC will be consistent with the P waves of all other junctional arrhythmias. Because atrial depolarization is retrograde, the P wave will be _____, and can fall before, during, or after the _____ complex.

inverted; QRS

23. If the P wave of the PJC precedes the QRS complex, the PRI will be less than _____ seconds.

.12

24. Conduction through the ventricles should be normal with a PJC. Therefore, the QRS complex should have a normal duration of _____.

less than .12 seconds

25. The rules for PJCs are:
    Regularity: depends on rhythm of underlying arrhythmia
        Rate: depends on rate of underlying arrhythmia
    P Wave: will be inverted; can fall before, during, or after the QRS complex
        PRI: can only be measured if the P wave precedes the QRS complex; if measurable will be less than .12 seconds
        QRS: less than .12 seconds

26. The normal, inherent rate for the AV junction is 40–60 beats per minute. A PJC occurs when the junction becomes irritable and overrides higher sites. But the junction can also take over pacemaking responsibility if higher sites fail. The junction would then "escape" and assume pacemaking functions at its own inherent rate of _____–_____ beats per minute.

40–60

27. As you recall, a premature beat is a sign of irritability, whereas an _____ beat comes later than you would expect it, and is a fail-safe mechanism to protect the heart. When the AV junction is allowed to assume pacemaking functions at its inherent rate of 40–60 beats per minute, this is an example of _____ mechanism, rather than irritability.

escape

escape

28. When you see Junctional Escape Rhythm you would expect it to have a rate of _____–_____ beats per minute, since this is the inherent rate of the AV junction. Junctional Escape Rhythm is sometimes referred to as "Passive" Junctional Rhythm.

40–60

29. The AV junction is normally a very regular pacemaker. In a Junctional Escape Rhythm you would find a regular R–R interval. AV Junctional Escape Rhythm is a _____ rhythm with a rate of 40–60 beats per minute.

regular

30. As with other junctional arrhythmias, AV Junctional Escape Rhythm has inverted P waves, which can fall before or after the QRS

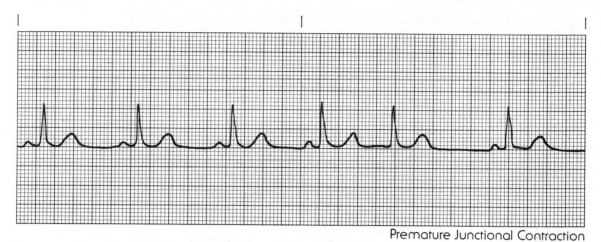

Premature Junctional Contraction

Figure 38. Rules for Premature Junctional Contraction

REGULARITY: **Since this is a single premature ectopic beat, it will inter-rupt the regularity of the underlying rhythm. The R–R interval will be irregular.**

RATE: **The overall heart rate will depend on the rate of the underlying rhythm.**

P WAVES: **The P wave can come before or after the QRS complex, or it can be lost entirely within the QRS complex. If visible, the P wave will be inverted.**

PRI: **If the P wave precedes the QRS complex, the PRI will be less than .12 seconds. If the P wave falls within the QRS complex or following it, there will be no PRI.**

QRS: **The QRS complex measurement will be less than .12 seconds.**

complex. It is also possible that there would be no P wave, since the P wave can be hidden within the QRS complex. Junctional Escape Rhythm always has inverted P waves, either before or after the QRS complex, or the P wave might be hidden within the _____ complex.

QRS

31. If the P wave precedes the QRS complex, the PRI will be less than _____ seconds. If the PRI is greater than .12 seconds, you would suspect that the rhythm originated in the _____.

.12
atria

32. As with other junctional arrhythmias, you would expect ventricular conduction to be _____, and thus the QRS measurement should be less than _____ seconds in a Junctional Escape Rhythm.

normal;
.12

33. The rules for Junctional Escape Rhythm are:
      Regularity: regular
            Rate: 40–60 beats per minute

P Wave: will be inverted; can fall before or after the QRS complex, or can be hidden within the QRS complex

PRI: can be measured only if the P wave precedes the QRS complex; if measurable will be less than .12 seconds

QRS: less than .12 seconds

34.   Junctional Escape Rhythm is a fail-safe mechanism, rather than an irritable arrhythmia. However, the AV junction is capable of irritability, and is known to produce an irritable arrhythmia called Junctional Tachycardia. This rhythm occurs when the junction initiates impulses at a rate _____ than its inherent rate of 40–60 beats per minute, thus overriding the SA node or other higher pacemaker sites for control of the heart rate. Junctional Escape Rhythm is an escape mechanism, whereas Junctional Tachycardia is an _____ rhythm.

faster

irritable

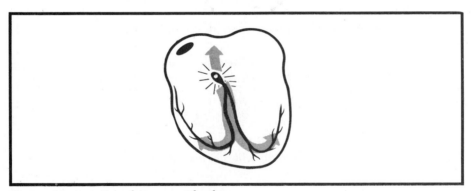

Figure 39. Junctional Escape Rhythm

When higher pacemaker sites fail, the AV junction is left with pacemaking responsibility. The atria are depolarized via retrograde conduction. Ventricular conduction is normal.

35.   Junctional Tachycardia is usually divided into two categories, depending on how fast the irritable site is firing. If the junction is firing between 60 and 100 beats per minute, the arrhythmia is termed an Accelerated Junctional Rhythm because a rate below 100 can't really be considered a tachycardia. When the junctional rate exceeds 100 beats per minute the rhythm is considered a Junctional Tachycardia. Junctional Tachycardia can be as fast as 180 beats per minute, but at this rapid rate it is extremely difficult to identify positively since P waves are superimposed on preceding T waves. When an AV junctional focus fires at a rate of 60–100 beats per minute, it is termed an _____ Junctional Rhythm. If the rate exceeds 100 beats per minute, up to a rate of 180 beats per minute, the rhythm is called a Junctional _____.

Accelerated

Tachycardia

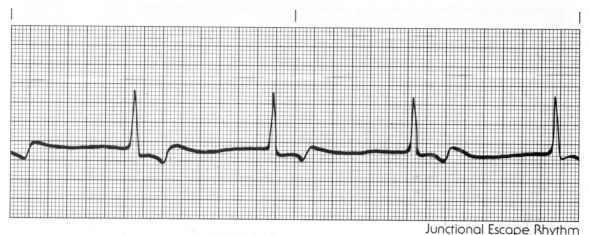

Junctional Escape Rhythm

Figure 40. Rules for Junctional Escape Rhythm

REGULARITY: **The R–R intervals are constant. The rhythm is regular.**

RATE: **Atrial and ventricular rates are equal. The inherent rate of the AV Junction is 40–60 beats per minute.**

P WAVES: **The P wave can come before or after the QRS complex, or it can be lost entirely within the QRS complex. If visible, the P wave will be inverted.**

PRI: **If the P wave precedes the QRS complex, the PRI will be less than .12 seconds. If the P wave falls within the QRS complex or following it, there will be no PRI.**

QRS: **The QRS complex measurement will be less than .12 seconds.**

36.   Let's take Accelerated Junctional Rhythm separately first. This is an irritable arrhythmia which originates in the AV junction and fires at a rate of _____–_____ beats per minute. It will have the inverted P wave typical of junctional arrhythmias, or may have no P wave if the atria and ventricles depolarize _____. If the P wave precedes the QRS complex, the PRI should be less than _____ seconds. Conduction through the ventricles is normal, so the QRS complex should have a _____ measurement of less than .12 seconds.

60–100

simultaneously;

.12
normal

37.   Here are the rules for Accelerated Junctional Rhythm:
    Regularity: regular
        Rate: 60–100 beats per minute
    P Wave: will be inverted; can fall before or after the QRS complex, or can be hidden within the QRS complex
        PRI: can be measured only if the P wave precedes the QRS complex; if measurable will be less than .12 seconds
    QRS: less than .12 seconds

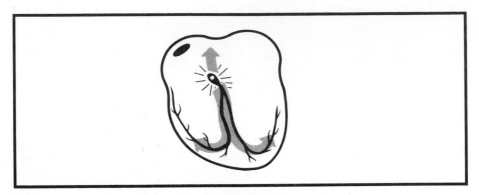

Figure 41. Accelerated Junctional Rhythm

An irritable focus in the AV junction speeds up to override the SA node for control of the heart. The atria are depolarized via retrograde conduction. Conduction through the ventricles is normal.

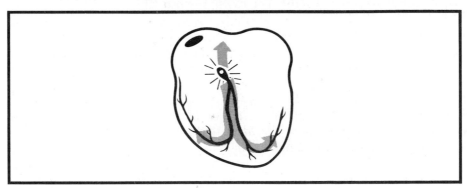

Figure 42. Junctional Tachycardia

An irritable focus in the AV junction speeds up to override the SA node for control of the heart. The atria are depolarized via retrograde conduction. Conduction through the ventricles is normal.

38.   When the AV junction fires in the tachycardia range (100–180 beats per minute) the rhythm will remain regular. The P waves will be inverted, and can fall before or after the QRS complex, or might be absent if they are _____ within the QRS complex. When the P wave precedes the QRS complex, the PRI will be _____ than .12 seconds. Since conduction through the ventricles is normal, the QRS complex will be less than _____ seconds.

hidden

less

.12

39.   The rules for Junctional Tachycardia are:
          Regularity: regular
               Rate: 100–180 beats per minute
          P Wave: will be inverted; can fall before or after the QRS complex, or can be hidden within the QRS complex

PRI: can be measured only if the P wave precedes the QRS complex; if measurable will be less than .12 seconds
QRS: less than .12 seconds

40. The only difference you will see on the EKG between Junctional Escape Rhythm, Accelerated Junctional Rhythm, and Junctional Tachycardia, is the rate. The rates are:

Junctional Escape Rhythm:	40–60 beats per minute
Accelerated Junctional Rhythm:	60–100 beats per minute
Junctional Tachycardia:	100–180 beats per minute

Each of these rhythms originates in the _____, and will thus produce an inverted P wave because of retrograde conduction. Depending on whether the atria or ventricles depolarize first, the P wave can come before, during, or after the QRS complex. If the P wave precedes the QRS complex, the PRI will be less than .12 seconds, and the QRS measurement will be normal. If the rate is 40–60 beats per minute, the rhythm is called _____ _____ Rhythm. If the rate is between 60 and 100 beats per minute, the rhythm is termed _____ Junctional Rhythm, and the rhythm is called Junctional Tachycardia if the rate is _____–_____ beats per minute.

AV junction

Junctional
Escape;
Accelerated;

100–180

41. A junctional impulse which reaches the atria before the ventricles will produce an inverted P wave which falls _____ the QRS complex. Such a beat would have a PRI of less than _____ seconds. If the PRI were greater than .12 seconds, you would suspect that the impulse originated in the _____.

before;
.12

atria

42. A regular rhythm with a QRS complex of less than .12 seconds and a rate of 50 beats per minute, which did not have any visible P waves, would fit the rules for a _____ _____ Rhythm.

Junctional
Escape

43. A single premature ectopic beat originating from an irritable focus in the AV junction would be called a PJC, or _____ _____ _____. Such a beat would have an inverted P wave _____, _____, or _____ the QRS complex.

Premature
Junctional
Contraction;
before;
during; after

44. All junctional arrhythmias have the same general characteristics, that is, they all have _____ P waves which can occur before, during, or after a QRS complex, and the PRI will be _____ and the QRS will be _____. However, not all junctional arrhythmias have the same mechanism. PJCs, Junctional Tachycardia, and Accelerated Junctional Rhythm are all caused by irritability, whereas a junctional rhythm within its inherent rate of 40–60 beats per minute would be an indication of an _____ mechanism.

inverted

shortened;
normal

escape

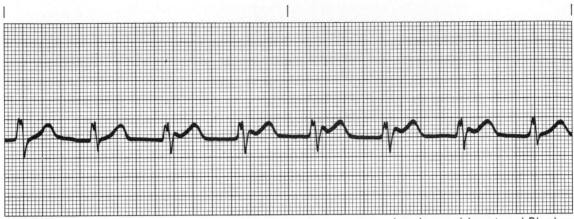

Accelerated Junctional Rhythm

Figure 43. Rules For Accelerated Junctional Rhythm

REGULARITY: The R–R intervals are constant. The rhythm is regular.

RATE: Atrial and ventricular rates are equal. The rate will be faster than the AV Junction's inherent rate, but not yet into a true tachycardia range. Usually in the 60–100 beats per minute range.

P WAVES: The P wave can come before or after the QRS complex, or it can be lost entirely within the QRS complex. If visible, the P wave will be inverted.

PRI: If the P wave precedes the QRS complex, the PRI will be less than .12 seconds. If the P wave falls within the QRS complex or following it, there will be no PRI.

QRS: The QRS complex will be less than .12 seconds.

45.   You have now learned several arrhythmias that are regular and beat at such a rapid rate that the P wave might not be discernible from the T wave. If you include Junctional Tachycardia, which might not have a visible P wave, you have a group of tachycardias which are regular and don't have visible P waves. The ventricular rates for these arrhythmias are:

- Sinus Tachycardia   100–160 beats per minute
- Atrial Tachycardia   150–250 beats per minute
- Atrial Flutter   150–250 beats per minute
- Junctional Tachycardia   100–180 beats per minute

From these rate ranges you can see that as the rate exceeds 150 or 160 beats per minute, a rate at which the P wave could very well be encroaching on the preceding _____ wave, you would have no way to distinguish between these arrhythmias. Since you can't accurately identify the rhythm, you would instead give it a descriptive identification. The term that's used to describe this category of indistinguishable arrhythmias is "Supraventricular Tachycardias."

T

46.   A Supraventricular Tachycardia (SVT) is not the name of a specific _____. It is a term that's used to _____ a   arrhythmia;
category of several regular tachyarrhythmias that can't be identified   describe
more accurately because they have indistinguishable _____   P;
waves and fall within a common _____ range.   rate

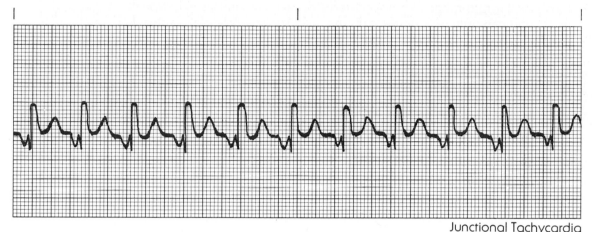

Junctional Tachycardia

Figure 44. Rules for Junctional Tachycardia

REGULARITY: **The R–R intervals are constant. The rhythm is regular.**

RATE: **Atrial and ventricular rates are equal. The rate will be in
the tachycardia range, but does not usually exceed 180
beats per minute. Usual range is 100–180 beats per
minute.**

P WAVES: **The P wave can come before or after the QRS complex, or
it can be lost entirely within the QRS complex. If visible,
the P wave will be inverted.**

PRI: **If the P wave precedes the QRS complex, the PRI will be
less than .12 seconds. If the P wave falls within the QRS
complex or following it, there will be no PRI.**

QRS: **The QRS complex measurement will be less than .12
seconds.**

47.   The rates at which you most commonly need to use the term
Supraventricular Tachycardia is the 150–250 range, although *sometimes* a slower rate will still have obscured P waves. An SVT is usually
a toss-up between Atrial Tachycardia and Junctional Tachycardia, although Sinus Tachycardia and, less commonly Atrial Flutter can also
be in the running. These arrhythmias can only be called SVT if they
cannot be identified more accurately. It is not a catch-all phrase. To
be called SVT, an arrhythmia must be _____, have no   regular;
visible _____ waves, and have a _____ range   P; rate
common to other arrhythmias, thereby making further and more accurate identification _____.   impossible

48.   You now know about four more arrhythmias: those that originate in the AV junction. You have learned the characteristics that these arrhythmias share, and how they differ from rhythms which originate in other pacemaker sites. You also learned that several of the tachycardias cannot always be differentiated, because they might have similar rate ranges and obscured P waves. When this situation exists you can only describe the rhythm as a Supraventricular Tachycardia, rather than giving it a specific name. Now you must practice applying this knowledge to actual interpretation of rhythm strips. Turn to Practice Sheet 7 and practice applying your new knowledge until you feel very comfortable in this area.

Practice
Sheet 7

Key Points – Junctional Rhythms

- Rhythms that originate in the AV junction include:

    Premature Junctional Contraction
    Junctional Escape Rhythm
    Accelerated Junctional Rhythm
    Junctional Tachycardia

- Junctional arrhythmias will create an inverted P wave because the atria are depolarized via retrograde conduction.

- A junctional impulse will depolarize the ventricles in a normal manner at the same time the atria are being depolarized with retrograde conduction.

- A junctional rhythm can have the inverted P wave occurring before, during, or after the QRS complex.

- All junctional arrhythmias will create an inverted P wave, but some low atrial impulses can also cause inverted P waves.

- All junctional arrhythmias will have a PRI of less than .12 seconds.

- Here are the rules for *Premature Junctional Contraction*:

    Regularity: depends on rhythm of underlying arrhythmia
    Rate: depends on rate of underlying arrhythmia
    P Waves: will be inverted; can fall before, during or after the QRS complex
    PRI: can only be measured if the P wave precedes the QRS complex;
        if measureable will be less than .12 seconds
    QRS: less than .12 seconds

- A PJC is an irritable ectopic.

- The normal inherent rate of the AV junction is 40–60 beats per minute.

- If higher pacemaker sites fail, a junctional escape pacemaker might take over control of the heart. This is called Junctional Escape Rhythm.

- The rules for *Junctional Escape Rhythm* are:

    Regularity: regular
    Rate: 40–60 beats per minute
    P Waves: will be inverted; can fall before, during, or after the QRS complex
    PRI: can be measured only if the P wave precedes the QRS complex;
        if measurable will be less than .12 seconds
    QRS: less than .12 seconds

- If the AV junction becomes irritable, it can speed up and override higher pacemaker sites. This arrhythmia is called Junctional Tachycardia.

- Junctional Tachycardia is usually divided into two categories depending on rate:

    60–100 beats per minute: Accelerated Junctional Rhythm
    100–180 beats per minute: Junctional Tachycardia

- Here are rules for *Accelerated Junctional Rhythm*:

    Regularity: regular
        Rate: 60–100 beats per minute
    P Waves: will be inverted; can fall before, during, or after the QRS complex
        PRI: can be measured only if the P wave precedes the QRS complex; if measurable will be less than .12 seconds
        QRS: less than .12 seconds

- Here are the rules for *Junctional Tachycardia*:

    Regularity: regular
        Rate: 100–180 beats per minute
    P Waves: will be inverted; can fall before, during, or after the QRS complex
        PRI: can be measured only if the P wave precedes the QRS complex; if measurable will be less than .12 seconds
        QRS: less than .12 seconds

- If a rapid arrhythmia is regular, has no visible P waves, and has a rate range common to other arrhythmias, thereby making more accurate identification impossible, the arrhythmia is termed Supraventricular Tachycardia.

Self-Test: Junctional Rhythms

Directions:

Complete this self-evaluation of the information you have learned from this chapter. If your answers are all correct and you feel comfortable with your understanding of the material, proceed to the next chapter. However, if you missed any of the questions you should review the referenced frames before proceeding. If you feel uncomfortable with any of your understanding, invest the time now to go back over the entire chapter. DO NOT PROCEED WITH THE NEXT CHAPTER UNTIL YOU ARE VERY COMFORTABLE WITH THE MATERIAL IN THIS CHAPTER.

Question	**Referenced Frames**	
1. What does the P wave look like in a Junctional Rhythm?	5; 6; 7; 8; 10; 11; 17; 44	The P is always inverted, even though it is often hidden in the QRS complex.
2. How do you explain the unusual configuration of the P wave in junctional rhythms?	2; 3; 4; 5; 6; 7	The atria are depolarized via retrograde conduction. Since the electrical flow will be traveling away from the positive electrode in Lead II, the wave form will be negative.
3. Will the QRS complex be normal in a junctional rhythm?	3; 5; 10	Yes, even though atrial depolarization is retrograde, ventricular depolarization will be

Question	Referenced Frames	
		normal. The QRS complex should measure less than .12 seconds.
4. Does an inverted P wave always indicate a junctional rhythm?	8; 9; 12; 13; 14	No; atrial rhythms can also have inverted P waves if the impulse originated low enough in the atria. You can differentiate between the two by looking at the PRI; in a junctional rhythm it will be less than .12 seconds.
5. Where will the P wave be located in a junctional rhythm?	6; 7; 10; 15; 16; 17; 41	It can fall before or after the QRS complex, or it can be hidden within the QRS complex. In the latter, it will appear as if the rhythm has no P wave at all.
6. What is the biggest clue to a junctional rhythm?	8	the inverted P wave
7. What is a PJC?	19; 20; 21; 25; 43	A premature junctional contraction is a single beat

Question	Referenced Frames	
		which originates from an irritable focus in the AV junction.
8. Will a PJC have a P wave?	22; 23; 25	Yes; the P wave will be inverted, either before or after the QRS complex, or it can be hidden within the QRS complex.
9. What will the PRI be for a PJC?	23; 25	If the P wave is in front of the QRS complex, the PRI will be less than .12 seconds. Otherwise, there will be no PRI.
10. Does a PJC come earlier or later than expected in the cardiac cycle?	19; 20; 25	earlier
11. What will the QRS measurement be for a PJC?	24; 25	Since conduction through the ventricles is normal, the QRS measurement should be less than .12 seconds.
12. What is the normal, inherent rate for the AV junction?	26; 27; 28; 44	40–60 beats per minute

Question	Referenced Frames	
13. What is a Junctional Escape Rhythm?	26; 27; 28; 33; 34; 42	An escape mechanism that occurs when a higher pacemaking site fails and the AV junction has to take over at its own inherent rate of 40–60 beats per minute.
14. Is Junctional Escape Rhythm regular or irregular?	29; 33	regular
15. What will the P waves look like for this arrhythmia?	30; 33	they will be inverted; they can fall before or after the QRS complex, or can be hidden within the QRS complex
16. Will the PRI measurement be normal for a Junctional Escape Rhythm?	31; 33	No; if the P wave precedes the QRS the PRI will be less than .12 seconds. If it falls within the QRS or after the QRS, there will be no PRI.
17. What is the rate range for an Accelerated Junctional Rhythm?	35; 36; 37; 40	60–100 beats per minute
18. Is Accelerated Junctional Rhythm regular or irregular?	37; 40	regular
19. What is the P wave like in Accelerated Junctional Rhythm?	36; 37; 40	just like the P wave in

Question	**Referenced Frames**	
		all other junctional rhythms: it is inverted, and can fall before, during, or after the QRS complex
20. Is the QRS measurement normal for Accelerated Junctional Rhythm?	36; 37; 40	Yes; since the conduction through to the ventricles is normal, the QRS should measure less than .12 seconds.
21. What is the rate range for Junctional Tachycardia?	35; 39; 40	100–180 beats per minute
22. Is a Junctional Tachycardia regular or irregular?	38; 39; 40	regular
23. What does the P wave look like in Junctional Tachycardia?	38; 39; 40	Probably not visible, since the rate is so fast that it might be hidden in the T waves, or it might be occurring within the QRS complex. If it is visible, it will be inverted either before or after the QRS complex.
24. Is the QRS measurement normal for Junctional Tachycardia?	38; 39; 40	Yes, it should be less than .12 seconds.

Question	Referenced Frames	
25. Is the PRI measurement normal for Junctional Tachycardia?	38; 39; 40	No; if the P wave precedes the QRS complex, the PRI will be less than .12 seconds. Otherwise, there will be no PRI.
26. When can you call an arrhythmia a Supraventricular Tachycardia?	45; 46; 47; 48	only when you have a regular rhythm, in a tachycardia range with no visible P waves, and at a rate that is common to more than one arrhythmia, thereby making more accurate identification impossible
27. Which arrhythmias commonly need to be described as Supraventricular Tachycardias?	45; 46; 47; 48	the most common ones are Atrial Tachycardia and Junctional Tachycardia, although it is also used to describe Sinus Tachycardia and Atrial Flutter

Question	**Referenced Frames**	
28. At what rate would you expect to have trouble discerning P waves, and might consider calling an arrhythmia Supraventricular Tachycardia?	47	usually 150–250 beats per minute, although you may lose the P waves at slower rates

Practice Sheet 7: Junctional Rhythms

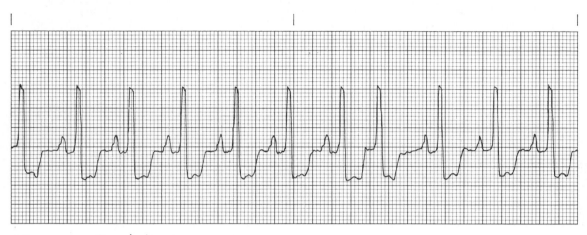

7.1   Regularity: _____
                      Rate: _____
                      P Waves: _____
                      PRI: _____
                      QRS: _____
                      Interp: _____

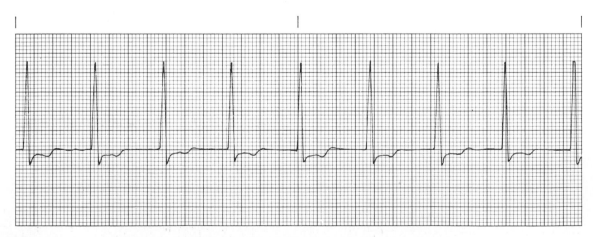

7.2   Regularity: _____
                      Rate: _____
                      P Waves: _____
                      PRI: _____
                      QRS: _____
                      Interp: _____

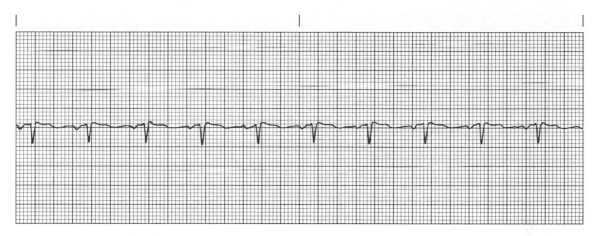

7.3   Regularity: _____
           Rate: _____
           P Waves: _____
           PRI: _____
           QRS: _____
           Interp: _____

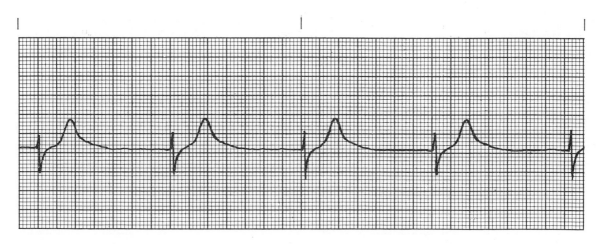

7.4   Regularity: _____
           Rate: _____
           P Waves: _____
           PRI: _____
           QRS: _____
           Interp: _____

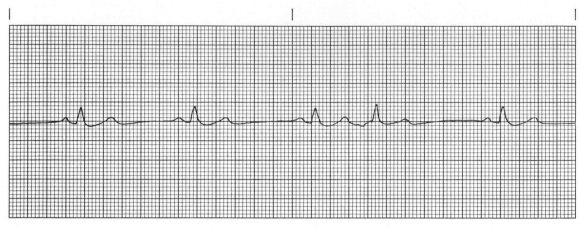

7.5   Regularity: _____
           Rate: _____
           P Waves: _____
           PRI: _____
           QRS: _____
           Interp: _____

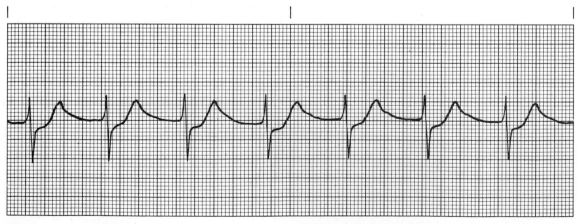

7.6   Regularity: _____
           Rate: _____
           P Waves: _____
           PRI: _____
           QRS: _____
           Interp: _____

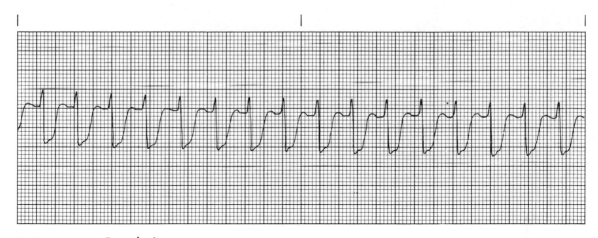

7.7   Regularity: _____
            Rate: _____
            P Waves: _____
            PRI: _____
            QRS: _____
            Interp: _____

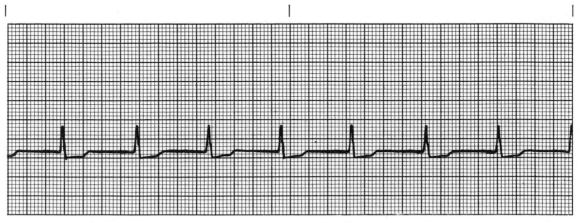

7.8   Regularity: _____
            Rate: _____
            P Waves: _____
            PRI: _____
            QRS: _____
            Interp: _____

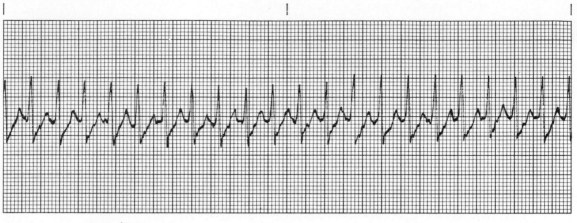

7.9   Regularity: _____
         Rate: _____
         P Waves: _____
         PRI: _____
         QRS: _____
         Interp: _____

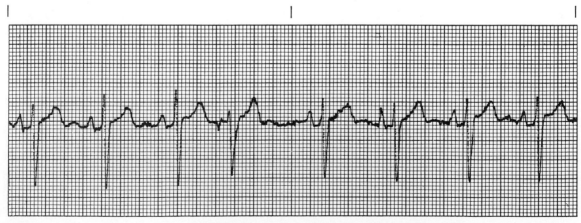

7.10   Regularity: _____
         Rate: _____
         P Waves: _____
         PRI: _____
         QRS: _____
         Interp: _____

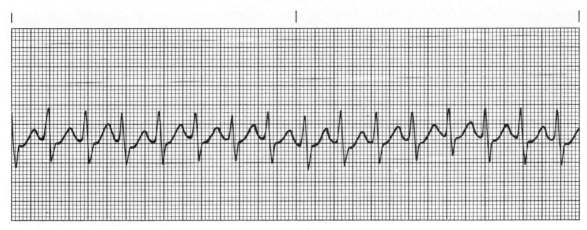

7.11   Regularity: _____
            Rate: _____
            P Waves: _____
            PRI: _____
            QRS: _____
            Interp: _____

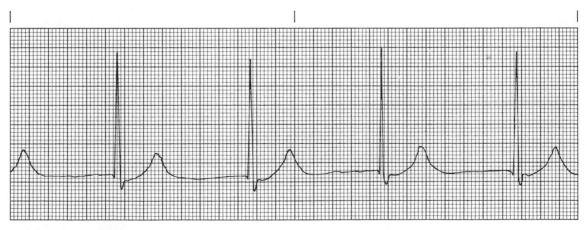

7.12   Regularity: _____
            Rate: _____
            P Waves: _____
            PRI: _____
            QRS: _____
            Interp: _____

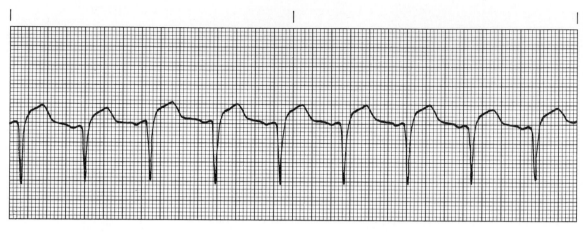

7.13   Regularity: _____
            Rate: _____
            P Waves: _____
            PRI: _____
            QRS: _____
            Interp: _____

7

Heart Blocks

1.   You are now familiar with four arrhythmias that originate in the AV junction. You will next learn about four different arrhythmias that don't actually originate in the AV junction, but are the result of conduction disturbances within the AV node. Each of these arrhythmias is caused by an impulse originating above the AV node, usually in the Sinus Node, that then has trouble getting through the node to the ventricles. This category of arrhythmias is most commonly called "heart blocks" because of the obstructed conduction at the AV node. Heart blocks are arrhythmias caused when a supraventricular impulse is unable to be conducted normally through to the ventricles because of a conduction disturbance at the _____ _____.   **AV node**
(Note: You may hear people refer to another type of heart block, called "bundle branch block." This is a disturbance in conduction within the ventricles, and is normally interpreted using a 12-lead EKG, rather than the single-lead rhythm strips we are discussing here. Bundle branch block is only mentioned here so that you will realize it is a totally different type of problem than AV heart block. We will not discuss it in this book at all.)

2.   The different types of heart blocks are categorized according to the severity of the obstruction at the AV node. A First Degree Block indicates that the obstruction at the _____ _____ is not   **AV node**
complete; all impulses are conducted but each undergoes a delay before being transmitted to the _____. A Second Degree   **ventricles**
Block means that there is an actual block, but it is intermittent; some of the impulses will be conducted through to the ventricles, but others will not. A Third Degree Block means that the block is complete; that is, none of the impulses will be conducted through to the ventricles. The First Degree Block is the mildest, because it is a delay rather than an actual block. In a First Degree Block, each impulse is delayed but all are conducted through to the _____. A   **ventricles;**
Second Degree Block is more serious, because some impulses are actually _____, while others are allowed to be conducted   **blocked**
through to the ventricles. Third degree is the most serious, since _____ of the impulses is conducted; the Third Degree   **none**
Block is also called a Complete Heart Block (CHB).

3.   In this chapter you will learn about four types of heart block:
   • first degree
   • second degree (Wenckebach)
   • second degree (classical)
   • third degree (complete heart block)
Each of these is considered a heart block because there is a disturbance in conduction through the AV _____.   **node**

4.   A First Degree Heart Block is not really a true block at all, since each impulse is conducted through to the ventricles. But it is included with the blocks because a partial block exists which causes a _____ in transmission of each impulse to the ventricles.   **delay**

5. Both types of Second Degree Heart Block exhibit some type of intermittent block at the AV node. Both types allow some impulses through to the ventricles while others are _____.   blocked

6. As a point of interest, both types of Second Degree Heart Block have other names also. Wenckebach is known as Mobitz I, and Classical Second Degree Heart Block is known as Mobitz II. This is just another way of differentiating between the two types of _____ Degree Heart Block.   Second

7. Third-Degree Block is called _____ Heart Block (CHB) because all impulses are completely _____ at the AV node; no impulses are allowed through to the ventricles.   Complete; blocked

8. Now that you have a general idea of the types of heart blocks and the mechanisms of each, let us take each one individually and examine it in more detail. We will start with First Degree Heart Block, since it is the least serious. First Degree Heart Block is the least _____ of all the heart blocks because, even though it does cause a _____ in conduction, it still allows _____ impulses through to the ventricles.   serious; delay; all

9. As you recall, atrial depolarization is depicted on the EKG by the _____ _____ and the delay in the AV node is shown by the _____ segment. Together, these make up the PR _____. Thus, if a heart block causes an increased delay in the AV node, you would expect the PRI to become prolonged. This is one of the foremost clues to a First Degree Heart Block. In First Degree Heart Block, the PRI is _____ than usual.   P wave; PR; interval

longer

	Mechanism of Block
First Degree Heart Block	• not a true block • delay at the AV node • each impulse is eventually conducted
Second Degree Heart Blocks • Wenckebach	• intermittent block • delay gets progressively longer, until . . . • one beat is eventually blocked
• Classical	• some beats are conducted • others are intermittently blocked
Third Degree Heart Block	• atria and ventricles are completely dissociated • there is a total block at the AV node

Figure 45. The Heart Blocks

10.   It's important to keep in mind with First Degree Heart Blocks that each sinus impulse, even though delayed in the AV node, does eventually reach the ventricles to depolarize them. Thus, the PRI will be _____, but will be the same duration from one beat to the next. This is because each pacemaker impulse is coming from the same site (the SA node usually) and is being conducted in the same manner through the AV node. So, each impulse takes the same time to pass through the atria, and is delayed the same amount of time in the AV node. Even though the PRI is _____ in First Degree Heart Block, all of the PRIs will be the same length because they all come from the same site and are conducted in the same manner.

| prolonged |
| prolonged |

11.   Thus, by definition, the PRI in First Degree Heart Block must be longer than .20 seconds, and must be constant from one beat to the next. This is the only abnormality to this arrhythmia. Ventricular conduction is normal, producing a QRS complex of less than _____ seconds. Since the SA node is the usual pacemaker, the rhythm is usually regular, although this can change if the underlying rhythm is something other than NSR. First Degree Heart Block is usually regular, has a PRI greater than _____ seconds, and each PRI is the same as all other _____ across the strip. Since ventricular conduction is normal, the QRS will be less than _____ seconds.

.12

.20;
PRIs;
.12

12.   At this point it should be apparent that First Degree Heart Block is not really a rhythm itself, but is actually a condition which is superimposed on another arrhythmia. This is an important feature to keep in mind, since you will also need to identify the underlying arrhythmia. For example, if you have a rhythm that fits all of the rules for Sinus Tachycardia except that the PRI is prolonged and constant, you would call the rhythm Sinus Tachycardia with _____ Degree Heart Block. In the same way, if the underlying rhythm fits the definition for NSR except that the PRI was greater than .20 seconds, you would call the arrhythmia a Sinus Rhythm with _____ _____ Block.

First

First
Degree

13.   First Degree Heart Block is not a rhythm in itself. It is a feature that helps explain a prolonged PRI in an otherwise normal rhythm. Thus, in addition to recognizing that a First Degree Heart Block exists, you must also identify the _____ rhythm.

underlying

14.   Here are the rules for First Degree Heart Block:
        Regularity: depends on underlying rhythm
            Rate: depends on underlying rhythm
        P Waves: upright and uniform; each P wave will be followed by a QRS complex
            PRI: greater than .20 seconds; constant across the strip
            QRS: less than .12 seconds

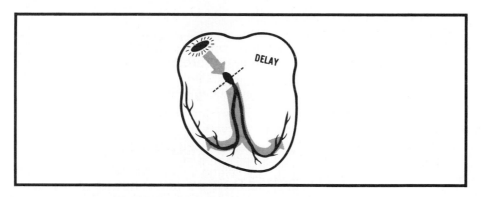

Figure 46. First Degree Heart Block

The AV node holds each sinus impulse longer than normal before conducting it through to the ventricles. Each impulse is eventually conducted. Once into the ventricles, conduction proceeds normally.

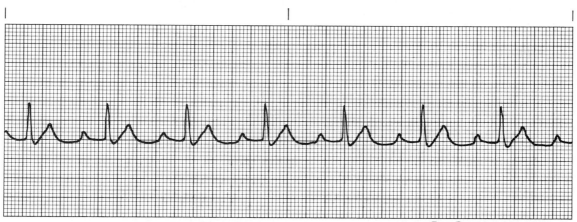

First Degree Heart Block

Figure 47. Rules for First Degree Heart Block

REGULARITY: This will depend on the regularity of the underlying rhythm.

RATE: The rate will depend on the rate of the underlying rhythm.

P WAVES: The P waves will be upright and uniform. Each P wave will be followed by a QRS complex.

PRI: The PRI will be constant across the entire strip, but it will always be greater than .20 seconds.

QRS: The QRS complex measurement will be less than .12 seconds.

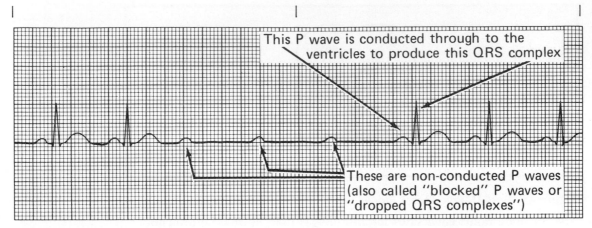

This P wave is conducted through to the ventricles to produce this QRS complex

These are non-conducted P waves (also called "blocked" P waves or "dropped QRS complexes")

Figure 48. Blocked P Waves

15.   There are two types of Second Degree Heart Block. Both occur when the AV node begins selectively blocking impulses that are being initiated in the SA node. On the EKG this will be seen as normal P waves, but not every one will be followed by a QRS complex. This indicates that the atria are being depolarized normally, but that not every impulse is being conducted through to the ventricles. Hence, you will see more _____ depolarizations than _____ depolarizations. In Second Degree Heart Block, you will always see more _____ waves than _____ complexes.

atrial;
ventricular
P; QRS

16.   A key feature of Second Degree Heart Blocks is that not every P wave is followed by a QRS complex. Sometimes you will see P waves without an associated ventricular depolarization. The appearance of P waves without a subsequent QRS complex indicates that the atria were depolarized by a pacemaker impulse, but that impulse was not conducted through to the _____ because it was blocked at the _____ _____.

ventricles;
AV node

17.   An important distinction is that some of the impulses are being conducted to the ventricles. Therefore, the QRS complexes you do see were conducted normally from the same impulse that produced the immediately preceding P wave. Thus, ventricular conduction will follow normal pathways, and the QRS measurement will be _____. Since the QRS complexes were produced in a normal manner, the QRS measurements will be less than _____ seconds.

normal
.12

18.   In both types of Second Degree Heart Block you should see a _____ complex with a normal measurement, because the conduction disturbance at the AV node is not a complete block. Even though some of the pacemaker impulses are blocked at the AV node, some *do* get through to depolarize the ventricles.

QRS

19.   There are two categories of Second Degree Heart Block. One is called Wenckebach and the other is called Classical Second Degree Block. In both types, the impulses originating in the sinus node are conducted through the AV node in an intermittent fashion. That is, not every P wave will be followed by a QRS complex. These two arrhythmias are classified as Second Degree Heart Block because some of the impulses are conducted through the AV node, but others are not. In Second Degree Heart Block, the AV node is unreliable in conducting impulses. Conduction to the ventricles is only accomplished on an _____ basis.

intermittent

20.   The difference between Wenckebach and Classical Second Degree Block is the *pattern* in which the P waves are blocked. Since the activity of the AV node is depicted by the _____ interval, the PRI is the most important clue to distinguishing between these two arrhythmias. When attempting to distinguish between a Wenckebach and a Classical Second Degree Heart Block, you should concentrate on the _____ intervals.

PR

PR

21.   Now, let's take Classical Second Degree Heart Block and look at it more closely. In Classical Second Degree Heart Block, the AV node selectively chooses to either conduct or block individual impulses from the SA node. This results in a pattern of _____ P waves than QRS complexes. Sometimes the AV node will allow every other P wave to be conducted, resulting in a 2:1 ratio, or it might be every third, or even every fourth P wave. It is also possible for the ratio to vary, that is, 2:1, 4:1, 2:1, 4:1, etc. This is called variable conduction. On the EKG, this will be seen as 2, 3, 4, or even more P waves between the _____ complexes.

more

QRS

22.   Regardless of the conduction ratio, there will always be more P waves than QRS complexes. However, when you do see QRS complexes, the PR intervals preceding them will all have the same measurement because conduction through the node proceeds uniformly on conducted beats. Hence, the PRI in a Classical Second Degree Block will always be *constant* from one complex to the next across the entire strip. This is probably the most important feature about a Classical Second Degree Heart Block. The PRI will always be _____ on those complexes that were conducted.

constant

23.   It is also possible for a Classical Second Degree Heart Block to have a prolonged PRI. That is, the PRI will be constant across the strip, there will be more than one P wave for every QRS complex, and the PRI will be greater than .20 seconds on the conducted beats. However, even though this fits the rules for calling the arrhythmia a Second Degree Heart Block with a First Degree Heart Block, this is a redundant distinction, and should be eliminated. Such an arrhythmia would simply be called a Classical Second Degree Heart Block, and the PRI duration could be noted separately. A Classical Second Degree Heart Block must have a _____ PRI on conducted beats, and the PRI may even be _____. Regardless, it is not

constant;
prolonged

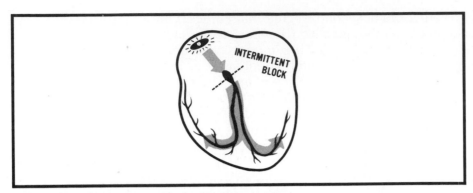

Figure 49. Classical Second Degree Heart Block

The AV node selectively conducts some beats while blocking others. Those that are not blocked are conducted through to the ventricles, although they may encounter a slight delay in the node. Once in the ventricles, conduction proceeds normally.

called a First Degree Heart Block, but is simply called a _____ | Classical
Second Degree Heart Block.

24.   Since the normal rate for the sinus node is _____–_____ | 60–100
beats per minute, and a Second Degree Heart Block conducts only
some of them, the ventricular rate for Classical Second Degree Block
will generally be in the bradycardia range. Often, the rate will be
one half to one third the normal rate, depending on the ratio of conduction. In Classical Second Degree Heart Block, the ventricular
rate will be _____ than normal because many of the im- | slower
pulses are blocked at the AV node.

25.   The regularity of the R–R intervals will depend on the manner
in which the AV node is blocking the impulses. If it is a regular ratio
of block, e.g., 2:1, 3:1, or 4:1, the ventricular rhythm will be regular. However, if the ratio is variable, e.g., 2:1, 4:1, 2:1, 4:1, the
ventricular rhythm will be irregular. Classical Second Degree Block
can be regular or irregular, depending on the _____ of | ratio
block at the AV node.

26.   Here are the rules for Classical Second Degree Heart Block:
     Regularity: R–R interval can be regular or irregular; P–P in-
          terval is regular
          Rate: usually in the bradycardia range; can be ½ to ⅓
               the normal rate
     P Waves: upright and uniform; more than one P wave for
          every QRS
          PRI: always constant across the strip; can be greater
               than .20 seconds
          QRS: less than .12 seconds

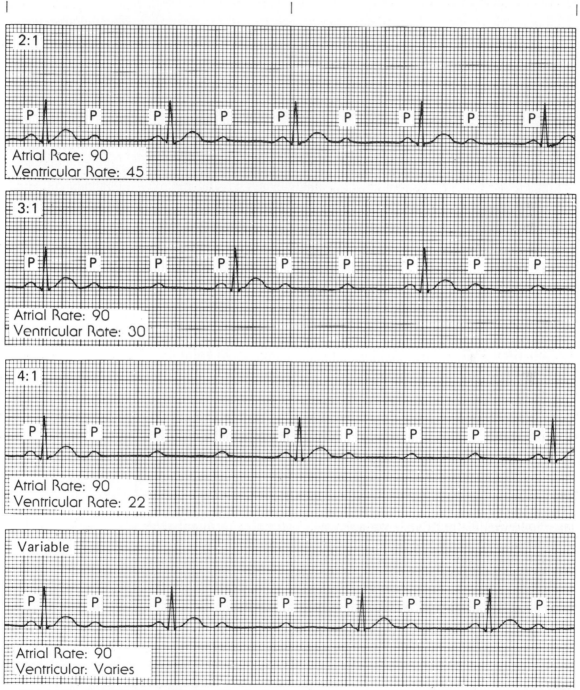

Figure 50. Conduction Ratios in Classical Second Degree Heart Block

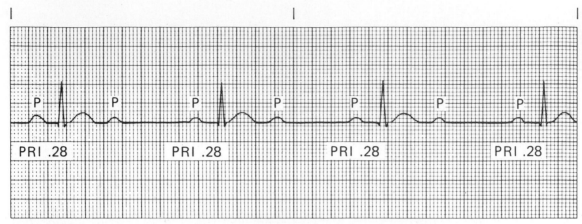

Figure 51. Classical Second Degree Heart Block with a Prolonged PRI

When a classical second degree heart block has a prolonged PRI on the conducted beats, it is still called a second degree heart block, *not* a second degree heart block with a first degree heart block.

27.   In Wenckebach, the conduction disturbance is different from Classical Second Degree, even though they both result in some "blocked" (non-conducted) beats. The difference is that Wenckebach consists of *progressive* delays at the AV node. Each impulse is held at the node a little longer than the preceding one, until eventually an impulse is blocked completely. Then the cycle starts over. Wenckebach is a cyclic pattern that results from _____ delays at the AV node.

progressive

28.   As with Classical Second Degree Heart Block, the key to recognizing a Wenckebach is in the PR intervals. Each PRI will get progressively longer, until you see a P wave without a resultant QRS complex. Then the cycle starts again with the shortest PRI. As you measure the PRIs across the strip you will notice a pattern of "long PRI, longer PRI, longer PRI, blocked P Wave." This cycle runs continuously across the strip. Wenckebach is characterized by increasingly long PRIs followed by a _____ P wave.

blocked

29.   The classic cycle seen with Wenckebach does not have to adhere to the ratio of three conducted beats to one blocked beat as illustrated in the preceding frame. It can be "long, longer, blocked" representing a 2:1 ratio, or a 4:1 ratio, or even a variable ratio. However, it will consistently follow a pattern of increasing PRIs followed by a blocked P wave. Regardless of the conduction ratio, a Wenckebach will always have progressively longer _____ intervals with blocked P waves.

PR

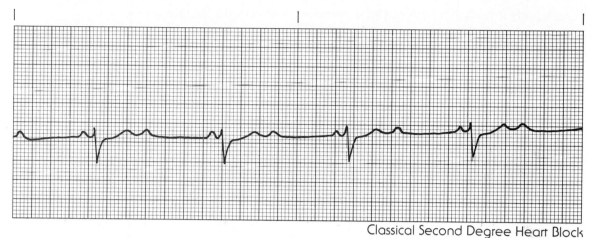

Classical Second Degree Heart Block

Figure 52. Rules for Classical Second Degree Block

REGULARITY: If the conduction ratio is consistent, the R–R interval will be constant, and the rhythm will be regular. If the conduction ratio varies, the R–R will be irregular.

RATE: The atrial rate is usually normal. Since many of the atrial impulses are blocked, the ventricular rate will usually be in the bradycardia range, often one half, one third, or one fourth of the atrial rate.

P WAVES: P waves are upright and uniform. There are always more P waves than QRS complexes.

PRI: The PRI on conducted beats will be constant across the strip, although it might be longer than a normal PRI measurement.

QRS: The QRS complex measurement will be less than .12 seconds.

30.   As with Classical Second Degree, those P waves that are conducted produce normal QRS complexes. This means that the QRS measurements in a Wenckebach should be less than _____ seconds.

.12

31.   Since the PR intervals are changing in Wenckebach, and some of the QRS complexes are being dropped, the R–R intervals will be irregular. As the PRI is getting longer, the R–R will get shorter, creating a cyclic pattern to the irregularity. Wenckebach has an _____ R–R interval which inversely corresponds to the changes in the PR intervals.

irregular

32.   However, Wenckebach does not usually block out as many P waves as Classical Second Degree Heart Block. Therefore, the rate of a Wenckebach is generally faster than a Classical Second Degree, but probably in the low/normal range. Since Wenckebach usually

conducts 2 out of 3, or 3 out of 4 impulses, the ventricular rate will be somewhat slower than normal, but still _____ than a Classical Second Degree Heart Block. | faster

33.   Here are the rules for Wenckebach:
       Regularity: irregular; the R–R interval gets shorter as the PRI gets longer
       Rate: usually slightly slower than normal
       P Waves: upright and uniform; some P waves are not followed by QRS complexes
       PRI: progressively lengthens until one P wave is blocked
       QRS: less than .12 seconds

34.   You now know that First Degree Heart Block is simply a _____ in conduction of the impulses from the SA node | delay
through the AV node, but each of the impulses *is* conducted. The Second Degree Heart Blocks both have *intermittent* AV conduction, where some impulses are conducted but others are _____. | blocked
We'll now look at Third Degree Heart Block, where *none* of the impulses is conducted because of a total block at the AV node. Third Degree Heart Block is also called Complete Heart Block because the block at the _____ is complete. | AV node

35.   The pathology of CHB is within the AV node. Therefore, the higher pacemaker in the SA node is not affected. The P waves will be normal, and atrial activity will be within a normal rate range. However, none of the P waves is conducted. This means that the ventricles won't be _____, nor will they _____ to | depolarized;

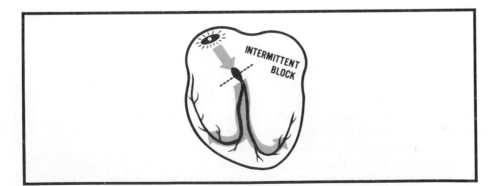

Figure 53. Wenckebach

As the sinus node initiates impulses, each one is delayed in the AV node a little longer than the preceding one, until one is eventually blocked completely. Those impulses that are conducted travel normally through the ventricles.

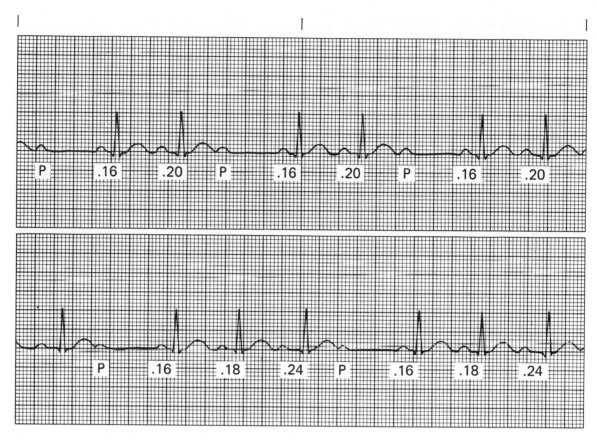

Figure 54. Conduction Pattern in Wenckebach

pump blood, unless one of the heart's fail-safe mechanisms comes into play. Since CHB involves a total block at the AV node, a lower escape mechanism will have to take over to _____ the ventricles.

36.   If possible, a junctional focus below the block site will take over pacemaking responsibilities by initiating a junctional _____ rhythm to depolarize the ventricles. However, if damage to the node extends into the junction, a ventricular focus may have to assume pacemaking responsibility. In either case, the ventricles are controlled by a lower escape focus. In CHB, the SA node functions normally, but cannot get past the block at the AV node, so a lower escape focus in either the AV junction or the _____ takes over to control ventricular activity.

37.   This means that ventricular activity will fall into one of two categories. If it originates in the AV junction, the rate will be in the _____–_____ beats per minute range, and the QRS complex will measure less than .12 seconds. But if a ventricular focus initiates

contract

depolarize

escape

ventricles

40–60

the escape rhythm, the rate will be _____–_____ beats per minute, and the QRS will be wider than .12 seconds, because of a longer conduction time within the ventricles. This information can help you determine the source of the ventricular pacemaker. If the rate is 20–40 and the QRS complex is greater than .12 seconds, you know the impulse is _____ in origin. But if the junction initiated the rhythm, the QRS complex is usually less than .12 seconds and the rate will be _____–_____ beats per minute. Remember, though, that since lower sites are less reliable than higher sites, these ranges are guidelines rather than concrete rules.

20–40

ventricular

40–60

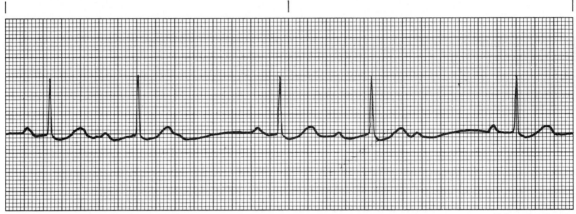

Wenckebach

Figure 55. Rules for Wenckebach

REGULARITY: **The R–R interval is irregular in a pattern of grouped beating. The R–R interval gets progressively shorter as the PRI gets progressively longer.**

RATE: **Since some beats are not conducted, the ventricular rate is usually slightly slower than normal. The atrial rate is normal.**

P WAVES: **The P waves are upright and uniform. Some P waves are not followed by QRS complexes.**

PRI: **The PR intervals get progressively longer, until one P wave is not followed by a QRS complex. After the blocked beat, the cycle starts again.**

QRS: **The QRS complex measurement will be less than .12 seconds.**

38. The mechanism depicted here is called atrioventricular (AV) dissociation. Simply speaking, this means that the atria and the ventricles are dissociated: they are functioning totally independent of each other. AV dissociation is not a rhythm in itself. It is merely a condition that exists in some arrhythmias. On the EKG you will see normal P waves marching regularly across the strip. You will also see QRS complexes at regular intervals. But the two wave forms will not

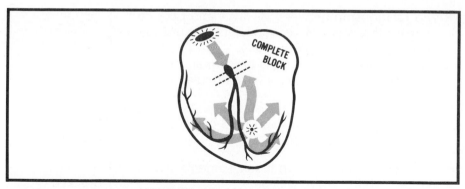

Figure 56. Complete Heart Block

The block at the AV node is complete. The sinus beats cannot penetrate the node, and thus, are not conducted through to the ventricles. An escape mechanism from either the junction or the ventricles will take over to pace the ventricles. The atria and the ventricles function in a totally dissociated fashion.

have any _____ to each other. The PRIs will be totally | relation
inconsistent, and you may even see P waves superimposed in the
middle of QRS complexes. There will be more P waves than QRS
complexes, because the intrinsic rate of the sinus node is _____ | faster
than either the junctional or ventricular rate. In CHB, the _____ | P
waves will have absolutely no relation to the QRS complexes, and
you may even see P waves superimposed on QRS complexes.

39.   As with other forms of AV block, the PRI is one of your most
important clues to interpretation. In CHB, the PRIs are totally inconsistent across the strip. The P waves have no relation to the QRS
complexes, thus the PR intervals will *not* be _____. | constant

40.   Another important feature about CHB is that the R–R interval is
regular. This is an important item to remember because the PRIs can
occasionally appear to be progressively lengthening, and can be
confused with Wenckebach. This is purely coincidental, however,
since the atria and the ventricles are completely _____ in | dissociated
Third Degree Heart Block. If you are trying to distinguish a Wencke-
bach from a CHB, you should recall that CHB has a _____ | regular
R–R interval, whereas Wenckebach has an _____ R–R | irregular
interval.

41.   Here are the rules for Third Degree Heart Block (CHB):
        Regularity: regular
              Rate: AR – usually normal (60–100 beats/minute);
                    VR – 40–60 if the focus is junctional,
                    20–40 if the focus is ventricular
        P Waves: upright and uniform; more P waves than QRS
                    complexes

PRI: no relationship between P waves and QRS complexes; P waves can occasionally be found superimposed on the QRS complex
QRS: less than .12 sec if focus is junctional
.12 sec or greater if focus is ventricular

42.   CHB is a *total* block at the AV node, resulting in AV dissociation. On the EKG, this is seen as P waves and QRS complexes that have no _____ to each other.

relation

43.   In both types of Second Degree Heart Block, some P waves will initiate QRS complexes, while others will be _____ at the AV node. There will be some P waves that are not followed by QRS complexes, but the QRS complexes that do exist were initiated by the preceding P waves.

blocked

44.   In First Degree Heart Block there is no real block. Instead, there is a delay in conduction at the AV _____, resulting in a _____ PR interval. But all P waves are conducted through to the ventricles.

node;
prolonged

45.   In Wenckebach the delay at the AV node gets increasingly longer, resulting in progressively longer _____ intervals. Those impulses that are conducted through produce normal QRS complexes.

PR

46.   Classical Second Degree Heart Block intermittently conducts some impulses through the AV node while others are blocked. This means that some P waves will not produce a QRS complex, but those that do will have a _____ PR interval.

constant

47.   First Degree Heart Block is actually a feature within a rhythm, rather than an arrhythmia itself. Therefore, a rhythm with First Degree Heart Block can be regular or irregular, depending on the _____ rhythm.

underlying

48.   Wenckebach always has an _____ R–R interval due to the progressively lengthening PRIs and the dropped QRS complexes. This type of second degree heart block often has a visible pattern of "grouping" of the QRS complexes, emphasized by the missing QRS complex. This is frequently the feature which separates Wenckebach from a CHB, since CHB has _____ R–R intervals.

irregular

regular

49.   You now have a very good foundation for approaching the heart blocks. As you go over the arrhythmias in Practice Sheet 8 remember to use your systematic approach for gathering all of the data available from each strip. To make the distinctions, pay particular attention to the PR intervals, since this will give you the most information about AV nodal activity.

Practice
Sheet 8

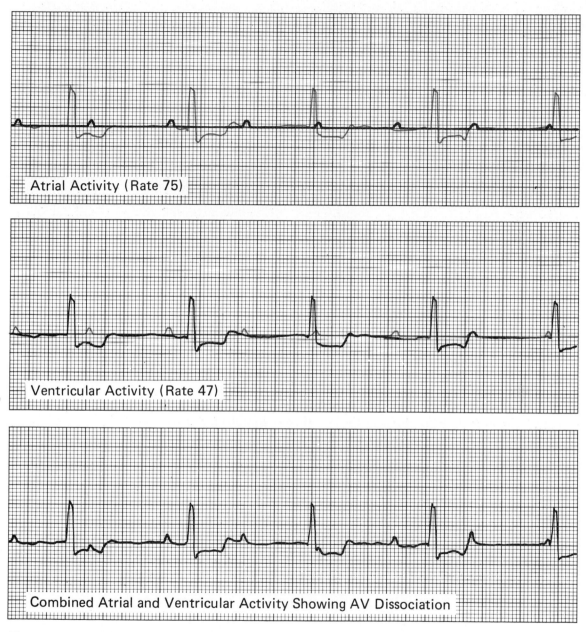

Atrial Activity (Rate 75)

Ventricular Activity (Rate 47)

Combined Atrial and Ventricular Activity Showing AV Dissociation

Figure 57. A–V Dissociation in CHB.

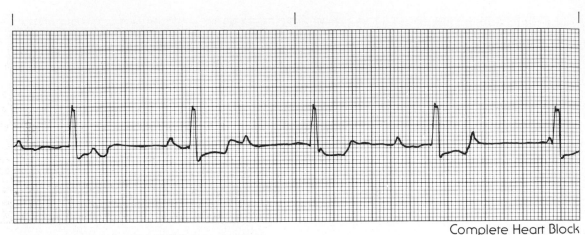

Complete Heart Block

Figure 58. Rules for Complete Heart Block

REGULARITY: **Both the atrial and the ventricular foci are firing regularly, thus the P–P intervals and the R–R intervals are regular.**

RATE: **The atrial rate will usually be in a normal range. The ventricular rate will be slower. If a junctional focus is controlling the ventricles, the rate will be 40–60 beats per minute. If the focus is ventricular, the rate will be 20–40 beats per minute.**

P WAVES: **The P waves are upright and uniform. There are more P waves than QRS complexes.**

PRI: **Since the block at the AV node is complete, none of the atrial impulses is conducted through to the ventricles. There is no PRI. The P waves have no relationship to the QRS complexes. You may occasionally see a P wave superimposed on the QRS complex.**

QRS: **If the ventricles are being controlled by a junctional focus, the QRS complex will measure less than .12 seconds. If the focus is ventricular, the QRS will measure .12 seconds or greater.**

	PRI	R–R	Conduction
1st Degree	Greater than .20 seconds constant	Usually regular (depending on underlying rhythm)	One P for every QRS
Wenckebach	Increasingly longer until one P is blocked	Irregular	More than one P for some QRSs
2nd Degree Classical	Constant on conducted beats (can be greater than .20 seconds)	Usually regular (can be irregular if conduction ratio varies)	More than one P for every QRS
3rd Degree	PRI not constant no relation of Ps to QRSs (Ps march through)	Regular	More Ps than QRSs

Figure 59. The Heart Blocks

Key Points – Heart Blocks

- The arrhythmias categorized as heart blocks are caused by conduction disturbances at the AV node.

- The four types of heart block are:

    First Degree: not actually a block; merely a delay in conduction

    Second Degree: an intermittent block; each beat is progressively delayed until
    (Wenckebach) one is blocked

    Second Degree: an intermittent block; the node selectively lets some beats
    (Classical)   through and blocks others

    Third Degree: a complete block; none of the supraventricular pacemaker
    (CHB)   impulses are conducted through the node to the ventricles;
                         the ventricles are depolarized by a dissociated pacemaker
                         from below the site of the block.

- A First Degree Heart Block is not a rhythm itself, but is a condition which is super-imposed on another rhythm. Therefore, when identifying a First Degree Heart Block, you must also identify the underlying rhythm.

- Here are the rules for *First Degree Heart Block*:

    Regularity: depends on underlying rhythm
    Rate: depends on underlying rhythm
    P Waves: upright and uniform; each P wave will be followed by a QRS complex
    PRI: greater than .20 seconds; constant across the strip
    QRS: less than .12 seconds.

- Wenckebach is a characteristic cyclic pattern in which the PRIs get longer and longer until one P wave does not produce a QRS complex. This cycle repeats itself, producing grouping of the R waves.

- The rules for *Wenckebach* are:

    Regularity: irregular; R–R interval gets progressively shorter as PR interval gets
                    longer; characteristic grouped beating
    Rate: usually slightly slower than normal
    P Waves: upright and uniform; some P waves are not followed by QRS
                 complexes
    PRI: progressively lengthens until one P wave is not conducted
    QRS: less than .12 seconds.

- In Classical Second Degree Heart Block, there can be two, three, or four P waves for every QRS complex, because the AV node blocks out many of the impulses.

- Here are the rules for *Classical Second Degree Heart Block*:

    Regularity: can be regular or irregular, depending on whether the conduction
                    ratio varies or is constant
    Rate: usually in the bradycardia range; can be one half to one third the
            normal rate

P Waves: upright and uniform; more than one P wave for every QRS complex; P–P interval is regular
PRI: always constant across the strip; can be greater than .20 seconds
QRS: less than .12 seconds.

- In Complete Heart Block (CHB) there is a total obstruction at the AV node, resulting in AV dissociation: the atria and ventricles are totally dissociated from each other.

- In CHB the ventricles can be controlled by either a junctional or a ventricular escape rhythm. The lower pacemaker site can be identified by looking at the width of the QRS and the ventricular rate.

- The rules for *Complete Heart Block* are:

Regularity: regular
Rate: 40–60 if the focus is junctional
20–40 if the focus is ventricular
P Waves: upright and uniform; more P waves than QRS complexes
PRI: no relationship between P waves and QRS complexes; P waves can occasionally be found superimposed on the QRS complex
QRS: less than .12 seconds if focus is junctional
.12 seconds or more if focus is ventricular.

Self-Test: Heart Blocks

Directions:

Complete this self-evaluation of the information you have learned from this chapter. If your answers are all correct and you feel comfortable with your understanding of the material, proceed to the next chapter. However, if you missed any of the questions, you should review the chapter before proceeding. If you feel uncomfortable with any of your understanding, invest the time now to go back over the entire chapter. DO NOT PROCEED WITH THE NEXT CHAPTER UNTIL YOU ARE VERY COMFORTABLE WITH THE MATERIAL IN THIS CHAPTER.

Question	Referenced Frames	
1. What kind of disturbance causes the arrhythmias you learned in this chapter?	1	conduction disturbances in the AV node
2. Which of the arrhythmias you learned in this chapter is not a true block?	2; 3; 4; 44	First Degree Heart Block is not a true block; it is a delay in conduction.
3. Which of the wave patterns on the EKG will yield information about the AV node?	9	the PR interval (specifically the PR segment) since it will tell you the relationship between the atria and the ventricles
4. What will the PRI be like in a First Degree Heart Block?	4; 9; 10; 11; 14; 44	it will be longer than normal; greater than .20 seconds
5. What is the rate of a First Degree Heart Block?	12; 14	First Degree Heart Block is

Question	**Referenced Frames**	
		not a rhythm in itself, thus it cannot have a rate; the rate of the rhythm will depend on the underlying rhythm.
6. Is a First Degree Heart Block regular or irregular?	11; 14; 47	again, this will depend on the regularity of the underlying rhythm
7. In addition to identifying a First Degree Heart Block, what other information must you provide in order for your interpretation to be complete?	12; 13	the identity of the underlying rhythm
8. Does the PRI in First Degree Heart Block vary from one beat to the next?	10; 11; 14	no, it remains constant across the strip
9. In First Degree Heart Block, how many P waves will you see for every QRS complex?	14	one; all beats are eventually conducted through to the ventricles, even though each one encounters a delay at the AV node
10. Is the QRS measurement also prolonged in First Degree Heart Block?	11; 33	no, once the impulse passes through the AV node, conduction through the ventricles is normal

Question	Referenced Frames	
11. In Wenckebach, do any of the sinus impulses get through the AV node to depolarize the ventricles?	2; 5; 15; 17 18; 19; 27; 30; 43; 45	yes, most of them do; but the AV node holds each one a little longer than the preceding one, until one is blocked completely. Then the cycle starts over
12. What is the ventricular rate of a Wenckebach?	32; 33	it's usually just a little bit slower than normal, since most of the impulses are conducted
13. Is the R–R interval regular in a Wenckebach?	31; 33; 48	no; as the PRI gets longer, the R–R gets shorter
14. Does a Wenckebach have a regular P–P interval?	27; 33	yes, even though the PRIs and the R–Rs change, the P–P remains regular
15. Is the R–R interval grossly irregular in a Wenckebach?	31; 33; 48	no; it has a distinctive cyclic pattern of grouped beating
16. Does a Wenckebach produce one P wave for every QRS complex?	5; 15; 19; 27; 28; 29; 33; 43	No; most P waves are followed by QRS complexes,

Question	**Referenced Frames**	
		but some P waves are not conducted through to the ventricles
17. What is the key feature of a Wenckebach?	20; 28	progressively lengthening PRIs with eventual blocked impulses
18. Does a Classical Second Degree Heart Block have an equal number of P waves and QRS complexes?	16; 19; 20; 21; 22; 26; 43; 46	No; a Classical Second Degree Heart Block will always have more P waves than QRS complexes.
19. Is the PRI of a Classical Second Degree Heart Block constant, or does it vary between beats?	22; 23; 26; 46	it's constant; this is a key diagnostic feature that helps distinguish it from Wenckebach and CHB
20. Is the PRI measurement normal in Classical Second Degree Heart Block?	23; 26	It can be normal, or it can be prolonged. Whatever the measurement, however, it will always be constant.
21. What is the usual rate range for a Classical Second Degree Heart Block?	24; 26	Since most of the P waves are being

Question	Referenced Frames	
		blocked, it will be in the bradycardia range; usually ½ to ⅓ the normal rate.
22. What is meant by a variable conduction ratio?	25	It means that the AV node is varying the pattern in which sinus impulses are being conducted to the ventricles. It changes from one beat to the next, e.g., 2:1, 4:1, 3:1, 2:1, etc.
23. Is the R–R interval regular or irregular in a Classical Second Degree Heart Block?	25; 26	It will be regular, unless the conduction ratio is variable, in which case the rhythm will be irregular.
24. Is the QRS measurement normal or abnormal in a Classical Second Degree Heart Block?	17; 18; 26	It should be normal, since those impulses that are allowed to pass through the AV node continue on through the ventricles in a normal way.

Question	Referenced Frames	
25. In Third Degree Heart Block (CHB), do any of the impulses from the SA node penetrate the AV node to depolarize the ventricles?	34; 35; 38; 42	No. In CHB the block at the AV node is complete. None of the sinus impulses passes through to the ventricles.
26. In CHB, will there be more P waves or more QRS complexes on the EKG?	35; 41	there will be more P waves
27. If none of the sinus impulses is able to depolarize the ventricles, what focus is producing the QRS complexes?	36; 38	A lower site will take over at an escape rate. This rhythm can be either junctional or ventricular in origin.
28. How would you differentiate between a junctional focus and a ventricular focus in a CHB?	37; 38; 41	junctional focus – QRS complex of less than .12 seconds; rate, 40–60 beats per minute. With ventricular focus, QRS is .12 seconds or more, and rate 20–40 beats per minute.
29. Is CHB regular or irregular?	40; 41	regular; this will help you distinguish it from Wenckebach.

Question	Referenced Frames	
30. What will the PRI be in a CHB?	38; 41; 42	There is no PRI, as atria and ventricles are dissociated. The P waves have no relationship to the QRS complexes.

Practice Sheet 8: Heart Blocks

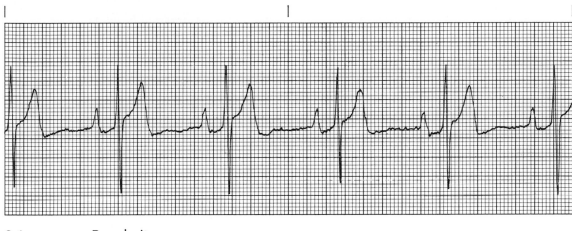

8.1

Regularity: _____

Rate: _____

P Waves: _____

PRI: _____

QRS: _____

Interp: _____

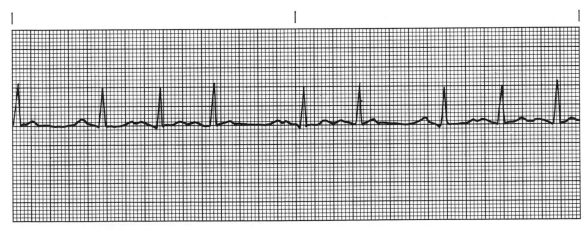

8.2

Regularity: _____

Rate: _____

P Waves: _____

PRI: _____

QRS: _____

Interp: _____

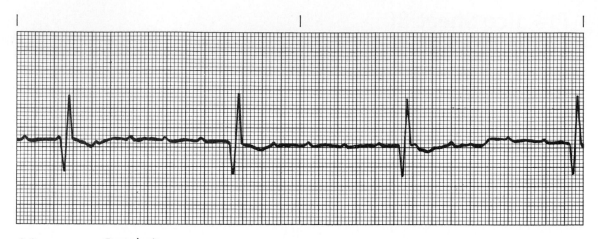

8.3   Regularity: _____
       Rate: _____
       P Waves: _____
       PRI: _____
       QRS: _____
       Interp: _____

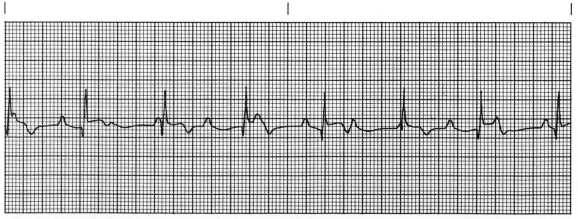

8.4   Regularity: _____
       Rate: _____
       P Waves: _____
       PRI: _____
       QRS: _____
       Interp: _____

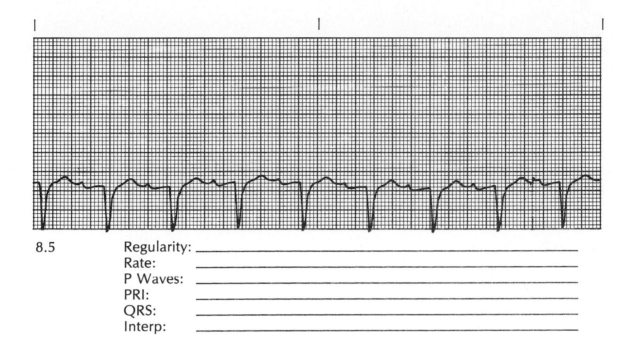

8.5   Regularity: _____
           Rate: _____
           P Waves: _____
           PRI: _____
           QRS: _____
           Interp: _____

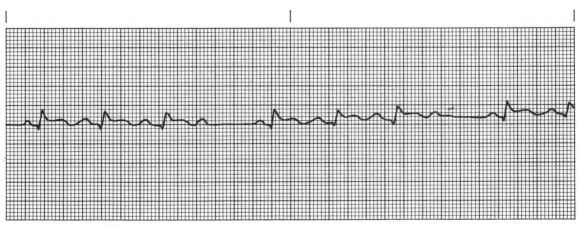

8.6   Regularity: _____
           Rate: _____
           P Waves: _____
           PRI: _____
           QRS: _____
           Interp: _____

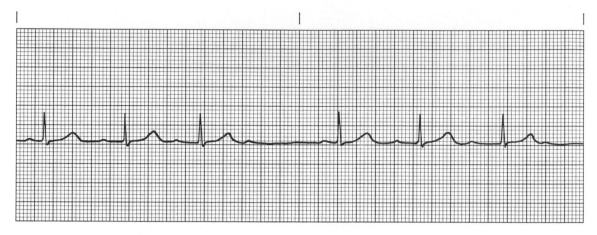

8.7   Regularity: _____
       Rate: _____
       P Waves: _____
       PRI: _____
       QRS: _____
       Interp: _____

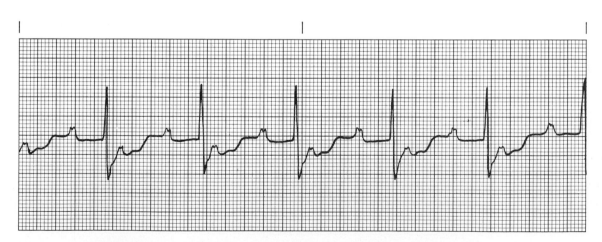

8.8   Regularity: _____
       Rate: _____
       P Waves: _____
       PRI: _____
       QRS: _____
       Interp: _____

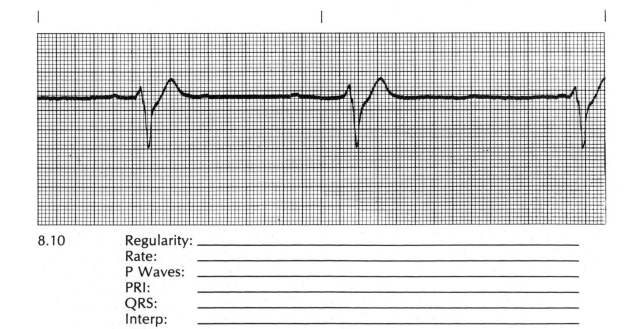

8.9   Regularity: _____
        Rate: _____
        P Waves: _____
        PRI: _____
        QRS: _____
        Interp: _____

8.10   Regularity: _____
        Rate: _____
        P Waves: _____
        PRI: _____
        QRS: _____
        Interp: _____

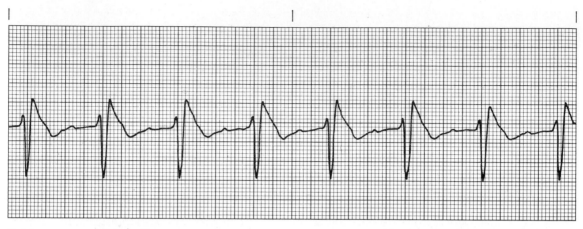

8.11   Regularity: _____
            Rate: _____
            P Waves: _____
            PRI: _____
            QRS: _____
            Interp: _____

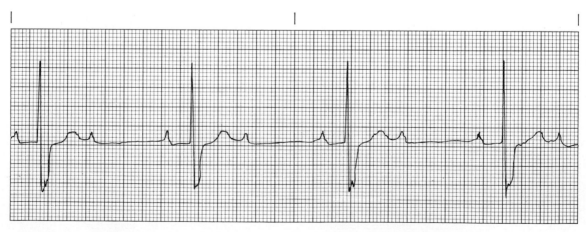

8.12   Regularity: _____
            Rate: _____
            P Waves: _____
            PRI: _____
            QRS: _____
            Interp: _____

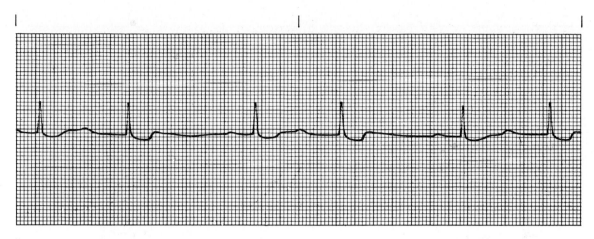

8.13   Regularity: _____
            Rate: _____
            P Waves: _____
            PRI: _____
            QRS: _____
            Interp: _____

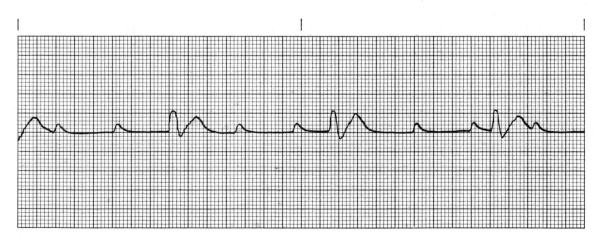

8.14   Regularity: _____
            Rate: _____
            P Waves: _____
            PRI: _____
            QRS: _____
            Interp: _____

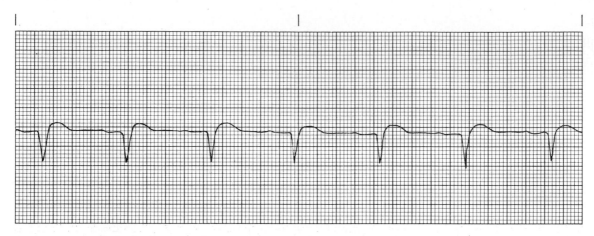

8.15   Regularity: _____
        Rate: _____
        P Waves: _____
        PRI: _____
        QRS: _____
        Interp: _____

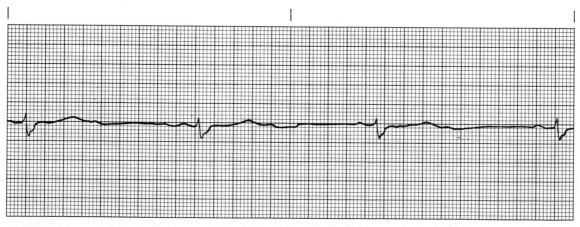

8.16   Regularity: _____
        Rate: _____
        P Waves: _____
        PRI: _____
        QRS: _____
        Interp: _____

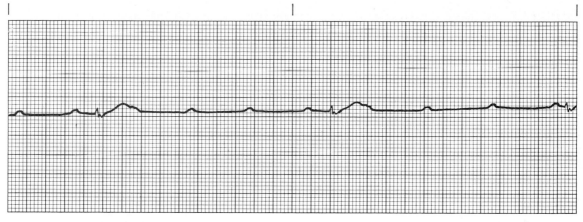

8.17   Regularity: _____
        Rate: _____
        P Waves: _____
        PRI: _____
        QRS: _____
        Interp: _____

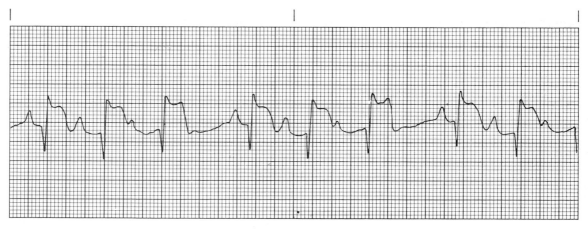

8.18   Regularity: _____
        Rate: _____
        P Waves: _____
        PRI: _____
        QRS: _____
        Interp: _____

8

Ventricular Rhythms

1. All of the arrhythmias you have learned so far are classified as supraventricular arrhythmias, because they originate above the ventricles. All supraventricular arrhythmias have one thing in common: they all have QRS complexes of less than _____ seconds duration. This classification has a very scientific basis. We know from physiological measurements that an impulse originating above the ventricles, which follows the normal conduction pathways, can depolarize the ventricles in less than .12 seconds. We also learned that it is possible for a supraventricular impulse to produce a QRS which is wider than .12 seconds, but that this would indicate some kind of delay in _____ through the ventricles, and thus would be considered an abnormality to be noted. Generally speaking, a normal supraventricular complex will have a _____ measurement of less than _____ seconds.

.12

conduction

QRS
.12

2. We say that a supraventricular arrhythmia should have a QRS complex of less than .12 seconds, but we also acknowledge that an abnormality could cause the QRS to be wider than that. However, we can say with certainty that an impulse which originated in the ventricles cannot depolarize the ventricles in less than .12 seconds. Hence, a basic rule for ventricular arrhythmias is that the QRS measurement will be .12 seconds or greater. If a complex measures less than .12 seconds, we know that it must have been initiated by a _____ impulse. But if it is .12 seconds or greater, it could either have originated above the ventricles and encountered a conduction disturbance, or it must have originated in the _____.

supraven-
tricular
ventricles

3. Ventricular arrhythmias are very serious for several reasons. First, the heart was intended to depolarize from the top down. The _____ were meant to contract before the _____ in order to effectively pump blood. When an impulse originates in the ventricles, this process is reversed, and the heart's efficiency is greatly reduced. Further, since the ventricles are the lowest site in the conduction system, there are no more fail-safe mechanisms to back up a ventricular arrhythmia. Ventricular arrhythmias are the most serious arrhythmias because the heart has lost its _____, and because it is functioning on its last level of backup support.

atria; ventricles

effectiveness

4. In this section we will be learning five ventricular arrhythmias:

  • premature ventricular contraction (PVC)
  • ventricular tachycardia
  • ventricular fibrillation
  • idioventricular rhythm
  • asystole

Although their mechanisms differ, each of these arrhythmias originates in the _____, and thus will have a QRS measurement of _____ seconds or more.

ventricles;
.12

5.   The first arrhythmia is not a rhythm, but instead is a single ectopic beat originating from an irritable ventricular focus. Since it arises from an irritable focus, the complex will come _____ than expected in the cardiac cycle, and will interrupt the regularity of the underlying rhythm. PVCs are single _____ that come earlier than expected and interrupt the underlying _____.

earlier

ectopics
rhythm

6.   Because PVCs originate in the ventricles, the QRS will be _____ than normal. But a second feature of a ventricular focus is that there is no P wave preceding the QRS complex. This is logical, since the SA node did not precipitate the ventricular depolarization. On the EKG you will see a very wide, bizarre QRS complex which is *not* preceded by a _____ wave.

wider

P

7.   One of the things that gives a PVC such a bizarre appearance, in addition to the width of the QRS complex, is the tendency for PVCs to produce a T wave which extends in the opposite direction of the QRS complex (Fig. 61). That is, if the QRS complex is upright, the T wave will be inverted, and if the QRS is negative, the T wave will be _____. This is not a hard-and-fast rule, but is a very frequent finding which contributes to an overall _____ appearance of a PVC.

upright;
bizarre

8.   PVCs are usually easy to spot because they are wide and bizarre, with a QRS complex measurement of _____ seconds or more, and they are not preceded by a _____ wave. Another feature common to many PVCs is that the T wave is in the opposite direction of the _____ wave.

.12;
P

QRS

9.   Another frequent feature that may be helpful in identifying a PVC is the compensatory pause that usually follows a ventricular ectopic. A compensatory pause is created when a PVC comes early, but since it doesn't conduct the impulse retrograde through the AV

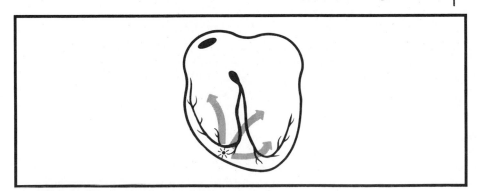

Figure 60. Premature Ventricular Contraction

A PVC is a single irritable focus within the ventricles that fires prematurely to initiate an ectopic complex.

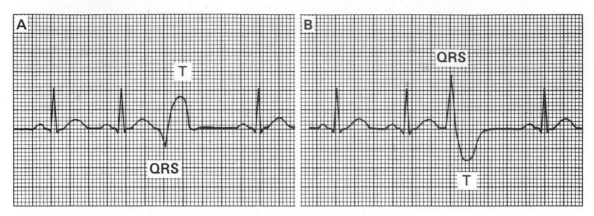

Figure 61. T Wave Configuration in PVCs

node, the atria are not depolarized. This leaves the sinus node undisturbed and able to discharge again at its next expected time. The result is that the distance between the complex preceding the PVC and the complex following the PVC is exactly twice the distance of one R–R interval (Fig. 63). If an ectopic is followed by a _____ pause, it is a good indication that the ectopic was a _____.

compensatory;
PVC

10.   Although it is most common for PVCs to be followed by compensatory pauses, this is not a rigid requirement. Another configuration possibility is that the PVC be followed by no pause whatsoever. This occurs when the PVC squeezes itself in between two regular complexes, and does not disturb the regular pattern of the sinus node. This phenomenon is called an "interpolated" PVC, because the PVC inserts itself between two regular beats (Fig. 64). With an interpolated PVC, the R–R interval remains _____, since the PVC does not interrupt the sinus rhythm.

regular

11.   If a PVC is followed by a pause before the next sinus beat, leaving a distance between the sinus beat preceding the PVC and the sinus beat following the PVC which measures exactly twice the normal R–R interval, you would call this a _____ pause. However, if the PVC falls directly between two sinus beats, without interrupting the regularity of the underlying rhythm, you would call this an _____ PVC.

compensatory

interpolated

12.   As with other types of ectopics, a PVC will interrupt the underlying rhythm. In interpreting the rhythm strip, it is important to identify both the ectopic and the underlying arrhythmia. For example, the arrhythmia might be Sinus Tachycardia with a PVC. When you are reporting a PVC you should convey as much information about the disorder as possible, including the _____ rhythm.

underlying

13.   Several other items are important information about a PVC. Since PVCs are an indication of myocardial irritability, it is important

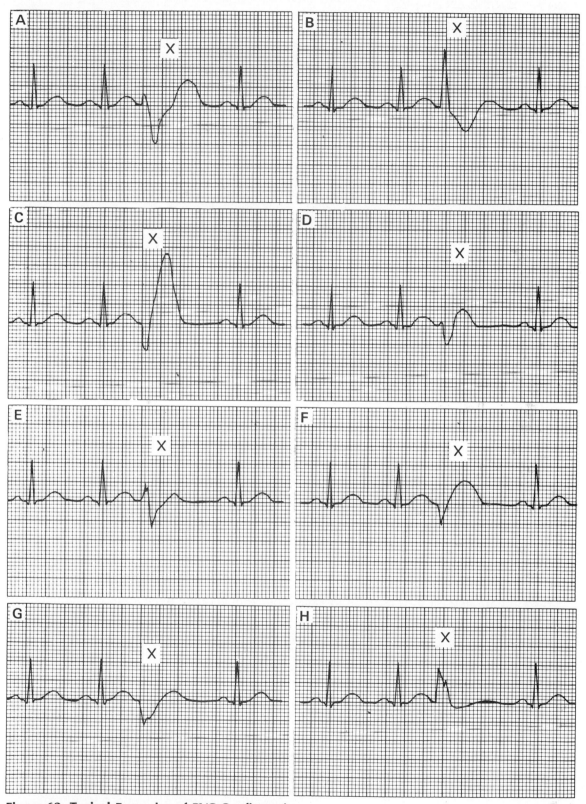

Figure 62. Typical Examples of PVC Configuration

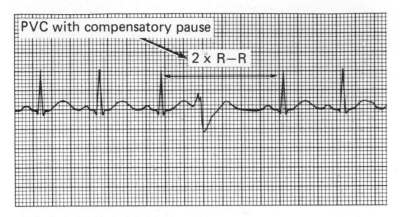

Figure 63. Compensatory Pause

to note how frequently they are occurring. If the patient is having only an occasional PVC this may be a normal rhythm for that person. But if the frequency picks up so that you are seeing 5–10 per minute, you would suspect that the ectopics were an indication of increasing _____. If the patient is experiencing chest pain of any | irritability
sort, even a single PVC could be considered ominous. It is important that you not only note the presence of PVCs, but also that you indicate the _____ of occurrence. | frequency

14. If a single focus within the ventricles has become irritable, and is the source of the PVCs, all of these ectopics will have an identical appearance. That is, if one first has a positive deflection, and then a wide negative deflection, all other PVCs from that single focus will have the same configuration. These are called "unifocal" (Fig. 65) PVCs, because they come from a _____ focus and are all | single
uniform in configuration. If all the PVCs on a rhythm strip had similar appearances you would assume they all originated from a _____ | single;
ectopic focus and would call them _____ PVCs. | unifocal

15. In cases of greater irritability, several ventricular foci might begin to initiate ectopics. In such an instance, the PVCs would have a variety of configurations (Fig. 66). If two foci were initiating PVCs, all of the PVCs would have one of two configurations. If more sites were irritable, there would be a greater variety of _____. In | configurations
this situation, the PVCs are called "multifocal" because the heart is so irritable that many foci are initiating the ectopics. Since they originate from many foci, _____ PVCs are more serious than | multifocal
unifocal PVCs because they are associated with a more irritable myocardium.

16. If the PVCs on a rhythm strip all had the same basic configuration, they would be considered _____. If the PVCs had | unifocal;
differing configurations, they would be considered _____. | multifocal

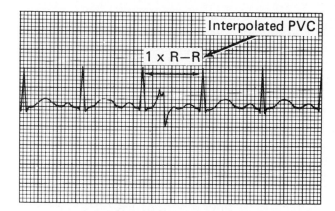

Figure 64. Interpolated PVC

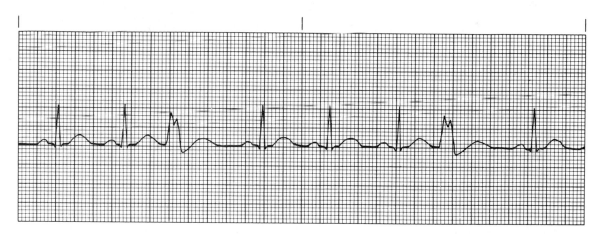

Figure 65. Unifocal PVCs

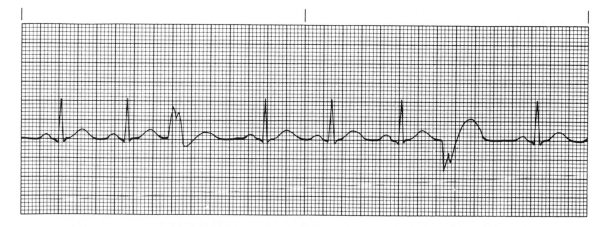

Figure 66. Multifocal PVCs

17.   PVCs represent a major electrical force, since they are a depiction of a premature depolarization of the ventricles. Because they come prematurely, they often fall near the end of the preceding QRS complex. If you recall, in Chapter 2 we learned that a portion of the T wave is considered a vulnerable area, because an electrical impulse could cause an aberrant depolarization of the heart if it should occur during that phase. If a PVC occurs during the _____ phase, it could throw the heart into an uncontrolled repetitive pattern. For this reason, it is important to note any PVC that is falling on or near the _____ wave of the preceding beat. This phenomenon is called "R on T" because the R wave of the PVC is hitting on the T wave (Fig. 67). If you see PVCs creeping up on the preceding T wave, you would call this an _____ phenomenon, and know that it represents a very serious situation.

vulnerable

T

R on T

18.   R on T phenomenon exists when the R wave of a _____ falls on or near the vulnerable phase of the cardiac cycle. The vulnerable phase, or relative refractory period, is located on the downslope of the _____ wave. (Note: If you have forgotten this material, turn back to Chapter 2 for a quick review.)

PVC

T

19.   Another sign of increasing myocardial irritability is when PVCs occur in immediate succession, without a normal beat intervening. If only two PVCs occur before the normal pattern resumes, you would see two PVCs attached to each other. This is called a "couplet," (Fig. 68) but if you see three or more PVCs occurring in succession, this would be called a "run of PVCs" (Fig. 69). The important distinction here is that several PVCs have fired without allowing the normal pacemaker to resume pacemaking responsibility. This is an indica-

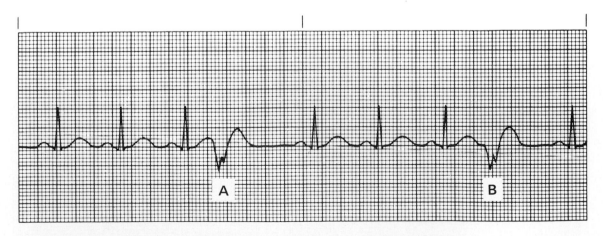

Figure 67. R on T Phenomenon: Ectopic A exhibits "R on T" Phenomenon; Exhibit B does not.

tion of significant _____. Regardless of whether you call | irritability
this pattern a couplet or a run of PVCs, you should note that the
PVCs are occurring in immediate succession, and indicate the number of PVCs observed. Technically, two successive PVCs would be
called a _____, but it is sufficient to call any number of | couplet;
successive PVCs a _____ of PVCs, and then indicate the | run
number of PVCs involved.

20.   A pair of PVCs in immediate succession could be called either
a _____ or a _____ of two PVCs. But if there | couplet; run
were three or more PVCs in a row, it should be called a _____ | run;
of three (or more) _____. | PVCs

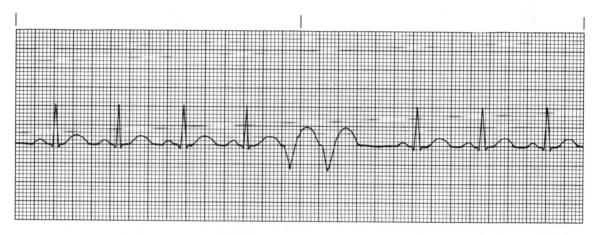

Figure 68. PVCs Occurring as a Couplet (Pair)

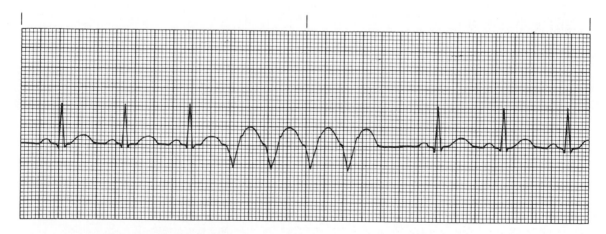

Figure 69. PVCs Occurring in a Run

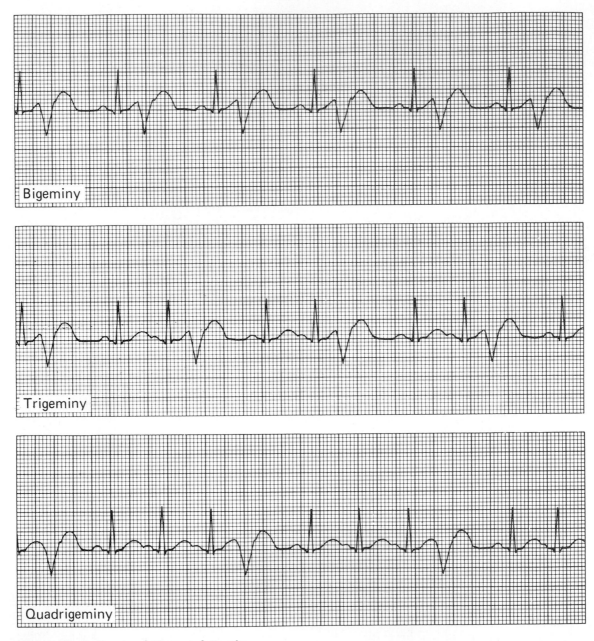

Figure 70. Patterns of Grouped Beating

21. Sometimes, frequently occurring PVCs will fall into a pattern with the surrounding normal beats. This is called "grouped beating." For example, you may see a PVC, then a normal beat, then a PVC, then a normal beat, and so on. When the PVCs are falling in a pattern of "every other beat" (Fig. 70) with the normal beats, this is called "bigeminy." Bigeminy refers to a repetitive pattern of grouped beat-

ing, e.g., one normal and one PVC, across the entire strip. When you see a pattern of one PVC, then one normal beat, then one PVC, then one normal beat, and this pattern continues across the strip, you would call the rhythm _____ of PVCs.

bigeminy

22. Don't forget, though, to include the identification of the underlying rhythm. For example, if you saw a sinus beat, then a PVC, then a sinus beat, then a PVC, across the strip, you would call this Sinus Rhythm with bigeminy of _____.

PVCs

23. Several other patterns of grouped beating that are very similar to bigeminy result from PVCs falling into a rhythm with normal beats. For example, if you saw a PVC followed by two sinus beats, then another PVC followed by two sinus beats, you would have a repetitive cycle of three beats, one PVC, and two sinus beats. This pattern is called trigeminy, since the cycle contains three beats. Such a rhythm would be called Sinus Rhythm with _____ of PVCs.

trigeminy

24. Another such pattern is quadrigeminy, where a pattern of four beats consists of one PVC and three normal beats. If you had a long enough rhythm strip, you could probably map out patterns of as many as eight, nine, or more beats to a cycle. However, the most common are bigeminy, a cycle consisting of one PVC and one normal beat; trigeminy, a cycle including one PVC and two normal beats; and _____, where there are four complexes to the cycle, one PVC, and three normal beats.

quadrigeminy

25. Patterns such as bigeminy, trigeminy, and quadrigeminy can be found with other ectopics, as well as PVCs. For example, you can have bigeminy of PACs, or quadrigeminy of PJCs. But to qualify as a true patterned beat, the grouping should continue across the entire strip. Just because you happen to have two PACs on the strip with a single normal beat between them, you could not necessarily call this bigeminy. But if the pattern continued regularly across the strip, you would call it Sinus Rhythm with bigeminy of _____.

PACs

26. You now know quite a few things about PVCs. They are wide and bizarre, with a QRS measurement of _____. Frequently, the T wave will be in the opposite direction of the _____. PVCs are a sign of myocardial _____, so you should note how frequently they are occurring. You should also note if they are all coming from a single focus, in which case you would call them _____. If they are coming from more than one focus you would call them _____.

.12 seconds
or more;
QRS Complex;
irritability

unifocal
multifocal

27. You should be very cautious of a PVC that is falling near the downslope of the _____ wave, since this is the vulnerable phase of the cardiac cycle. This is called _____ phenomenon, and is dangerous because it could throw the heart into an ineffective repetitive pattern.

T
R on T

28. If the myocardial irritability is sufficient, you may notice PVCs falling in succession, without an intervening normal beat. If there were several PVCs connected in this manner you would call it a _____ of PVCs, and would note how many ectopics were involved. If there were only two PVCs paired, you might call this a _____.

run

couplet

29. Finally, you know that PVCs can fall into patterns with the underlying normal beats. If it is a pattern of twos, i.e., one normal, one PVC, you would call this _____. If it is a pattern of threes, it is called _____, and it is called quadrigeminy if there are _____ complexes in the pattern.

bigeminy;
trigeminy;
four

30. Here are the rules for PVCs:

       Regularity: ectopics will disrupt regularity of underlying rhythm

       Rate: depends on underlying rhythm and number of ectopics

       P Waves: will not be preceded by a P wave; dissociated P wave may be seen near PVC

       PRI: since the ectopic comes from a lower focus, there will be no PRI

       QRS: wide and bizarre; .12 seconds or greater; T wave is usually in opposite direction from R wave

31. If the myocardium is extremely irritable, the ventricular focus could speed up and override higher pacemaker sites. This would create what is essentially a sustained run of PVCs. This rhythm is called ventricular tachycardia (VT). In fact, a run of PVCs is often called a short burst of VT. They both result from myocardial _____, and they both fit the same rules. However, PVCs are _____ ectopics, whereas VT is an actual arrhythmia. In VT you will see a succession of PVCs across the strip at a rate of about 150–250 beats per minute. This arrhythmia usually has a very uniform appearance, even though the R–R interval may be *slightly* irregular. It is possible for VT to occur at slower rates, but when it does it is qualified by calling it a slow VT. A true VT has a ventricular rate of _____–_____ beats per minute.

irritability;
single

150–250

32. Each of the other rules for a PVC also applies to VT. The QRS complex will be .12 seconds or greater, and the complex will be _____ and bizarre with the T wave usually in the opposite direction of the _____ wave. Since this rhythm originates from a _____ focus, you will not see a P wave in front of the QRS complex. However, this is another form of AV dissociation, so you may see an occasional P wave coincidentally occurring near the QRS complex. As with PVCs, VT will have a QRS measurement of _____ seconds or greater, with a bizarre

wide;
QRS;
ventricular

.12;

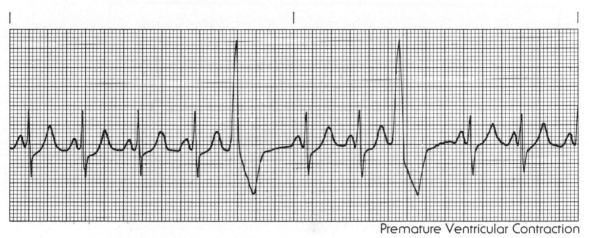

Premature Ventricular Contraction

Figure 71. Rules for Premature Ventricular Contractions

REGULARITY: The underlying rhythm can be regular or irregular. The ectopic PVC will interrupt the regularity of the underlying rhythm (unless the PVC is interpolated).

RATE: The rate will be determined by the underlying rhythm. PVCs are not usually included in the rate determination because they frequently do not produce a pulse.

P WAVES: The ectopic is not preceded by a P wave. You may see a coincidental P wave near the PVC, but it is dissociated.

PRI: Since the ectopic comes from a lower focus, there will be no PRI.

QRS: The QRS complex will be wide and bizarre, measuring at least .12 seconds. The configuration will differ from the configuration of the underlying QRS complexes. The T wave is frequently in the opposite direction from the QRS complex.

configuration of the _____ complex and T wave, and there will be no _____ waves preceding the QRS complexes.

QRS
P

33.   Ventricular tachycardia is caused by a _____ focus in the ventricles which fires at a tachycardia rate to override the higher pacemaker sites and take over control of the heart. It is also possible for the ventricular focus to change to a flutter mechanism, which would result in an arrhythmia very similar to VT, but with a ventricular rate of more than 300. When the ventricles depolarize at such a rapid rate, the resultant EKG pattern becomes a very uniform, regular tracing and looks almost like a coiled spring. There is very little difference between VT and ventricular flutter, except for the rate. Most clinicians choose to consider ventricular flutter in with VT, and eliminate this academic distinction. For our purposes, we will con-

single

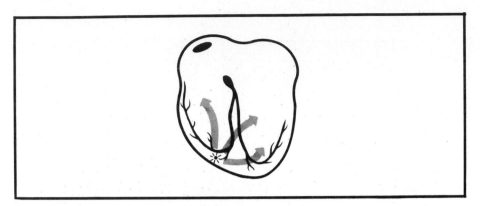

Figure 72. Ventricular Tachycardia

An irritable focus in the ventricles fires regularly at a rate of 150–250 beats per minute to override higher sites for control of the heart.

sider ventricular flutter a rapid form of VT. We will not make a distinction between the two, since the only real difference is in the ventricular _____.

rate

34.   Here are the rules for Ventricular Tachycardia:
  Regularity: usually regular; can be slightly irregular
      Rate: 150–250 beats per minute; can exceed 250 beats per minute if the rhythm progresses to ventricular flutter; may occasionally be slower than 150 beats per minute, in which case it is called slow VT
  P Waves: will not be preceded by P waves; dissociated P waves may be seen
      PRI: Since the focus is in the ventricles, there will be no PRI
      QRS: wide and bizarre; .12 seconds or greater; T wave is usually in opposite direction from R wave

35.   In extremely severe cases of ventricular irritability, the electrical foci in the ventricles can begin fibrillating. This means that many, many foci are firing in a chaotic, ineffective manner, and the heart muscle is unable to contract in response. Ventricular Fibrillation is a lethal arrhythmia, since the rhythm is very chaotic and _____.

ineffective

36.   Ventricular Fibrillation (VF) is probably the easiest of all the rhythmias to recognize. This is because there are no discernible complexes or intervals, and the entire rhythm consists of chaotic, irregular activity. Since there are no identifiable complexes or wave forms, the EKG pattern of VF is simply a grossly _____ fibrillatory pattern.

chaotic

37.   VT is distinguishable from VF because Ventricular Tachycardia has wide, bizarre complexes, but they are uniform and measurable. VF has no measurable waves or _____.

complexes

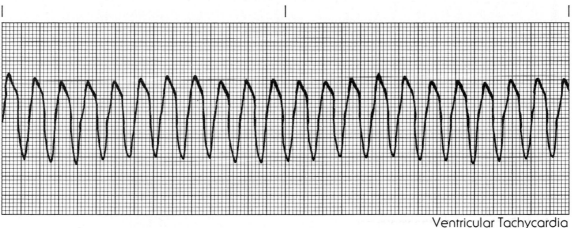

Ventricular Tachycardia

Figure 73. Rules for Ventricular Tachycardia

REGULARITY: **This rhythm is usually regular, although it can be slightly irregular.**

RATE: **Atrial rate cannot be determined. The ventricular rate range is 150–250 beats per minute. If the rate is below 150 beats per minute it is considered a slow VT. If the rate exceeds 250 beats per minute it's called Ventricular Flutter.**

P WAVES: **None of the QRS complexes will be preceded by P waves. You may see dissociated P waves intermittently across the strip.**

PRI: **Since the rhythm originates in the ventricles, there will be no PRI.**

QRS: **The QRS complexes will be wide and bizarre, measuring at least .12 seconds. It is often difficult to differentiate between the QRS and the T wave.**

38.   Here are the rules for Ventricular Fibrillation:

Regularity:
Rate:
P Wave: } totally chaotic with no discernible waves or complexes
PRI:
QRS:

39.   So far, you have learned three ventricular arrhythmias, all of which are the result of ventricular irritability. These are PVCs, Ventricular Tachycardia, and Ventricular Fibrillation. It is also possible for a ventricular rhythm to be produced by an escape mechanism. If a higher pacemaker site fails, a ventricular focus can step in to take over pacemaking responsibility. There are two ways a ventricular focus can assume control of the heart. One is irritability, and the other is _____ mechanism.   escape

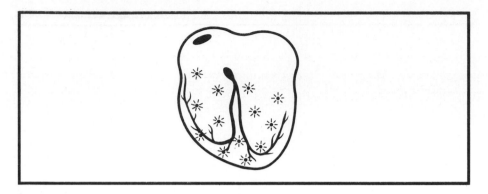

Figure 74. Ventricular Fibrillation

**Multiple foci in the ventricles become irritable and generate uncoordi-
nated, chaotic impulses that cause the heart to fibrillate rather than
contract.**

40.   A ventricular escape rhythm is one that takes over pacemaking
in the absence of a higher focus, and depolarizes the heart at the
inherent rate of the ventricles, which is _____–_____   20–40
beats per minute. This rhythm is called Idioventricular Rhythm, because the ventricles are initiating the rhythm on their own, without a
conducted stimulus from a higher focus. The rate for Idioventricular
Rhythm would be _____–_____ beats per   20–40
minute.

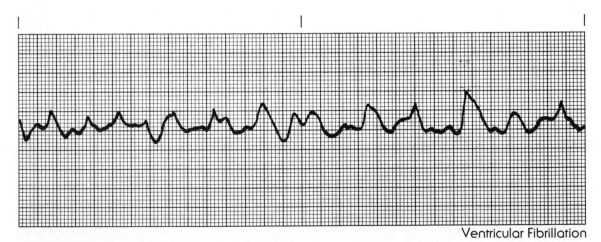

Ventricular Fibrillation

Figure 75: Rules for Ventricular Fibrillation

REGULARITY: **There are no waves or complexes that can be analyzed to
determine regularity. The baseline is totally chaotic.**

RATE: **The rate cannot be determined since there are no discernible waves or complexes to measure.**

P WAVES: **There are no discernible P waves.**

PRI: **There is no PRI.**

QRS: **There are no discernible QRS complexes.**

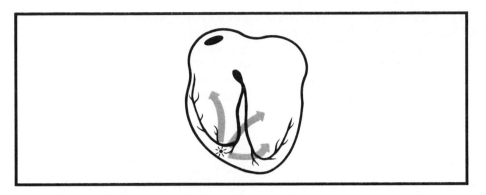

Figure 76. Idioventricular Rhythm

In the absence of a higher pacemaker, the Ventricles initiate a regular impulse at their inherent rate of 20–40 beats per minute.

41. You might consider Idioventricular Rhythm a ventricular escape rhythm, since it is a fail-safe rhythm that takes over when _____ pacemaker sites fail. A ventricular focus firing within the inherent rate range of the ventricles would produce a rhythm called _____ Rhythm.

higher

Idioventricular

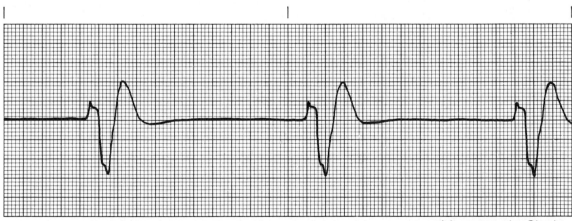

Idioventricular Rhythm

Figure 77. Rules for Idioventricular Rhythm

REGULARITY: **This rhythm is usually regular, although it can slow as the heart dies.**

RATE: **The ventricular rate is usually 20–40 beats per minute, but it can drop below 20 beats per minute.**

P WAVES: **There are no P waves in this arrhythmia.**

PRI: **There is no PRI.**

QRS: **The QRS complex is wide and bizarre, measuring at least .12 seconds.**

42.   You should not see P waves in an Idioventricular Rhythm, since the escape mechanism would only take over if the atrial pacemaker sites had failed. What you will see is a rhythm of very slow ventricular complexes, usually in a regular rhythm, although it is possible for such an unreliable pacemaker to discharge irregularly. An Idioventricular Rhythm will not have _____ waves. Instead, you will see ventricular complexes measuring at least _____ seconds, firing at a rate below 40 beats per minute.

P
.12

43.   Idioventricular Rhythm is initiated by the very last possible fail-safe mechanism within the heart. This means that it is frequently an unreliable focus. It may fire a little irregularly, and the rate may be less than 20 beats per minute, even though the intrinsic ventricular rate is supposed to be 20–40 beats per minute. When the rhythm is in its terminal stages, that is, as the patient is dying, the complexes can lose some of their form and be quite irregular. In this stage, the arrhythmia is said to be "agonal", or a dying heart. The word agonal is used to describe a terminal, lethal arrhythmia, especially when it has stopped beating in a reliable pattern. Idioventricular Rhythm is an _____ rhythm, especially when the rate drops below 20 beats per minute and the pattern loses its uniformity.

agonal

44.   Here are the rules for Idioventricular Rhythm:
       Regularity: usually regular
            Rate: 20–40 beats per minute; can drop below 20 beats
                  per minute
        P Waves: none
             PRI: none
            QRS: wide and bizarre; .12 seconds or more

45.   The last stage of a dying heart is when all electrical activity ceases. This results in a straight line on the EKG, an arrhythmia called "asystole" (pronounced ā-sis'-toe-lee). Asystole is a period of absent electrical activity, seen on the EKG as a _____ line. Asystole is a lethal arrhythmia which is very resistant to resuscitation efforts.

straight

46.   Here are the rules for Asystole:
       Regularity:
            Rate:
        P Wave: } straight line indicates no electrical activity
             PRI:
            QRS:

47.   A straight line on the EKG would suggest that there is no electrical activity left in the heart. This rhythm would be called _____.

asystole

48.   If the EKG only has ventricular complexes at a rate between 20 and 40 beats per minute, with no P waves, you would call the arrhythmia _____ Rhythm.

Idioventricular

49.   An EKG that is totally chaotic, with no discernible waves or complexes, and nothing but a lot of irregular undulations, would fit the rules of _____ _____.

Ventricular Fibrillation

50.   Ventricular Tachycardia is a very rapid rhythm with no _____ waves and wide, bizarre QRS complexes.

P

51.   A single ectopic with a QRS greater than .12 seconds, with a T wave in the opposite direction of the R wave, and having no P wave preceding it, would be called a Premature _____ Contraction.

Ventricular

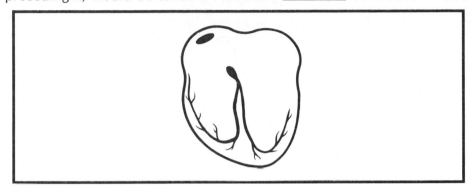

Figure 78. Asystole

The heart has lost its electrical activity. There is no electrical pacemaker to initiate electrical flow.

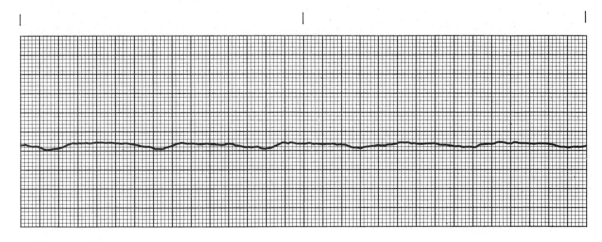

Figure 79. Rules for Asystole

REGULARITY:
RATE:
P WAVES: } **There is no electrical activity; only a straight line.**
PRI:
QRS:

Key Points – Ventricular Rhythms

- A QRS measurement of less than .12 seconds indicates a supraventricular pace-maker. If the QRS is .12 seconds or greater, it could be ventricular, or it could be supraventricular with a ventricular conduction defect.

- All ventricular impulses will have a QRS measurement of .12 seconds or greater.

- Ventricular arrhythmias are the most serious arrhythmias because the heart is less effective than usual, and because the heart is functioning on its last level of backup support.

- A PVC is a single ectopic beat arising from an irritable focus in the ventricles. It comes earlier than expected and interrupts the regularity of the underlying rhythm.

- PVCs are usually wide and bizarre, and usually have a T wave in the opposite direction of the QRS Complex. They are not preceded by a P wave.

- A compensatory pause usually follows a PVC. This means that the distance between the R wave of the complex preceding the PVC and the R wave of the complex following the PVC is exactly twice the R–R interval of the underlying rhythm.

- A PVC does not have to have a compensatory pause. It can be "interpolated" between two sinus beats without interrupting the underlying rhythm.

- PVCs are an indication of myocardial irritability. The frequency of PVCs should be noted because this suggests the degree of myocardial irritability.

- PVCs are considered unifocal if they all originate from a single ventricular focus, and thus have similar configurations.

- PVCs are considered multifocal if they arise from many foci and assume a variety of configurations.

- If a PVC lands during the vulnerable (relative refractory) phase of the cardiac cycle it can produce a lethal, repetitive arrhythmia. Thus, a PVC that falls on the downslope of the T wave is referred to as "R on T" phenomenon, and is considered very dangerous.

- With increasing irritability, the PVCs can occur in pairs, called couplets, or in runs of three or more consecutive ectopics.

- PVCs frequently occur in patterns of grouped beating. If every other beat is a PVC it is called bigeminy. If every third beat is a PVC it is called trigeminy. If every fourth beat is a PVC it is called a quadrigeminy. Bigeminy, trigeminy, and quadrigeminy can also describe patterns of PACs or PJCs.

- The rules for *Premature Ventricular Contractions* are:

    Regularity: ectopics will disrupt regularity of underlying rhythm
    Rate: depends on underlying rhythm and number of ectopics
    P Waves: will not be preceded by a P wave; dissociated P waves may be seen near PVC
    PRI: since the ectopic comes from a lower focus, there will be no PRI

QRS: wide and bizarre; .12 seconds or greater; T wave is usually in opposite direction from R wave.

- Ventricular Tachycardia is a rhythm originating from a single irritable focus within the ventricles. It looks very much like an uninterrupted series of PVCs.

- You may see some P waves in a VT, but they are dissociated from the QRS complexes.

- The rules for *Ventricular Tachycardia* are:

> Regularity: usually regular; can be slightly irregular
> Rate: 150–250 beats per minute; can exceed 250 beats per minute if the rhythm progresses to ventricular flutter; may occasionally be slower than 150 beats per minute, in which case it is called a slow VT
> P Waves: will not be preceded by P waves; dissociated P waves may be seen
> PRI: since the focus is in the ventricles, there will be no PRI
> QRS: wide and bizarre; .12 seconds or greater; T wave is usually in opposite direction from R wave.

- Ventricular Fibrillation is an indication of extreme myocardial irritability. Many ventricular foci initiate impulses in a chaotic fashion, causing the ventricles to fibrillate in an ineffective manner.

- In Ventricular Fibrillation, no waves or complexes are identifiable. All that is visible is a grossly chaotic baseline.

- The rules for *Ventricular Fibrillation* are:

> Regularity:
> Rate:
> P Waves: } totally chaotic with no discernible waves or complexes
> PRI:
> QRS:

- Idioventricular Rhythm is an escape rhythm that takes over pacemaking responsibility when higher centers fail.

- The rules for *Idioventricular Rhythm* are:

> Regularity: usually regular (it can be unreliable since it is such a low site)
> Rate: 20–40 beats per minute; can drop below 20 beats per minute
> P Waves: none
> PRI: none
> QRS: wide and bizarre; .12 seconds or greater

- Agonal is the term used to describe a terminal, lethal arrhythmia, especially when it has stopped beating in a reliable pattern; also called a dying heart.

- When all electrical activity within the heart ceases, it is seen on the EKG as a straight line, possibly with some undulations in it. This arrhythmia is called Asystole.

- The rules for *Asystole* are:

  Regularity:
        Rate:
  P Waves: } straight line indicates absence of electrical activity
        PRI:
      QRS:

Self-Test: Ventricular Rhythms

Directions:

Complete this self-evaluation of the information you have learned from this chapter. If your answers are all correct and you feel comfortable with your understanding of the material, proceed to the next chapter. However, if you missed any of the questions you should review the referenced frames before proceeding. If you feel uncomfortable with any of your understanding, invest the time now to go back over the entire chapter. DO NOT PROCEED WITH THE NEXT CHAPTER UNTIL YOU ARE VERY COMFORTABLE WITH THE MATERIAL IN THIS CHAPTER.

Question	Referenced Frames	
1. What is the minimum QRS measurement for a ventricular complex?	1; 4	.12 seconds
2. Are all wide QRS complexes ventricular in origin?	2	not necessarily — they might also be superventricular with a ventricular conduction defect
3. Why are ventricular arrhythmias so serious?	3	because the heart can't pump effectively if the ventricles contract first; also, the heart is relying on its final fail-safe mechanism.
4. What is a PVC?	5; 6; 7; 8; 26; 30; 51	a single premature ectopic arising from an irritable focus within the ventricles

Question	**Referenced Frames**	
5. How can you tell whether a PVC is unifocal or multifocal?	14; 15; 16; 26	unifocal PVCs will all have similar configurations; if they have a variety of shapes, they are multifocal
6. Are PVCs preceded by P waves?	6; 30; 51	No. These ectopics originate in the ventricles; they are not initiated by a sinus impulse.
7. What do you call two PVCs which are connected to each other without a normal beat in between?	19; 20; 28	a couplet, or a pair
8. What is a "run" of PVCs?	19; 20; 28	three or more PVCs occurring in rapid succession without an intervening normal beat; this might also be called a short burst of VT.
9. What is a compensatory pause?	9; 11	it's the pause that usually follows a PVC; it means that the distance between the R wave of the beat preceding the PVC and the R wave

Question	**Referenced Frames**	
		following the PVC is exactly twice the R–R interval of the underlying rhythm.
10. What is an interpolated PVC?	10; 11	a PVC that squeezes itself in between two normal beats without interrupting the underlying rhythm
11. How can you tell if the myocardium is irritable?	13; 19; 26; 28	The frequency of ventricular activity (PVCs, ventricular tachyarrhythmias) will increase with an increase in myocardial irritability.
12. What do you call the grouping of PVCs so that every other beat is an ectopic?	21; 23; 24; 29	bigeminy
13. Do patterns of grouped beats such as trigeminy occur only with ventricular ectopics, or can they occur with ectopics from other areas of the heart?	25	Bigeminy, trigeminy, and quadrigeminy can all occur with PACs, PJCs, and PVCs.
14. What is meant by "R on T"?	17; 18; 27	It means a PVC is falling on the down-slope of the preceding T wave, and thus is causing a stimulus

Question	Referenced Frames	
		during the vulnerable relative refractory phase. This is very dangerous, since it can cause the rhythm to change to VT or VF.
15. In addition to identifying a PVC, what other information must you provide in order for your interpretation of the rhythm to be complete?	12; 13; 22	the identity of the underlying rhythm
16. A PVC shouldn't have a P wave, but don't you sometimes see a P wave somewhere near the PVC?	32; 30	you may, but it is dissociated; it did not initiate the ventricular depolarization
17. Will a PVC have a PRI?	6; 8; 30	no, since it originates in the ventricles
18. What will the rate be for a PVC?	30	that will depend on the rate of the underlying rhythm
19. Are PVCs included when you calculate the heart rate?	3; 30	not usually, since PVCs frequently do not produce a pulse
20. What rhythm is produced if the irritable ventricular focus that produced a single PVC suddenly continued firing to produce a rapid succession of ventricular complexes at a rate of 150–250 beats per minute?	31; 34	Ventricular Tachycardia

Question	**Referenced Frames**	
21. Does Ventricular Tachycardia have P waves?	32; 34; 50	In VT, a P wave does not appear in front of every QRS complex. However, you may see dissociated P waves since the sinus node can still be firing.
22. Is VT regular or irregular?	31; 34	It is usually regular, although it can be slightly irregular.
23. Does VT ever occur at a rate below 150 beats per minute?	31; 34	Yes, it can, but it is then identified as a Slow VT.
24. Can VT exceed 250 beats per minute?	33; 34	Yes, it can. To be technically accurate, this rhythm is then called Ventricular Flutter. However, Ventricular Flutter is clinically identical to VT, and only differs in rate. Thus, both rhythms are frequently grouped in the category of VT.

Question	Referenced Frames	
25. What does the QRS complex look like in VT?	32; 34; 50	As in all ventricular rhythms, the QRS in VT is wide and bizarre and the T wave goes in the opposite direction from the QRS Complex. The measurement is .12 seconds or greater.
26. What is the PRI in a VT?	32; 34	VT does not have a PRI, since it originates in the ventricles.
27. What do the QRS complexes look like in Ventricular Fibrillation?	36; 37; 38; 49	VF does not have any identifiable waves or complexes. The QRS complex cannot be distinguished from other undulations.
28. Why is VF such an ominous rhythm?	35	The ventricles are not pumping, they are merely quivering. No blood is being pumped. The patient is clinically dead.

Question	**Referenced Frames**	
29. Is VF an irritable rhythm or an escape mechanism?	35	VF is a sign of extreme irritability
30. Is VF regular or irregular?	35; 36; 37; 38	Again, VF is grossly chaotic, with no discernible waves or complexes.
31. Can the ventricles produce an escape rhythm?	39	Yes. If higher pacemaker sites fail, the ventricles can initiate an Idioventricular Rhythm as a fail-safe escape mechanism.
32. What does Idioventricular Rhythm look like?	40; 41; 42; 44; 48	wide ventricular complexes at a rate of 20–40 beats per minute, with no P waves
33. What is the QRS measurement in an Idioventricular Rhythm?	44	at least .12 seconds
34. Is Idioventricular Rhythm regular or irregular?	42; 44	Idioventricular Rhythm is usually regular, but can be slightly irregular since it is a relatively unreliable pacemaker site.

Question	**Referenced Frames**	
35. What is the PRI in an Idioventricular Rhythm?	42; 44	Idioventricular Rhythm has no P waves, thus it has no PRI.
36. Can Idioventricular Rhythm be slower than 20 beats per minute?	43; 44	Yes it can. As the heart dies, the rate slows, and the rate can drop below the inherent rate of the ventricular pacemaker. At this point, the rhythm becomes less formed and is described as being "agonal," or a dying heart.
37. What does a straight line on the EKG indicate?	45; 47	Assuming that the machine is turned on and is functioning correctly, a straight line indicates that the heart is producing no electrical activity. This arrhythmia is called Asystole.

Question	**Referenced Frames**	
38. What is the QRS measurement for Asystole?	46	Asystole has no waves or complexes. It has no P waves, no QRS complexes, and no PRIs.

Practice Sheet 9:
Ventricular Rhythms

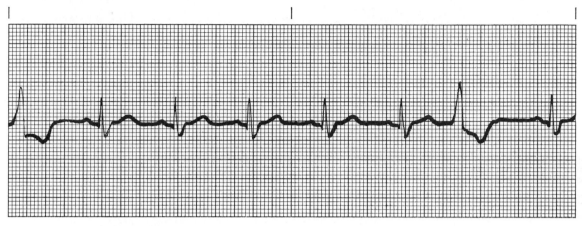

9.1   Regularity: _____
               Rate: _____
               P Waves: _____
               PRI: _____
               QRS: _____
               Interp: _____

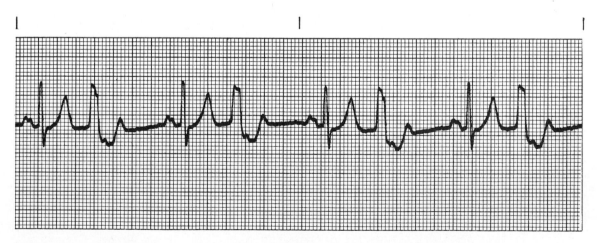

9.2   Regularity: _____
               Rate: _____
               P Waves: _____
               PRI: _____
               QRS: _____
               Interp: _____

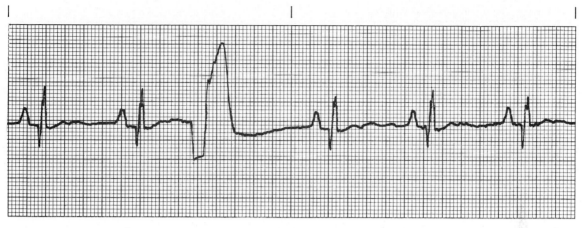

9.3   Regularity: _____
            Rate: _____
            P Waves: _____
            PRI: _____
            QRS: _____
            Interp: _____

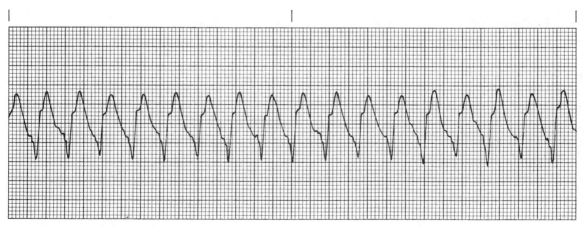

9.4   Regularity: _____
            Rate: _____
            P Waves: _____
            PRI: _____
            QRS: _____
            Interp: _____

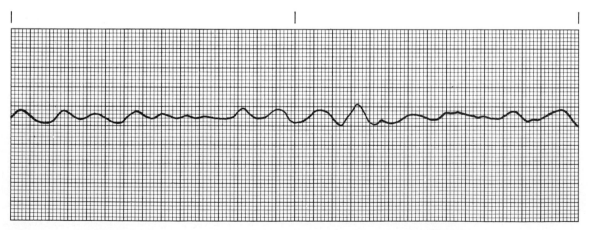

9.5

Regularity: _____

Rate: _____

P Waves: _____

PRI: _____

QRS: _____

Interp: _____

9.6

Regularity: _____

Rate: _____

P Waves: _____

PRI: _____

QRS: _____

Interp: _____

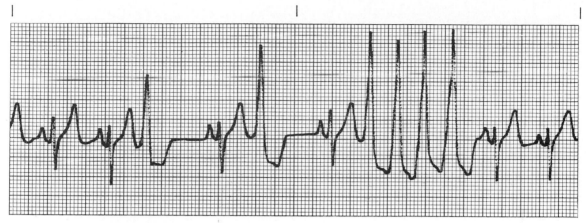

9.7   Regularity: _____
             Rate: _____
             P Waves: _____
             PRI: _____
             QRS: _____
             Interp: _____

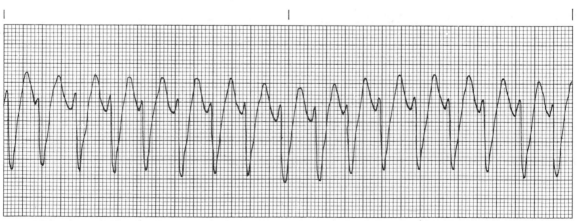

9.8   Regularity: _____
             Rate: _____
             P Waves: _____
             PRI: _____
             QRS: _____
             Interp: _____

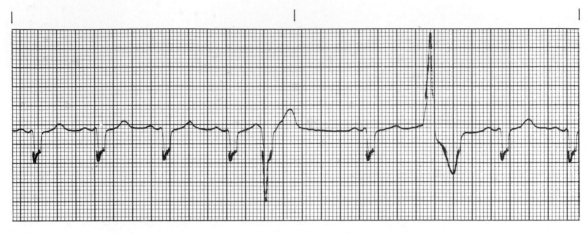

9.9   Regularity: _____
           Rate: _____
           P Waves: _____
           PRI: _____
           QRS: _____
           Interp: _____

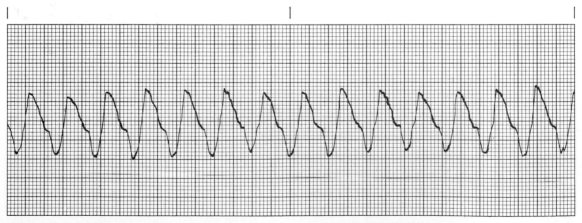

9.10   Regularity: _____
           Rate: _____
           P Waves: _____
           PRI: _____
           QRS: _____
           Interp: _____

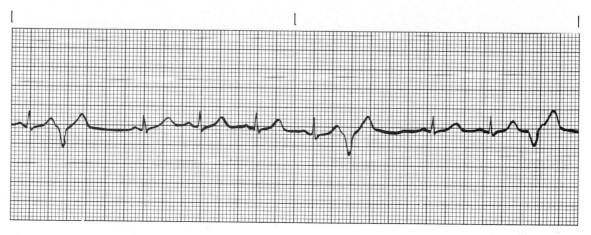

9.11   Regularity: _____
        Rate: _____
        P Waves: _____
        PRI: _____
        QRS: _____
        Interp: _____

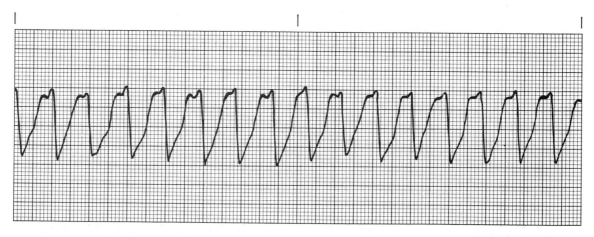

9.12   Regularity: _____
        Rate: _____
        P Waves: _____
        PRI: _____
        QRS: _____
        Interp: _____

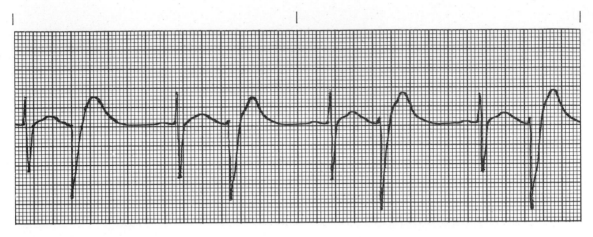

9.13   Regularity: _____
            Rate: _____
            P Waves: _____
            PRI: _____
            QRS: _____
            Interp: _____

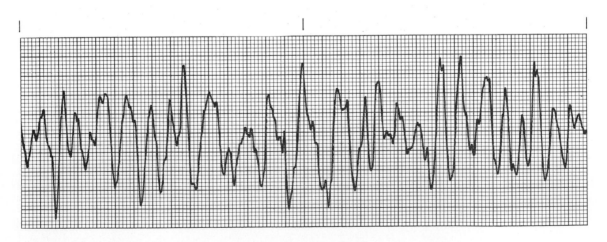

9.14   Regularity: _____
            Rate: _____
            P Waves: _____
            PRI: _____
            QRS: _____
            Interp: _____

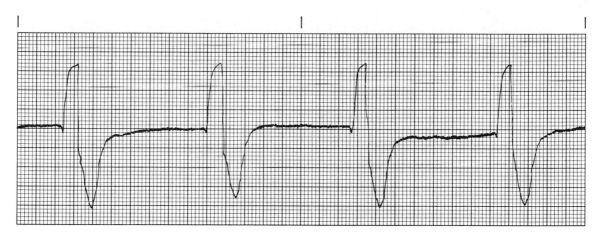

9.15   Regularity: _____
        Rate: _____
        P Waves: _____
        PRI: _____
        QRS: _____
        Interp: _____

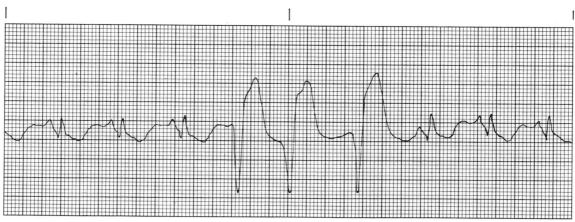

9.16   Regularity: _____
        Rate: _____
        P Waves: _____
        PRI: _____
        QRS: _____
        Interp: _____

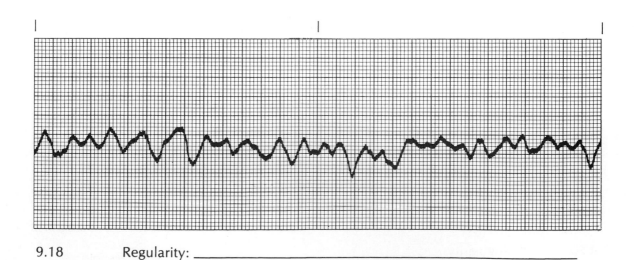

9.17   Regularity: _____
        Rate: _____
        P Waves: _____
        PRI: _____
        QRS: _____
        Interp: _____

9.18   Regularity: _____
        Rate: _____
        P Waves: _____
        PRI: _____
        QRS: _____
        Interp: _____

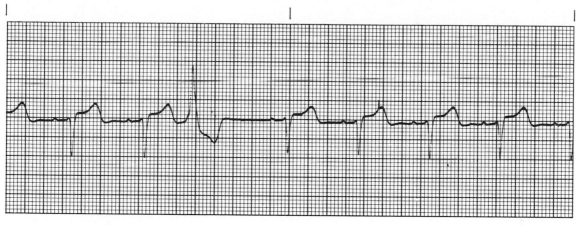

9.19   Regularity: _____

        Rate: _____

        P Waves: _____

        PRI: _____

        QRS: _____

        Interp: _____

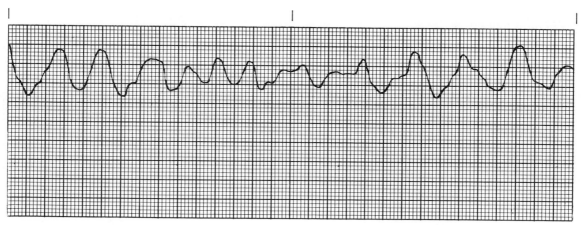

9.20   Regularity: _____

        Rate: _____

        P Waves: _____

        PRI: _____

        QRS: _____

        Interp: _____

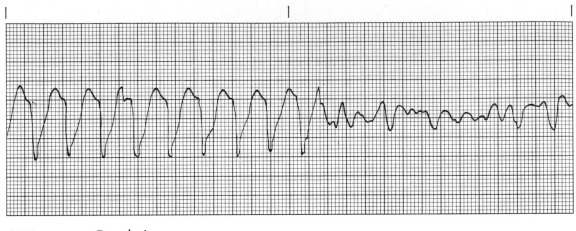

9.21   Regularity: _____
        Rate: _____
        P Waves: _____
        PRI: _____
        QRS: _____
        Interp: _____

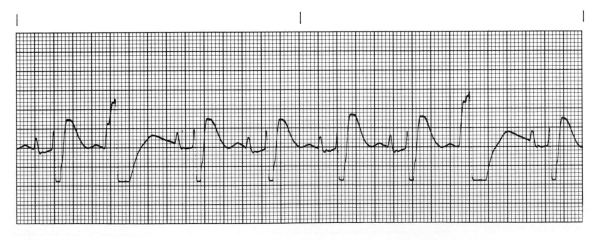

9.22   Regularity: _____
        Rate: _____
        P Waves: _____
        PRI: _____
        QRS: _____
        Interp: _____

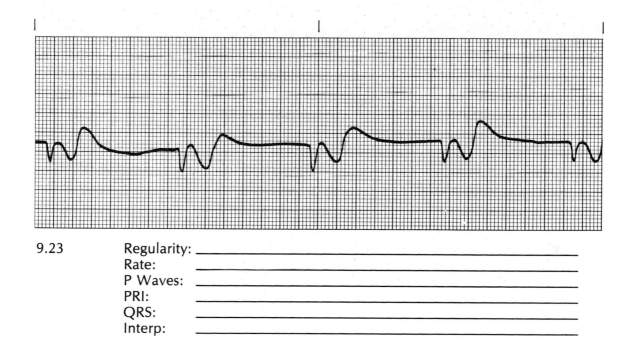

9.23   Regularity: _____
        Rate: _____
        P Waves: _____
        PRI: _____
        QRS: _____
        Interp: _____

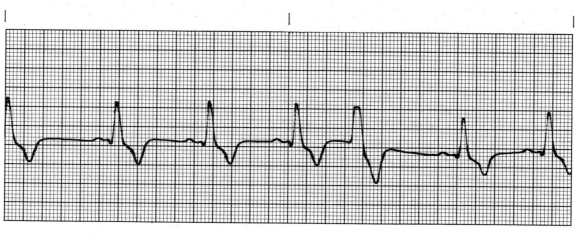

9.24   Regularity: _____
        Rate: _____
        P Waves: _____
        PRI: _____
        QRS: _____
        Interp: _____

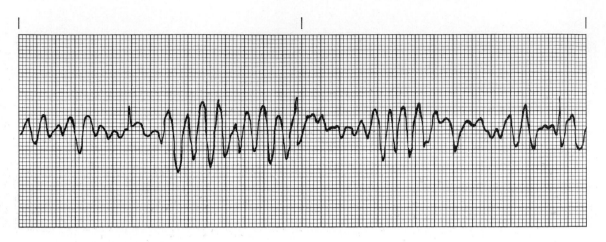

9.25   Regularity: _____
            Rate: _____
            P Waves: _____
            PRI: _____
            QRS: _____
            Interp: _____

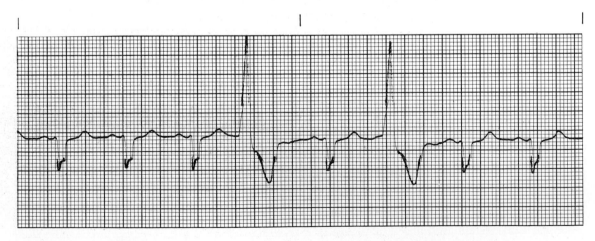

9.26   Regularity: _____
            Rate: _____
            P Waves: _____
            PRI: _____
            QRS: _____
            Interp: _____

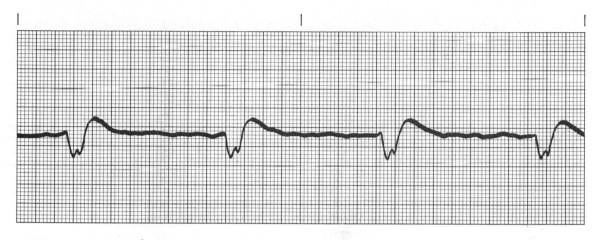

9.27   Regularity: _____
        Rate: _____
        P Waves: _____
        PRI: _____
        QRS: _____
        Interp: _____

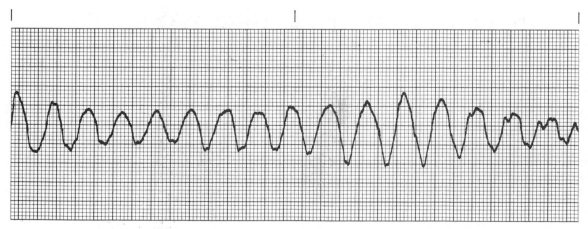

9.28   Regularity: _____
        Rate: _____
        P Waves: _____
        PRI: _____
        QRS: _____
        Interp: _____

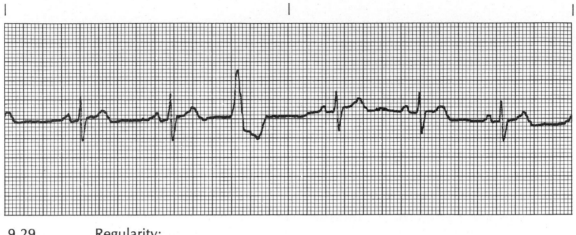

9.29   Regularity: _____

Rate: _____

P Waves: _____

PRI: _____

QRS: _____

Interp: _____

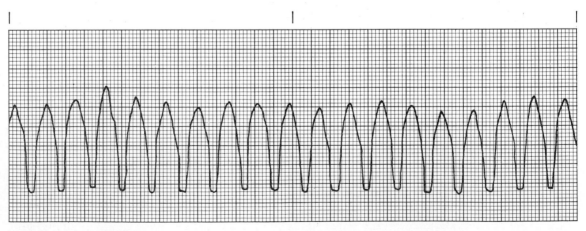

9.30   Regularity: _____

Rate: _____

P Waves: _____

PRI: _____

QRS: _____

Interp: _____

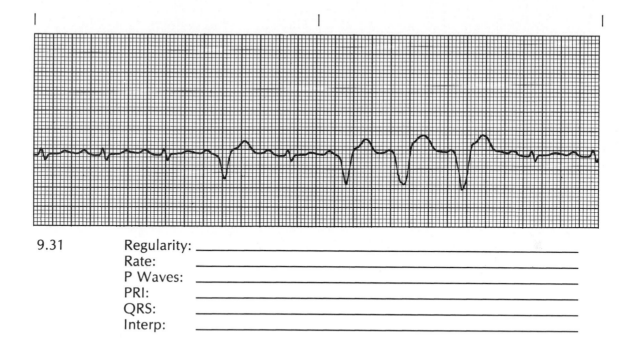

9.31   Regularity: _____
            Rate: _____
            P Waves: _____
            PRI: _____
            QRS: _____
            Interp: _____

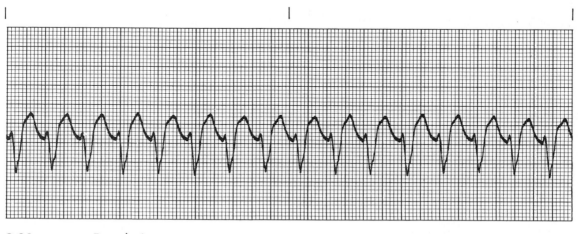

9.32   Regularity: _____
            Rate: _____
            P Waves: _____
            PRI: _____
            QRS: _____
            Interp: _____

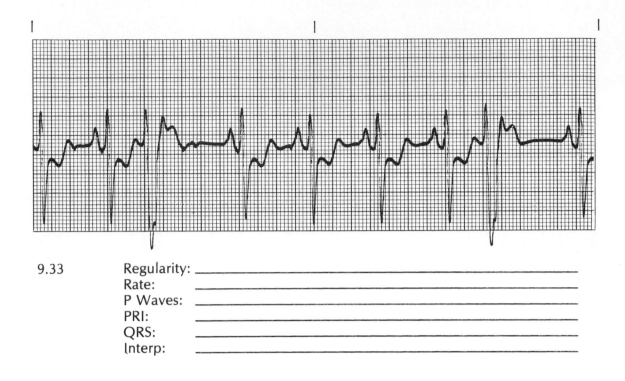

9.33   Regularity: _____
            Rate: _____
            P Waves: _____
            PRI: _____
            QRS: _____
            Interp: _____

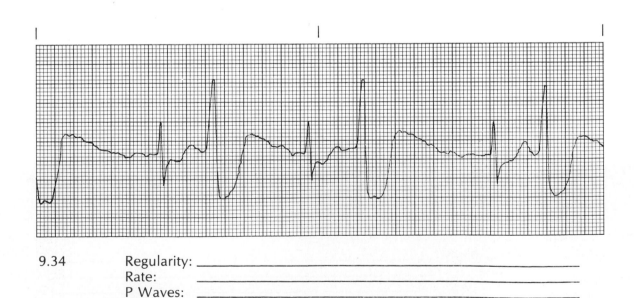

9.34   Regularity: _____
            Rate: _____
            P Waves: _____
            PRI: _____
            QRS: _____
            Interp: _____

9

Practice Makes Perfect

In this program you learned the basic principles of arrhythmia interpretation. You also learned the rules for 22 of the most common arrhythmias. This book has provided you with a format for analyzing any arrhythmia so that you can compare it to the rules and identify it. The format directs you to systematically inspect the regularity, rate, P waves, PR intervals, and QRS complexes, and to use all of that data to help you identify the arrhythmia.

As you practice on more and more rhythm strips, you will develop your interpretation skill. The more you practice, the easier this process will become, and you will find that you are conducting many of the format steps without really thinking about them. It will become almost second nature to you. At that point, you might begin to think that the format is no longer useful, or that it no longer applies. In actual fact, you have simply learned to perform the process quickly. The important issue is that you know the format, and if you ever need to interpret a very complex arrhythmia, you can always revert to the 5-step process. Once you are comfortable using this format, it will always be available to help you identify even the most intimidating arrhythmia.

For you to be truly comfortable in arrhythmia identification, you must practice, practice, practice! That's what this chapter is for. As you go through the practice strips, remember the analysis format, even if you only use it mentally most of the time. When you check your answers with the key, look to see how the answers were reached. If you repeatedly make errors in the same area, go back to the related chapter and review the key points. If possible, have an instructor or other knowledgeable person assist you.

This book was designed to provide you with a solid foundation of knowledge and skill in arrhythmia interpretation. As you complete the program you should be very capable of recognizing and understanding the most common uncomplicated arrhythmias. But this is only the tip of the iceberg in the field of electrocardiography. If you are interested in continuing to learn more about this field, you can add to the core of information you already have by attending higher level EKG classes, reading the many books that are available, or talking to people who work with EKGs every day. This is a fascinating area of study. Researchers are discovering new things daily that add to our understanding of electrocardiography. The most difficult step in the learning process is the very first phase of learning the basics, and now you have completed that phase. Now there is nothing to prevent you from becoming an expert in this field. Nothing but practice, that is. And practice begins here.

Practice Sheet 10:
General Practice

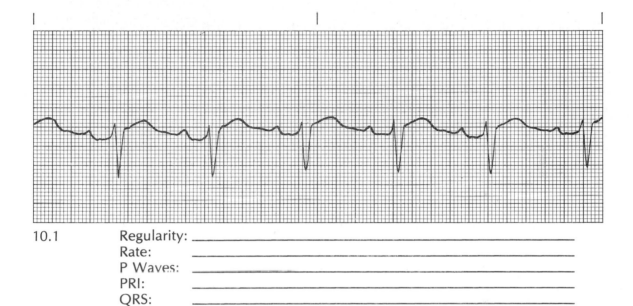

10.1   Regularity: _____
        Rate: _____
        P Waves: _____
        PRI: _____
        QRS: _____
        Interp: _____

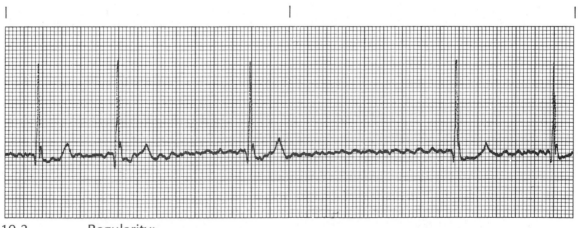

10.2   Regularity: _____
        Rate: _____
        P Waves: _____
        PRI: _____
        QRS: _____
        Interp: _____

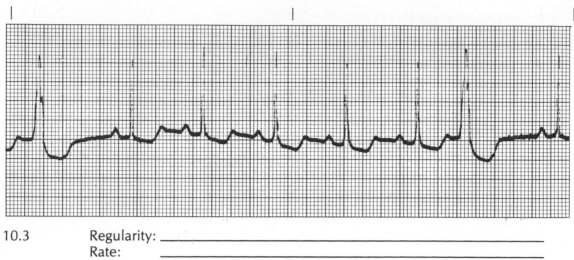

10.3   Regularity: _____
            Rate: _____
            P Waves: _____
            PRI: _____
            QRS: _____
            Interp: _____

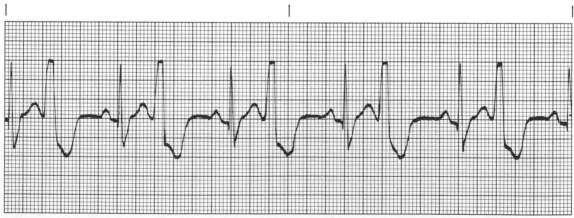

10.4   Regularity: _____
            Rate: _____
            P Waves: _____
            PRI: _____
            QRS: _____
            Interp: _____

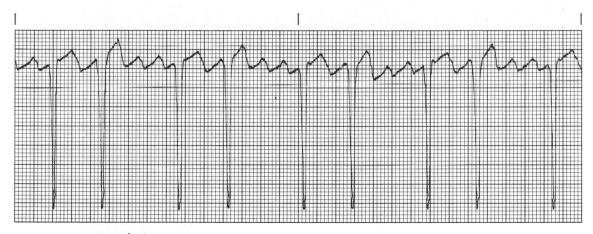

10.5   Regularity: _____
              Rate: _____
              P Waves: _____
              PRI: _____
              QRS: _____
              Interp: _____

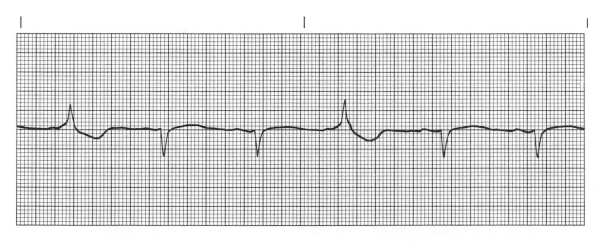

10.6   Regularity: _____
              Rate: _____
              P Waves: _____
              PRI: _____
              QRS: _____
              Interp: _____

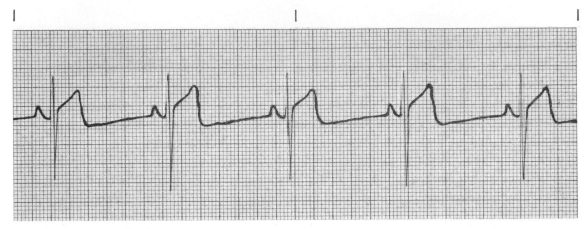

10.7   Regularity: _____
            Rate: _____
            P Waves: _____
            PRI: _____
            QRS: _____
            Interp: _____

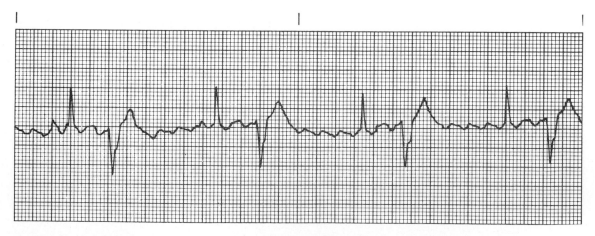

10.8   Regularity: _____
            Rate: _____
            P Waves: _____
            PRI: _____
            QRS: _____
            Interp: _____

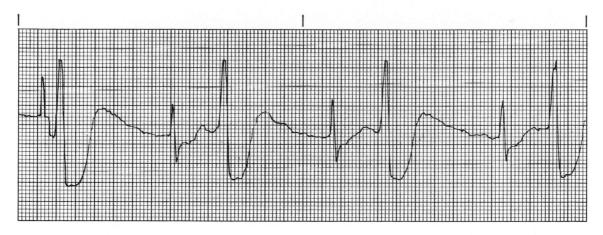

10.9   Regularity: _____
            Rate: _____
            P Waves: _____
            PRI: _____
            QRS: _____
            Interp: _____

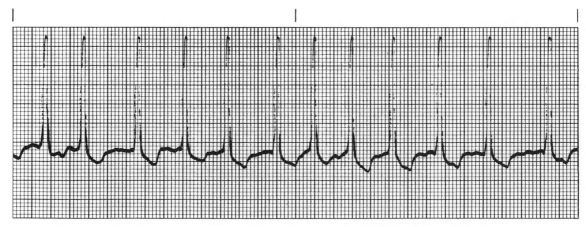

10.10   Regularity: _____
            Rate: _____
            P Waves: _____
            PRI: _____
            QRS: _____
            Interp: _____

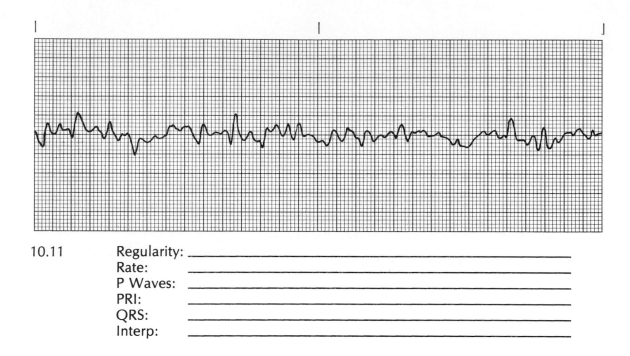

10.11   Regularity: _____
             Rate: _____
             P Waves: _____
             PRI: _____
             QRS: _____
             Interp: _____

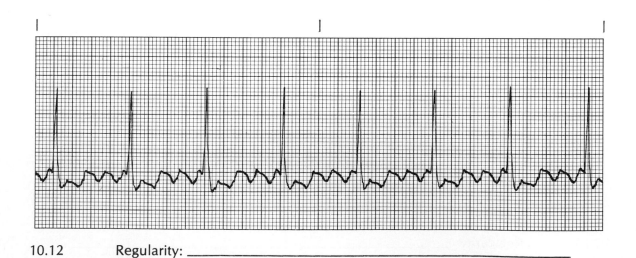

10.12   Regularity: _____
             Rate: _____
             P Waves: _____
             PRI: _____
             QRS: _____
             Interp: _____

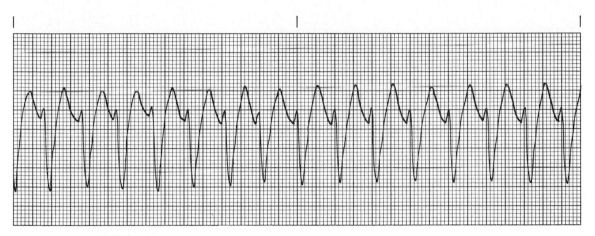

10.13   Regularity: _____
       Rate: _____
       P Waves: _____
       PRI: _____
       QRS: _____
       Interp: _____

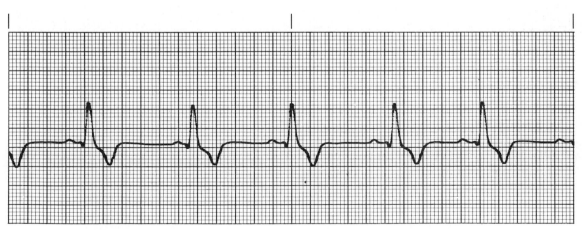

10.14   Regularity: _____
       Rate: _____
       P Waves: _____
       PRI: _____
       QRS: _____
       Interp: _____

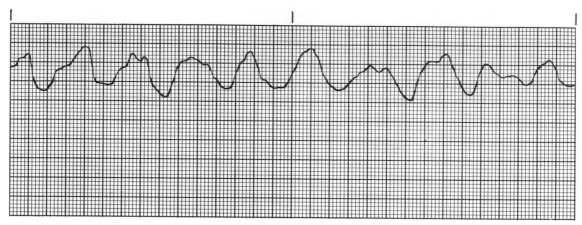

10.15   Regularity: _____
             Rate: _____
             P Waves: _____
             PRI: _____
             QRS: _____
             Interp: _____

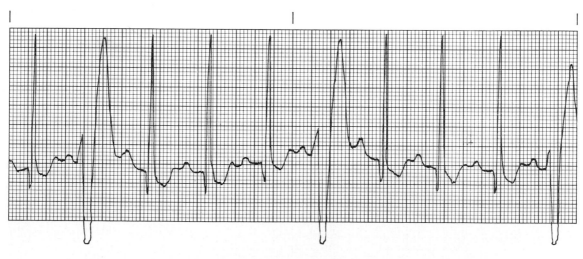

10.16   Regularity: _____
             Rate: _____
             P Waves: _____
             PRI: _____
             QRS: _____
             Interp: _____

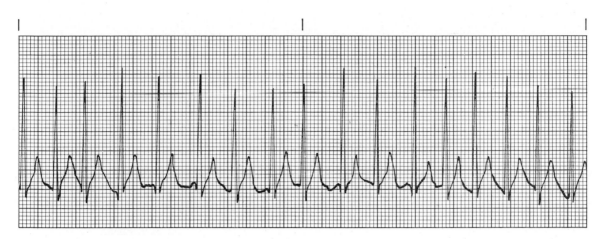

10.17   Regularity: _____
         Rate: _____
         P Waves: _____
         PRI: _____
         QRS: _____
         Interp: _____

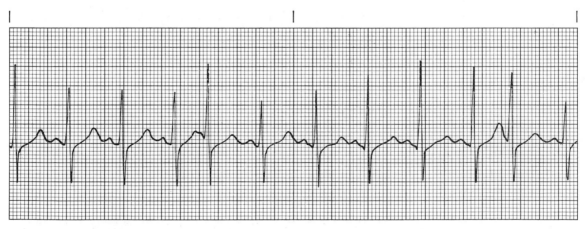

10.18   Regularity: _____
         Rate: _____
         P Waves: _____
         PRI: _____
         QRS: _____
         Interp: _____

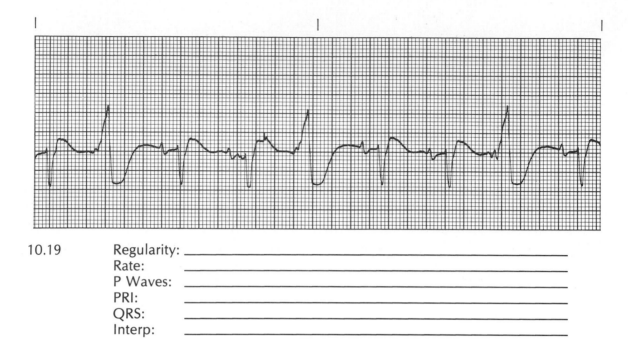

10.19   Regularity: _____
             Rate: _____
             P Waves: _____
             PRI: _____
             QRS: _____
             Interp: _____

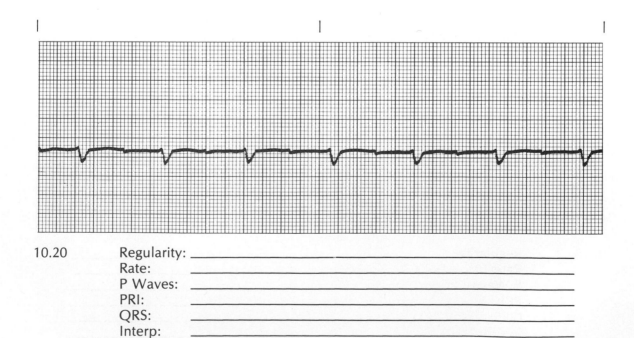

10.20   Regularity: _____
             Rate: _____
             P Waves: _____
             PRI: _____
             QRS: _____
             Interp: _____

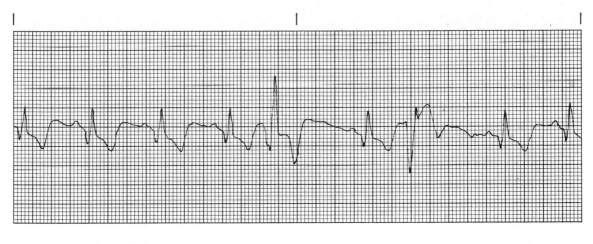

10.21   Regularity: _____
          Rate: _____
          P Waves: _____
          PRI: _____
          QRS: _____
          Interp: _____

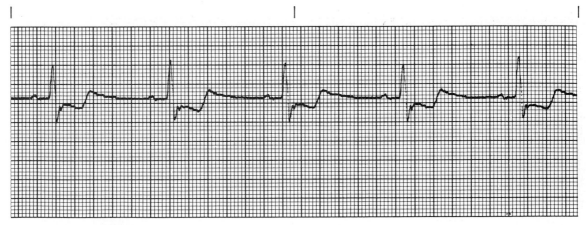

10.22   Regularity: _____
          Rate: _____
          P Waves: _____
          PRI: _____
          QRS: _____
          Interp: _____

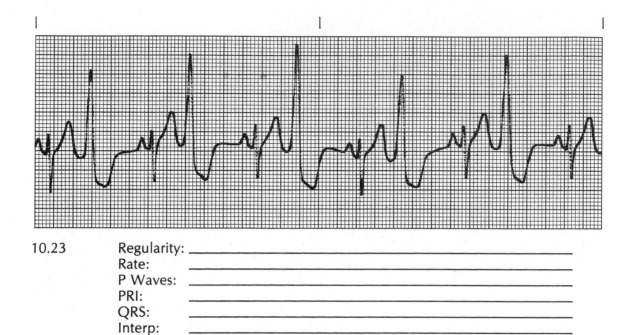

10.23   Regularity: _____
          Rate: _____
          P Waves: _____
          PRI: _____
          QRS: _____
          Interp: _____

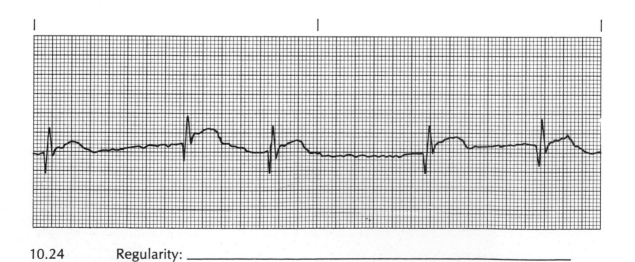

10.24   Regularity: _____
          Rate: _____
          P Waves: _____
          PRI: _____
          QRS: _____
          Interp: _____

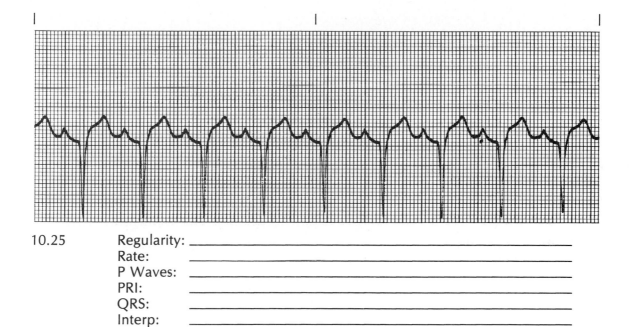

10.25   Regularity: _____
             Rate: _____
             P Waves: _____
             PRI: _____
             QRS: _____
             Interp: _____

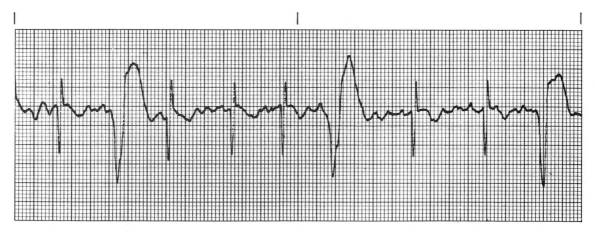

10.26   Regularity: _____
             Rate: _____
             P Waves: _____
             PRI: _____
             QRS: _____
             Interp: _____

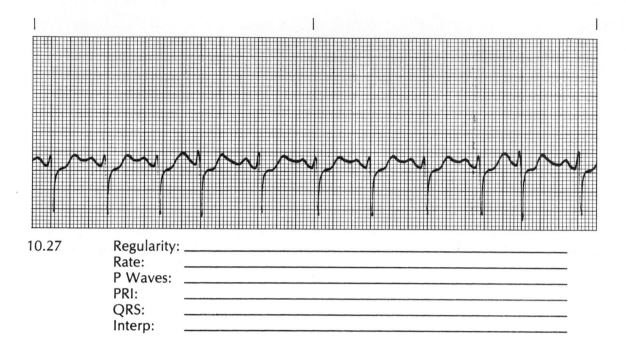

10.27   Regularity: _____

Rate: _____

P Waves: _____

PRI: _____

QRS: _____

Interp: _____

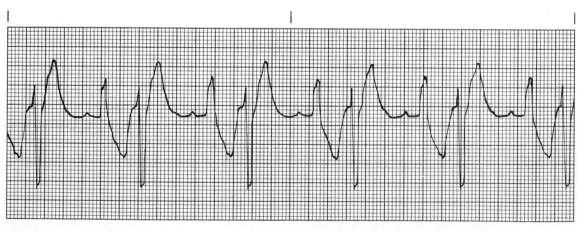

10.28   Regularity: _____

Rate: _____

P Waves: _____

PRI: _____

QRS: _____

Interp: _____

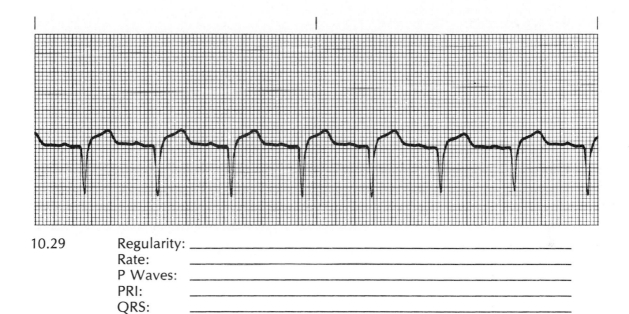

10.29   Regularity: _____
             Rate: _____
             P Waves: _____
             PRI: _____
             QRS: _____
             Interp: _____

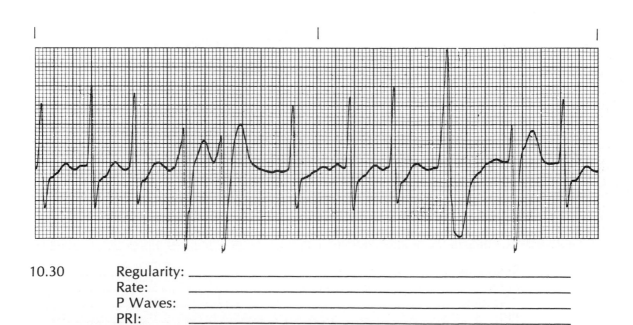

10.30   Regularity: _____
             Rate: _____
             P Waves: _____
             PRI: _____
             QRS: _____
             Interp: _____

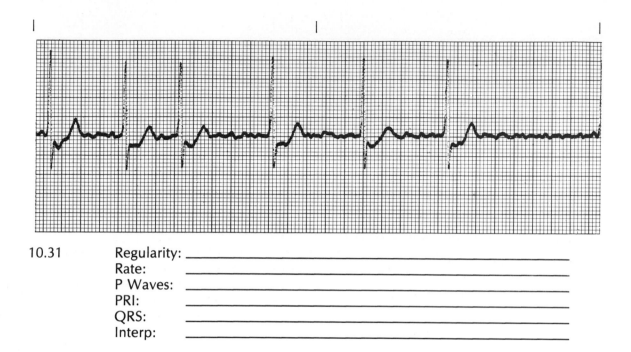

10.31   Regularity: _____
          Rate: _____
          P Waves: _____
          PRI: _____
          QRS: _____
          Interp: _____

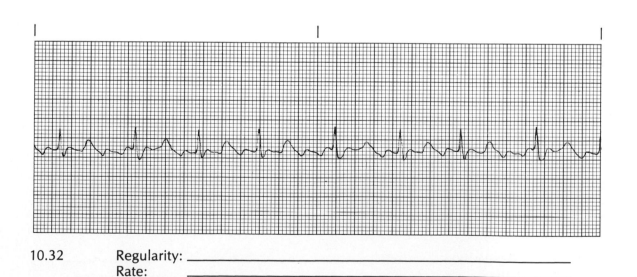

10.32   Regularity: _____
          Rate: _____
          P Waves: _____
          PRI: _____
          QRS: _____
          Interp: _____

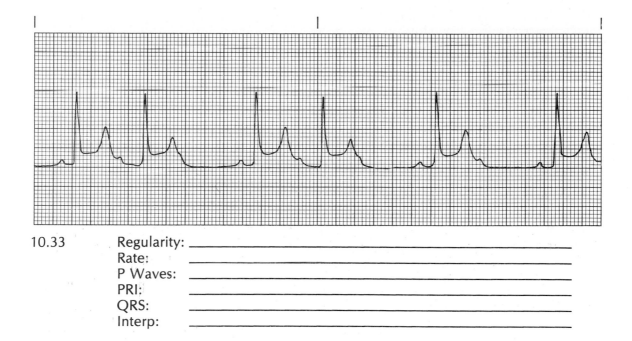

10.33   Regularity: _____
         Rate: _____
         P Waves: _____
         PRI: _____
         QRS: _____
         Interp: _____

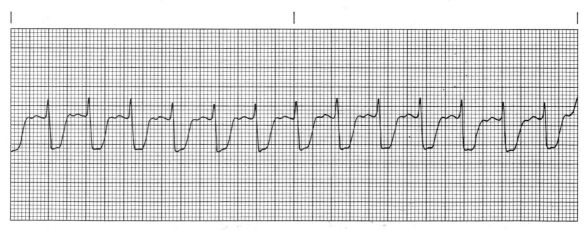

10.34   Regularity: _____
         Rate: _____
         P Waves: _____
         PRI: _____
         QRS: _____
         Interp: _____

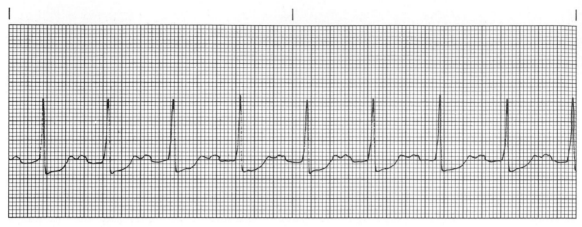

10.35   Regularity: _____
             Rate: _____
             P Waves: _____
             PRI: _____
             QRS: _____
             Interp: _____

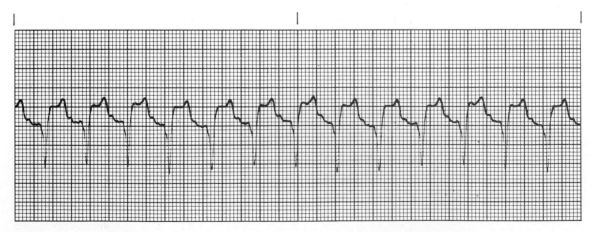

10.36   Regularity: _____
             Rate: _____
             P Waves: _____
             PRI: _____
             QRS: _____
             Interp: _____

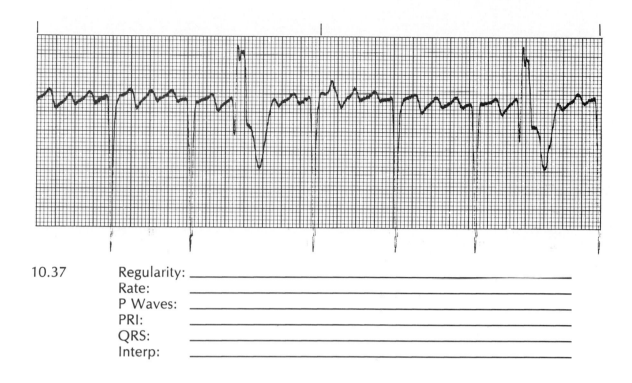

10.37   Regularity: _____
                Rate: _____
                P Waves: _____
                PRI: _____
                QRS: _____
                Interp: _____

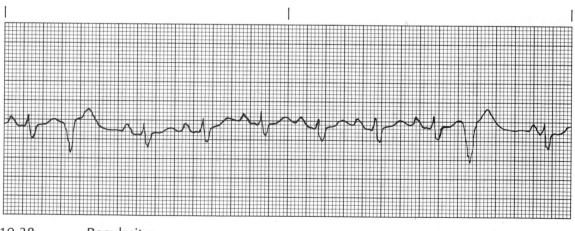

10.38   Regularity: _____
                Rate: _____
                P Waves: _____
                PRI: _____
                QRS: _____
                Interp: _____

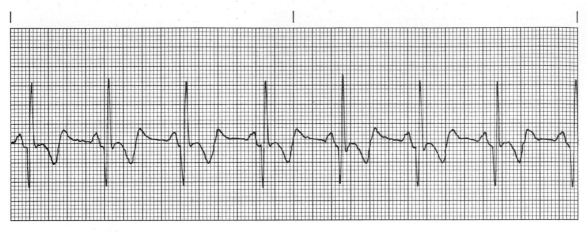

10.39   Regularity: _____
         Rate: _____
         P Waves: _____
         PRI: _____
         QRS: _____
         Interp: _____

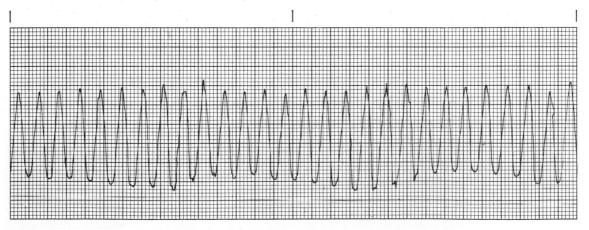

10.40   Regularity: _____
         Rate: _____
         P Waves: _____
         PRI: _____
         QRS: _____
         Interp: _____

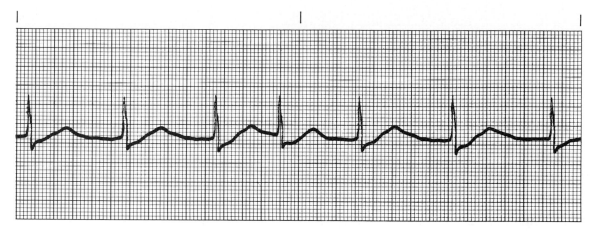

10.41   Regularity: _____
             Rate: _____
             P Waves: _____
             PRI: _____
             QRS: _____
             Interp: _____

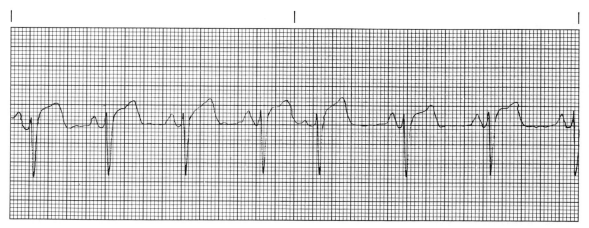

10.42   Regularity: _____
             Rate: _____
             P Waves: _____
             PRI: _____
             QRS: _____
             Interp: _____

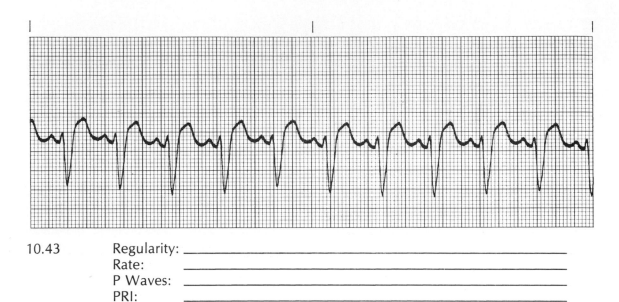

10.43   Regularity: _____
           Rate: _____
           P Waves: _____
           PRI: _____
           QRS: _____
           Interp: _____

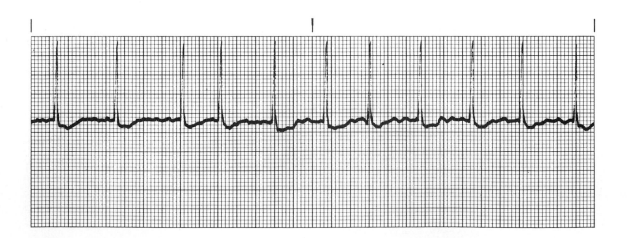

10.44   Regularity: _____
           Rate: _____
           P Waves: _____
           PRI: _____
           QRS: _____
           Interp: _____

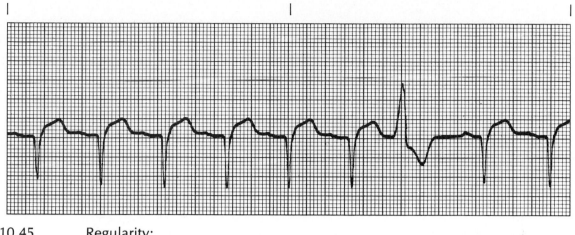

10.45   Regularity: _____
          Rate: _____
          P Waves: _____
          PRI: _____
          QRS: _____
          Interp: _____

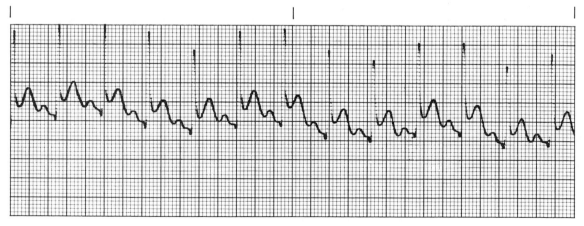

10.46   Regularity: _____
          Rate: _____
          P Waves: _____
          PRI: _____
          QRS: _____
          Interp: _____

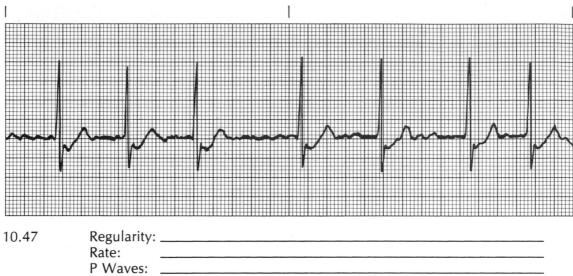

10.47   Regularity: _____
         Rate: _____
         P Waves: _____
         PRI: _____
         QRS: _____
         Interp: _____

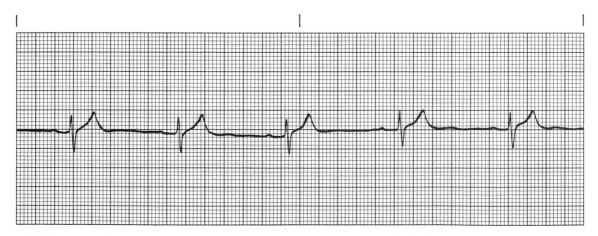

10.48   Regularity: _____
         Rate: _____
         P Waves: _____
         PRI: _____
         QRS: _____
         Interp: _____

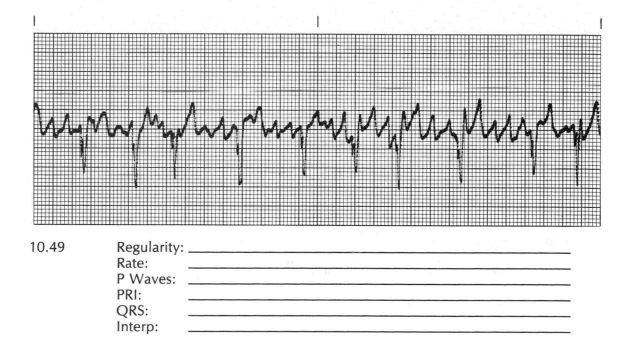

10.49   Regularity: _____
             Rate: _____
             P Waves: _____
             PRI: _____
             QRS: _____
             Interp: _____

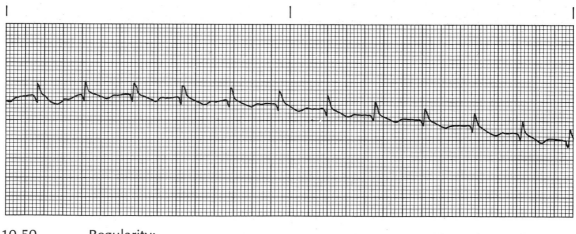

10.50   Regularity: _____
             Rate: _____
             P Waves: _____
             PRI: _____
             QRS: _____
             Interp: _____

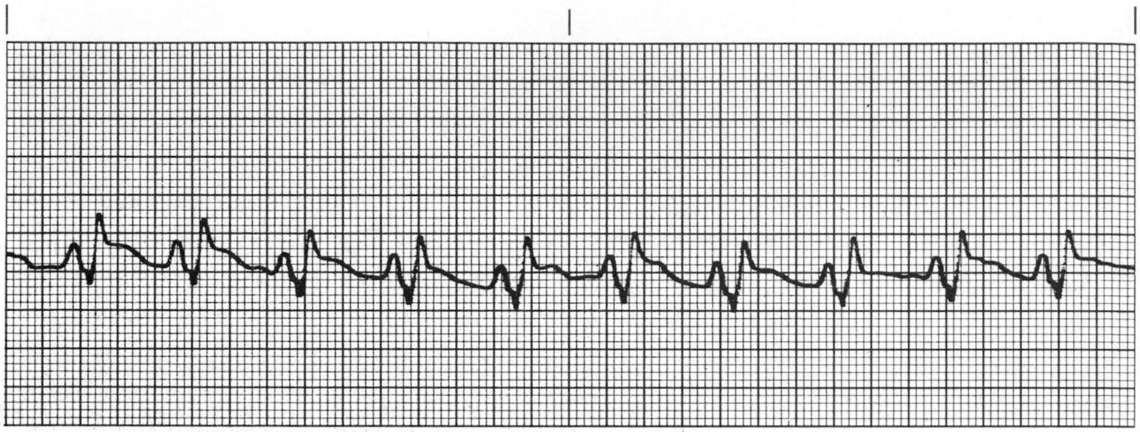

10.51   Regularity: _____
         Rate: _____
         P Waves: _____
         PRI: _____
         QRS: _____
         Interp: _____

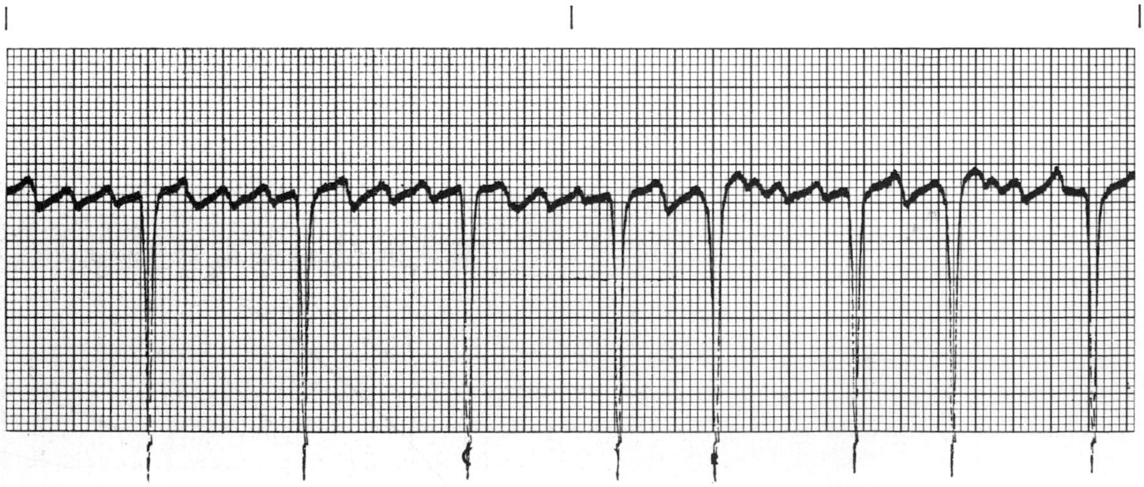

10.52   Regularity: _____
         Rate: _____
         P Waves: _____
         PRI: _____
         QRS: _____
         Interp: _____

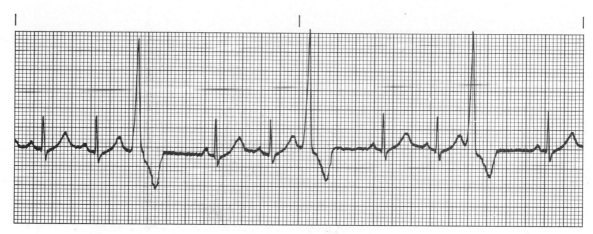

10.53   Regularity: _____
         Rate: _____
         P Waves: _____
         PRI: _____
         QRS: _____
         Interp: _____

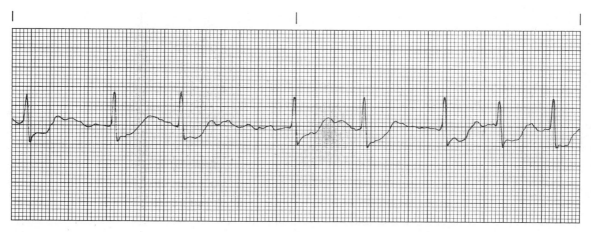

10.54   Regularity: _____
         Rate: _____
         P Waves: _____
         PRI: _____
         QRS: · _____
         Interp: _____

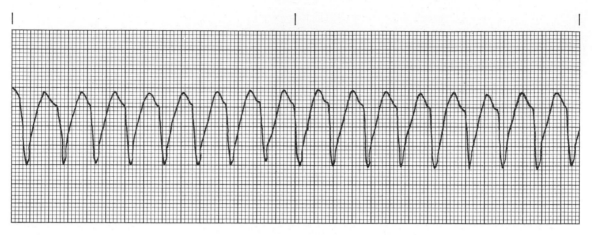

10.55   Regularity: _____
         Rate: _____
         P Waves: _____
         PRI: _____
         QRS: _____
         Interp: _____

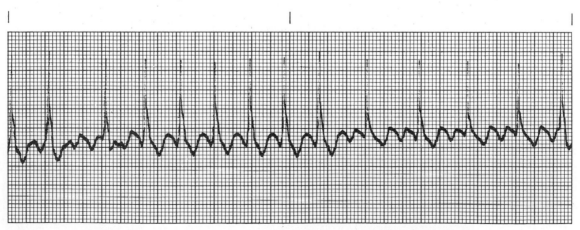

10.56   Regularity: _____
         Rate: _____
         P Waves: _____
         PRI: _____
         QRS: _____
         Interp: _____

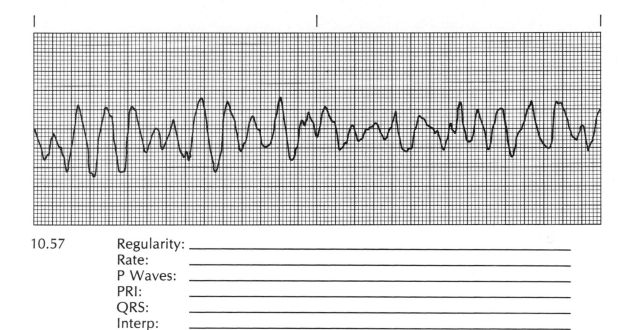

10.57   Regularity: _____
         Rate: _____
         P Waves: _____
         PRI: _____
         QRS: _____
         Interp: _____

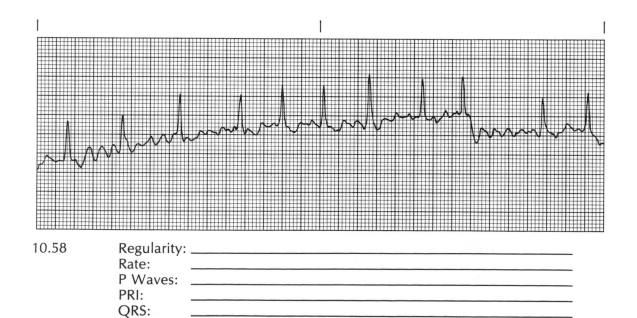

10.58   Regularity: _____
         Rate: _____
         P Waves: _____
         PRI: _____
         QRS: _____
         Interp: _____

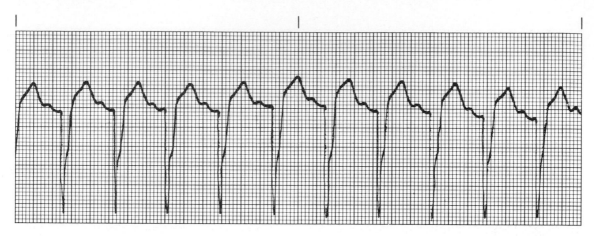

10.59   Regularity: _____
                 Rate: _____
                 P Waves: _____
                 PRI: _____
                 QRS: _____
                 Interp: _____

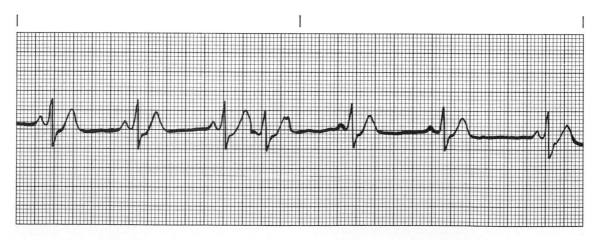

10.60   Regularity: _____
                 Rate: _____
                 P Waves: _____
                 PRI: _____
                 QRS: _____
                 Interp: _____

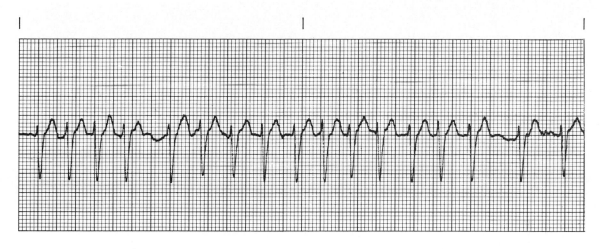

10.61   Regularity: _____
         Rate: _____
         P Waves: _____
         PRI: _____
         QRS: _____
         Interp: _____

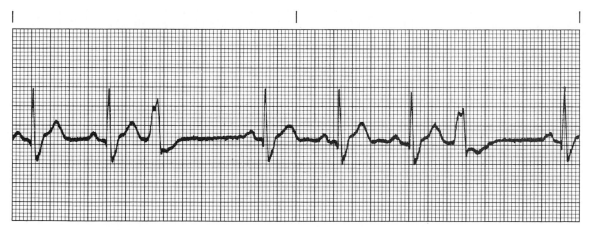

10.62   Regularity: _____
         Rate: _____
         P Waves: _____
         PRI: _____
         QRS: _____
         Interp: _____

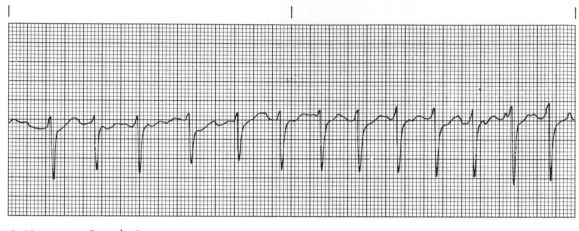

10.63   Regularity: _____
         Rate: _____
         P Waves: _____
         PRI: _____
         QRS: _____
         Interp: _____

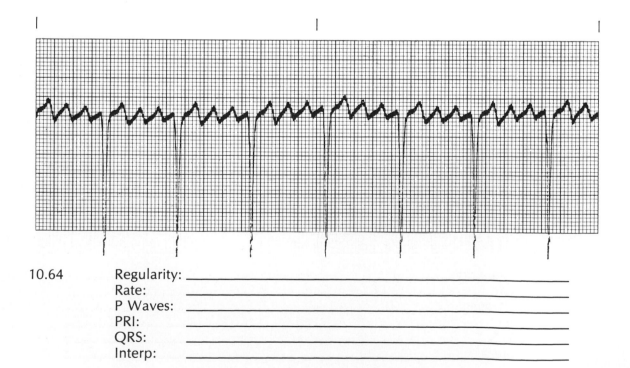

10.64   Regularity: _____
         Rate: _____
         P Waves: _____
         PRI: _____
         QRS: _____
         Interp: _____

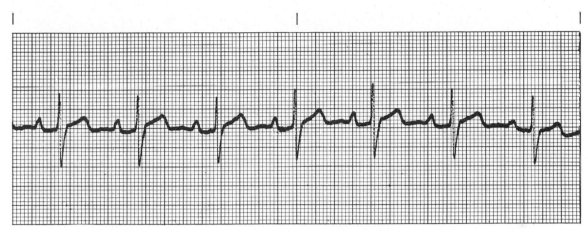

10.65   Regularity: _____
             Rate: _____
             P Waves: _____
             PRI: _____
             QRS: _____
             Interp: _____

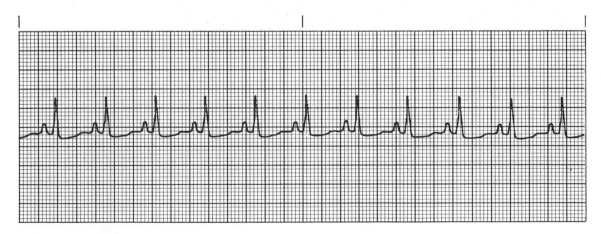

10.66   Regularity: _____
             Rate: _____
             P Waves: _____
             PRI: _____
             QRS: _____
             Interp: _____

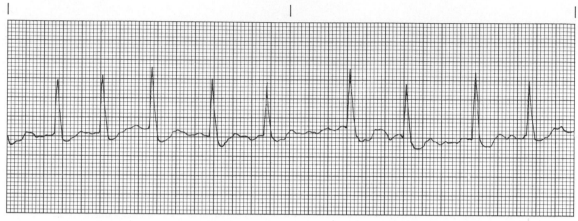

10.67   Regularity: _____

Rate: _____

P Waves: _____

PRI: _____

QRS: _____

Interp: _____

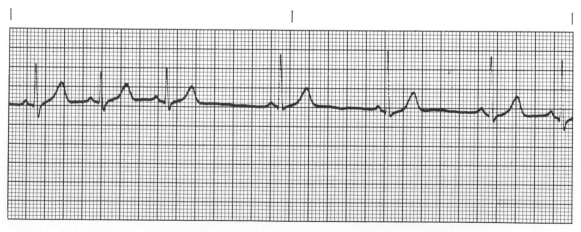

10.68   Regularity: _____

Rate: _____

P Waves: _____

PRI: _____

QRS: _____

Interp: _____

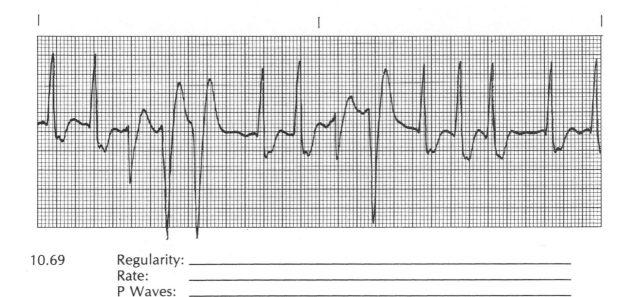

10.69   Regularity: _____
         Rate: _____
         P Waves: _____
         PRI: _____
         QRS: _____
         Interp: _____

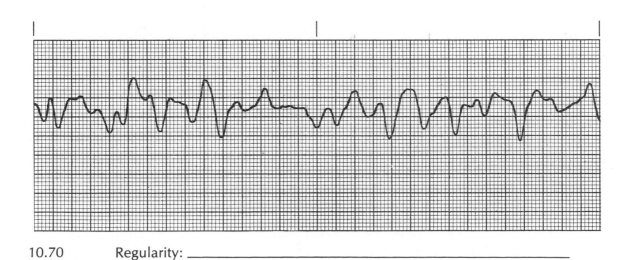

10.70   Regularity: _____
         Rate: _____
         P Waves: _____
         PRI: _____
         QRS: _____
         Interp: _____

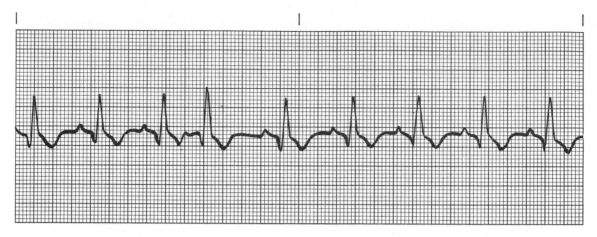

10.71   Regularity: _____
         Rate: _____
         P Waves: _____
         PRI: _____
         QRS: _____
         Interp: _____

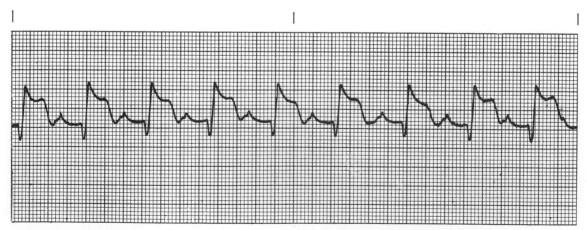

10.72   Regularity: _____
         Rate: _____
         P Waves: _____
         PRI: _____
         QRS: _____
         Interp: _____

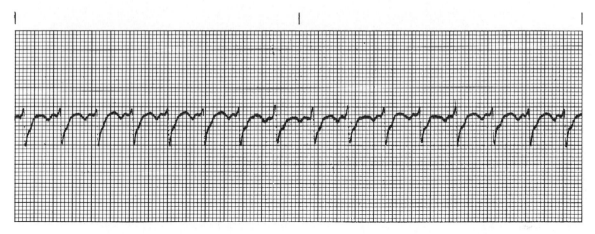

10.73   Regularity: _____

              Rate: _____

              P Waves: _____

              PRI: _____

              QRS: _____

              Interp: _____

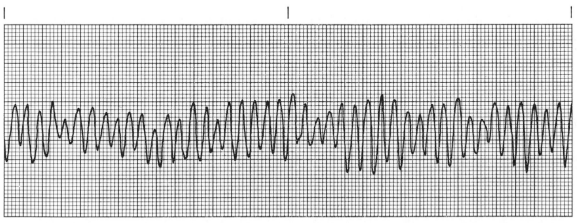

10.74   Regularity: _____

              Rate: _____

              P Waves: _____

              PRI: _____

              QRS: _____

              Interp: _____

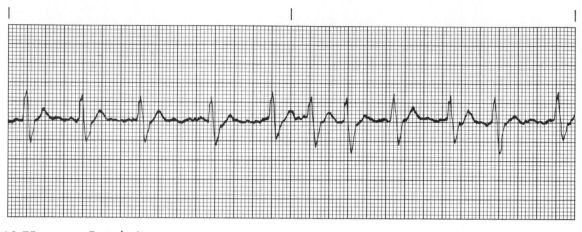

10.75   Regularity: _____
        Rate: _____
        P Waves: _____
        PRI: _____
        QRS: _____
        Interp: _____

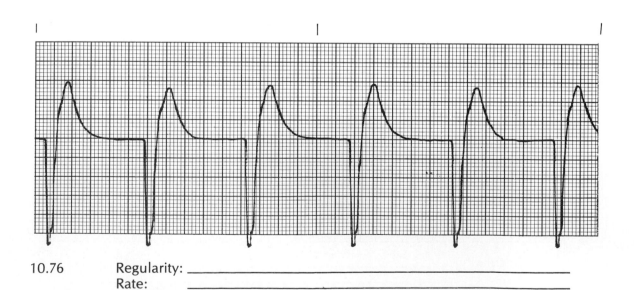

10.76   Regularity: _____
        Rate: _____
        P Waves: _____
        PRI: _____
        QRS: _____
        Interp: _____

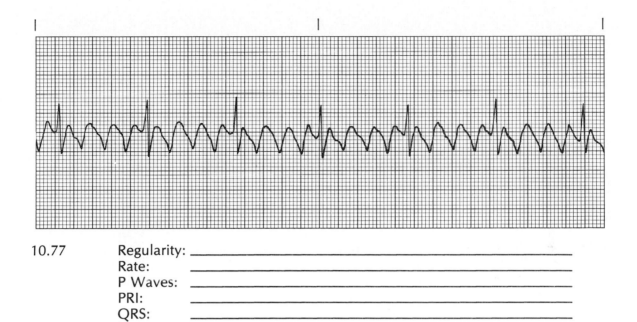

10.77   Regularity: _____

Rate: _____

P Waves: _____

PRI: _____

QRS: _____

Interp: _____

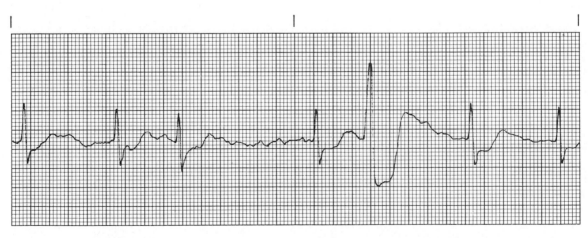

10.78   Regularity: _____

Rate: _____

P Waves: _____

PRI: _____

QRS: _____

Interp: _____

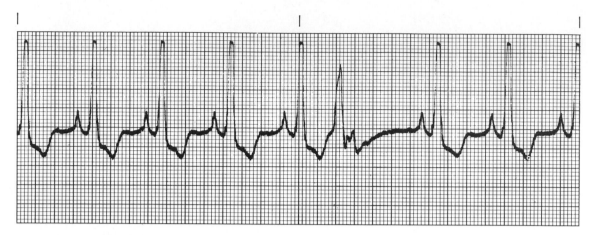

10.79   Regularity: _____
         Rate: _____
         P Waves: _____
         PRI: _____
         QRS: _____
         Interp: _____

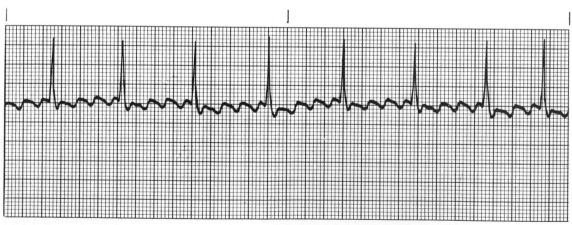

10.80   Regularity: _____
         Rate: _____
         P Waves: _____
         PRI: _____
         QRS: _____
         Interp: _____

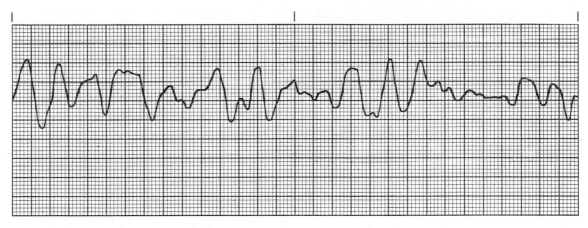

10.81   Regularity: _____
             Rate: _____
             P Waves: _____
             PRI: _____
             QRS: _____
             Interp: _____

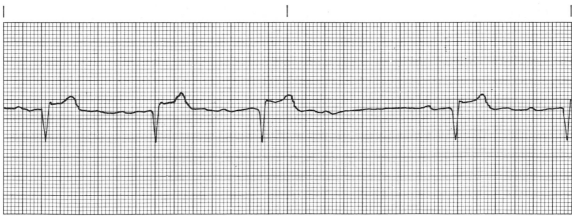

10.82   Regularity: _____
             Rate: _____
             P Waves: _____
             PRI: _____
             QRS: _____
             Interp: _____

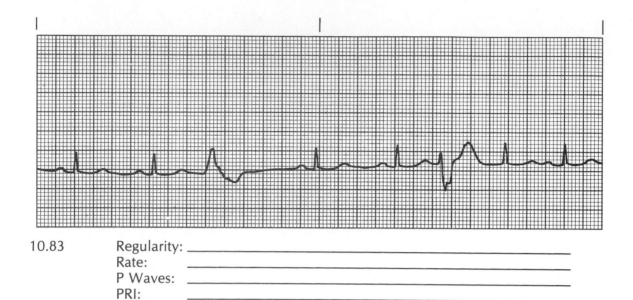

10.83   Regularity: _____
          Rate: _____
          P Waves: _____
          PRI: _____
          QRS: _____
          Interp: _____

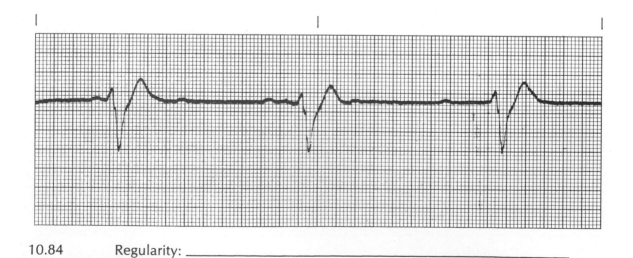

10.84   Regularity: _____
          Rate: _____
          P Waves: _____
          PRI: _____
          QRS: _____
          Interp: _____

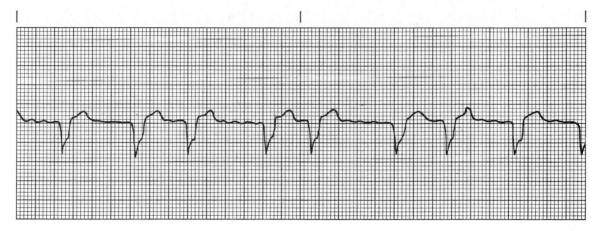

10.85   Regularity: _____
         Rate: _____
         P Waves: _____
         PRI: _____
         QRS: _____
         Interp: _____

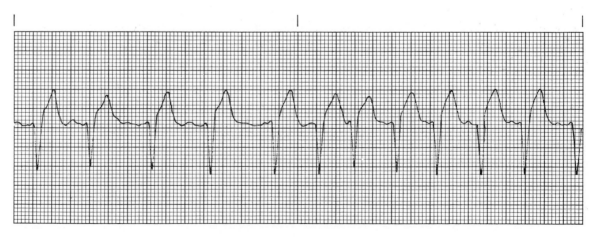

10.86   Regularity: _____
         Rate: _____
         P Waves: _____
         PRI: _____
         QRS: _____
         Interp: _____

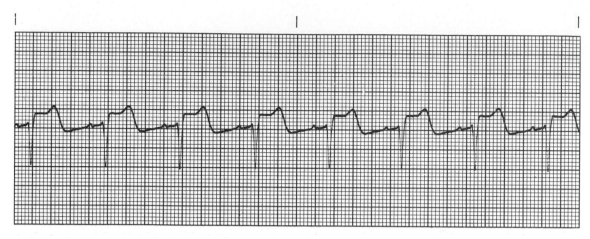

10.87   Regularity: _____

           Rate: _____

           P Waves: _____

           PRI: _____

           QRS: _____

           Interp: _____

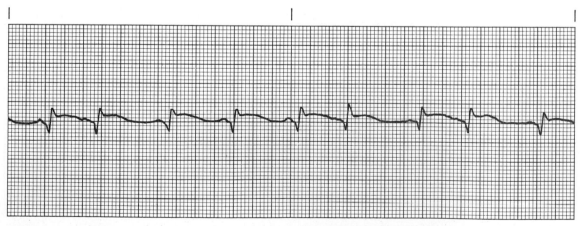

10.88   Regularity: _____

           Rate: _____

           P Waves: _____

           PRI: _____

           QRS: _____

           Interp: _____

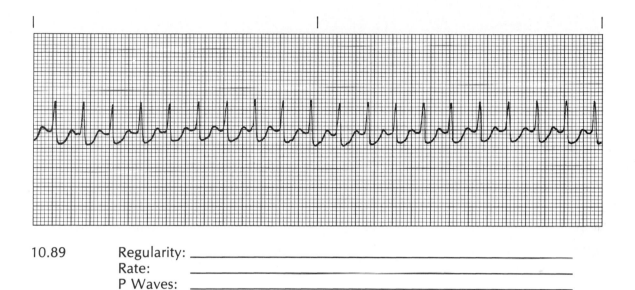

10.89   Regularity: _____
         Rate: _____
         P Waves: _____
         PRI: _____
         QRS: _____
         Interp: _____

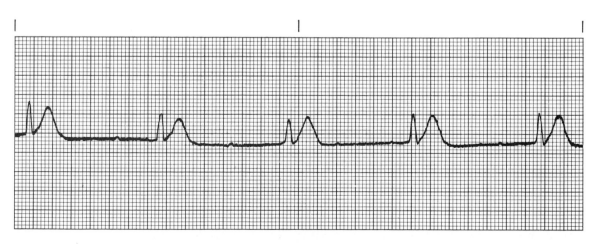

10.90   Regularity: _____
         Rate: _____
         P Waves: _____
         PRI: _____
         QRS: _____
         Interp: _____

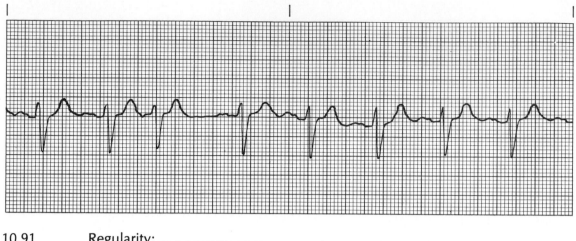

10.91   Regularity: _____
             Rate: _____
             P Waves: _____
             PRI: _____
             QRS: _____
             Interp: _____

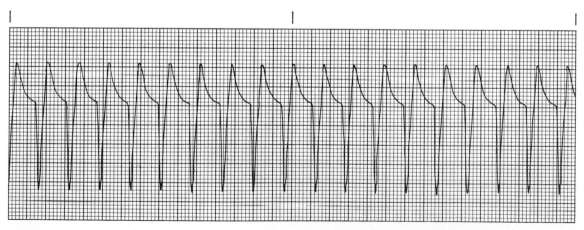

10.92   Regularity: _____
             Rate: _____
             P Waves: _____
             PRI: _____
             QRS: _____
             Interp: _____

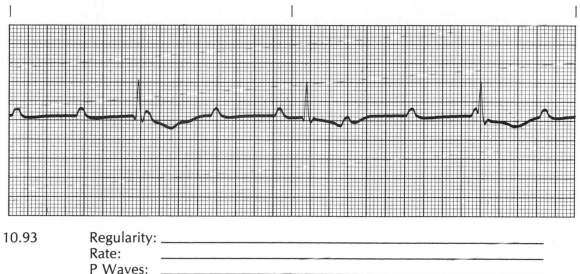

10.93   Regularity: _____
         Rate: _____
         P Waves: _____
         PRI: _____
         QRS: _____
         Interp: _____

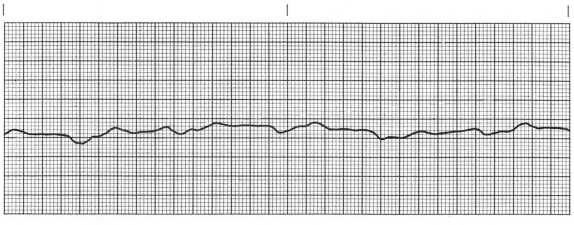

10.94   Regularity: _____
         Rate: _____
         P Waves: _____
         PRI: _____
         QRS: _____
         Interp: _____

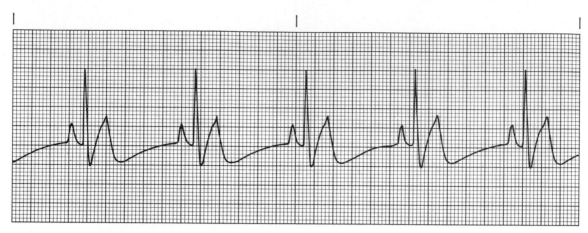

10.95   Regularity: _____
             Rate: _____
             P Waves: _____
             PRI: _____
             QRS: _____
             Interp: _____

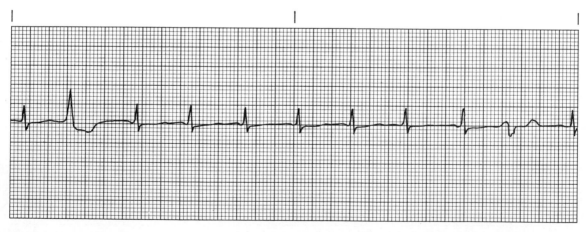

10.96   Regularity: _____
             Rate: _____
             P Waves: _____
             PRI: _____
             QRS: _____
             Interp: _____

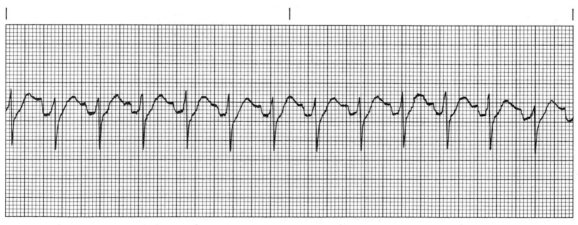

10.97   Regularity: _____

          Rate: _____

          P Waves: _____

          PRI: _____

          QRS: _____

          Interp: _____

10.98   Regularity: _____

          Rate: _____

          P Waves: _____

          PRI: _____

          QRS: _____

          Interp: _____

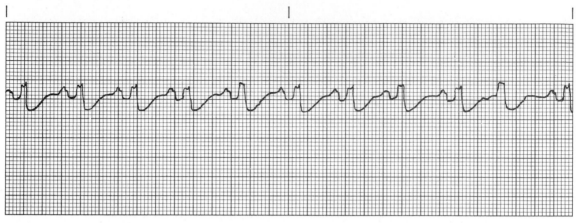

10.99   Regularity: _____
         Rate: _____
         P Waves: _____
         PRI: _____
         QRS: _____
         Interp: _____

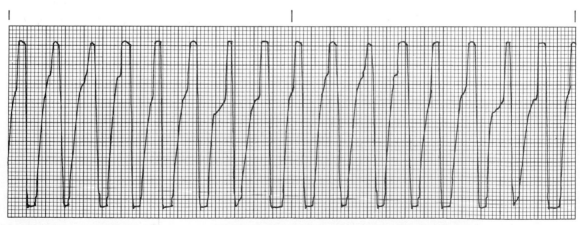

10.100   Regularity: _____
         Rate: _____
         P Waves: _____
         PRI: _____
         QRS: _____
         Interp: _____

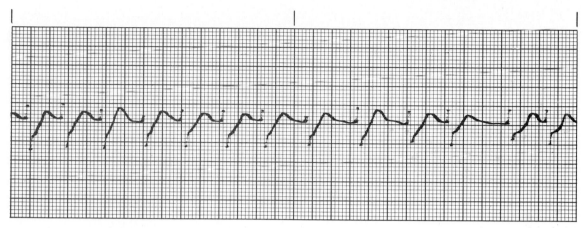

10.101   Regularity: _____
            Rate: _____
            P Waves: _____
            PRI: _____
            QRS: _____
            Interp: _____

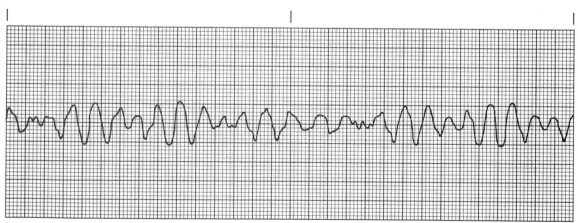

10.102   Regularity: _____
            Rate: _____
            P Waves: _____
            PRI: _____
            QRS: _____
            Interp: _____

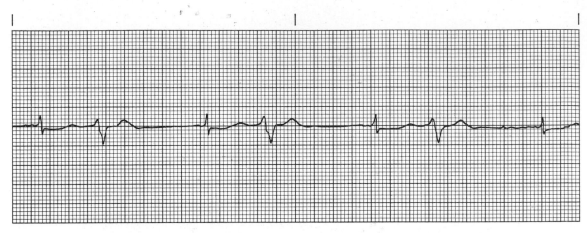

10.103   Regularity: _____
            Rate: _____
            P Waves: _____
            PRI: _____
            QRS: _____
            Interp: _____

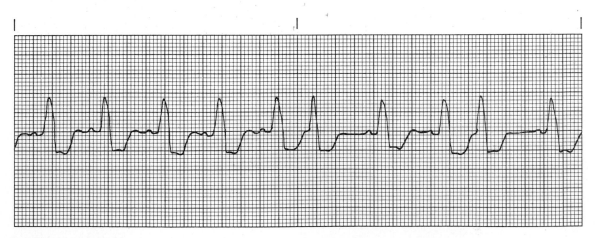

10.104   Regularity: _____
            Rate: _____
            P Waves: _____
            PRI: _____
            QRS: _____
            Interp: _____

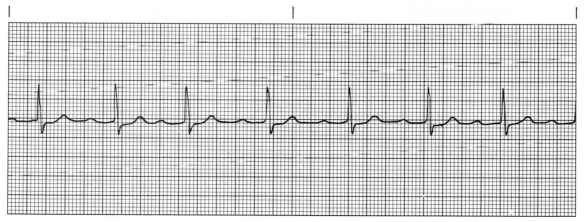

10.105   Regularity: _____
         Rate: _____
         P Waves: _____
         PRI: _____
         QRS: _____
         Interp: _____

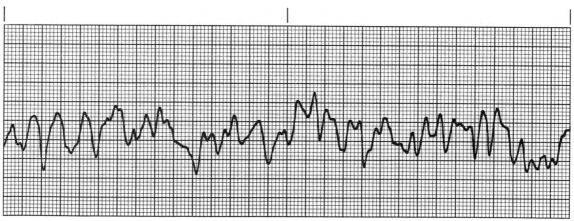

10.106   Regularity: _____
         Rate: _____
         P Waves: _____
         PRI: _____
         QRS: _____
         Interp: _____

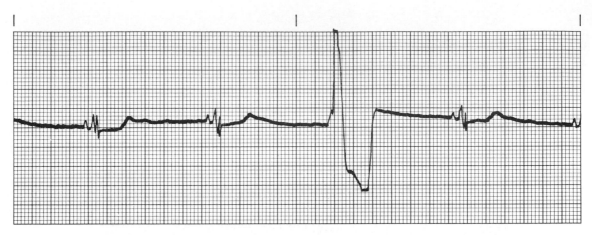

10.107   Regularity: _____
          Rate: _____
          P Waves: _____
          PRI: _____
          QRS: _____
          Interp: _____

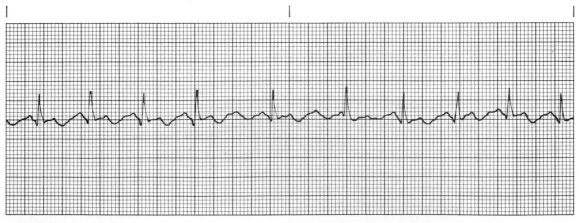

10.108   Regularity: _____
          Rate: _____
          P Waves: _____
          PRI: _____
          QRS: _____
          Interp: _____

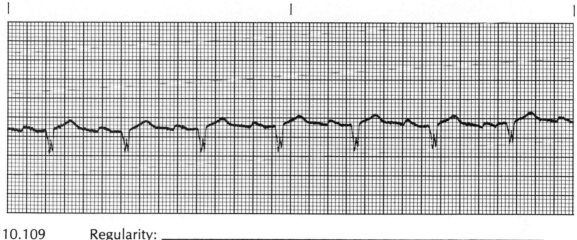

10.109   Regularity: _____

              Rate: _____

              P Waves: _____

              PRI: _____

              QRS: _____

              Interp: _____

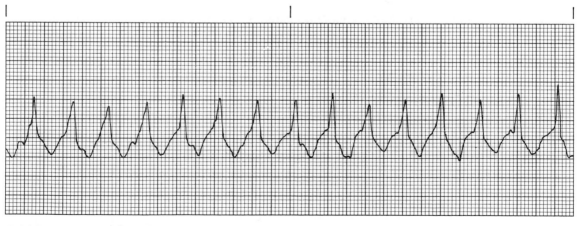

10.110   Regularity: _____

              Rate: _____

              P Waves: _____

              PRI: _____

              QRS: _____

              Interp: _____

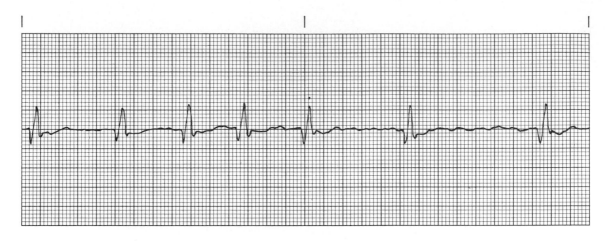

10.111   Regularity: _____
         Rate: _____
         P Waves: _____
         PRI: _____
         QRS: _____
         Interp: _____

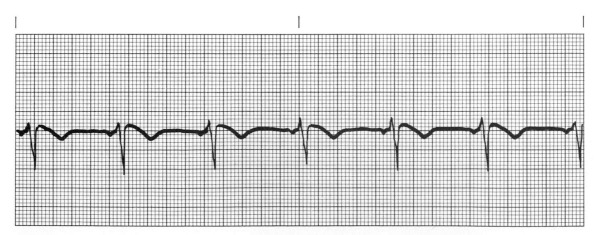

10.112   Regularity: _____
         Rate: _____
         P Waves: _____
         PRI: _____
         QRS: _____
         Interp: _____

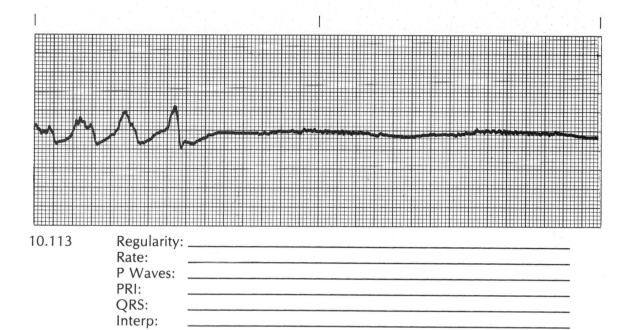

10.113   Regularity: _____

Rate: _____

P Waves: _____

PRI: _____

QRS: _____

Interp: _____

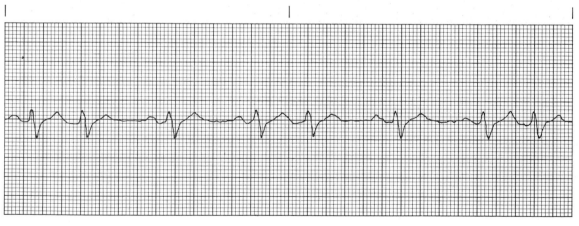

10.114   Regularity: _____

Rate: _____

P Waves: _____

PRI: _____

QRS: _____

Interp: _____

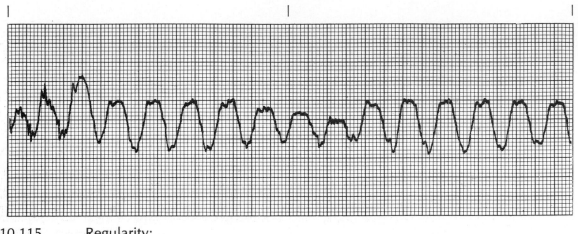

10.115   Regularity: _____
          Rate: _____
          P Waves: _____
          PRI: _____
          QRS: _____
          Interp: _____

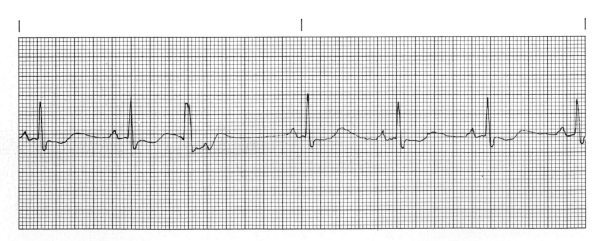

10.116   Regularity: _____
          Rate: _____
          P Waves: _____
          PRI: _____
          QRS: _____
          Interp: _____

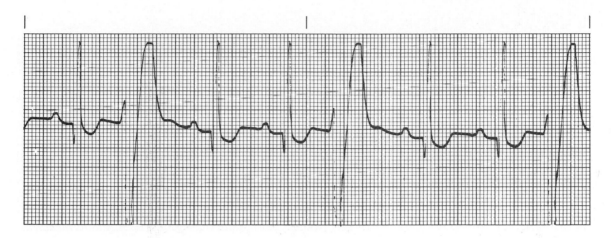

10.117   Regularity: _____

            Rate: _____

            P Waves: _____

            PRI: _____

            QRS: _____

            Interp: _____

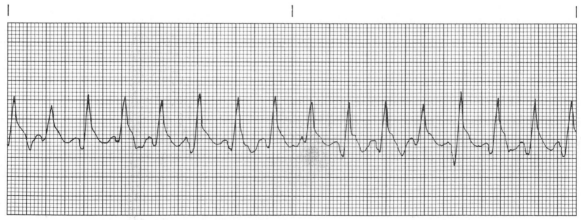

10.118   Regularity: _____

            Rate: _____

             P Waves: _____

            PRI: _____

            QRS: _____

            Interp: _____

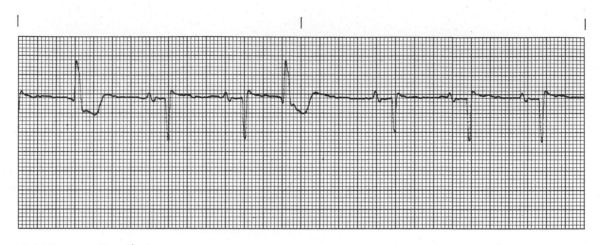

10.119   Regularity: _____

Rate: _____

P Waves: _____

PRI: _____

QRS: _____

Interp: _____

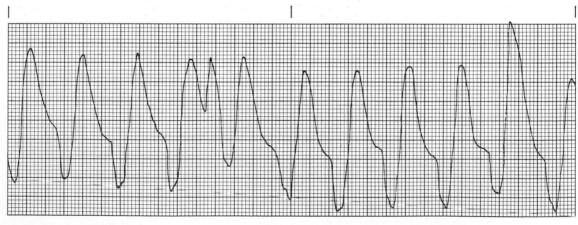

10.120   Regularity: _____

Rate: _____

P Waves: _____

PRI: _____

QRS: _____

Interp: _____

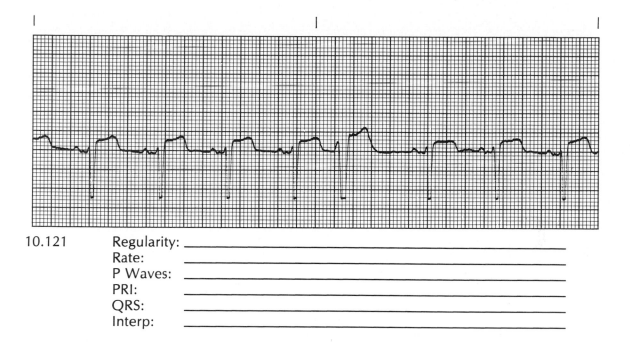

10.121   Regularity: _____
           Rate: _____
           P Waves: _____
           PRI: _____
           QRS: _____
           Interp: _____

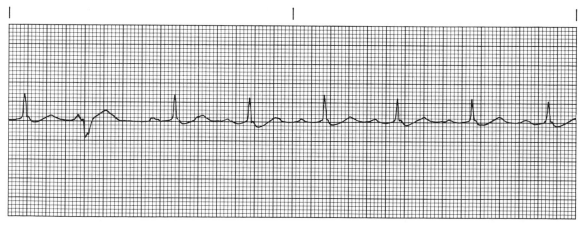

10.122   Regularity: _____
           Rate: _____
           P Waves: _____
           PRI: _____
           QRS: _____
           Interp: _____

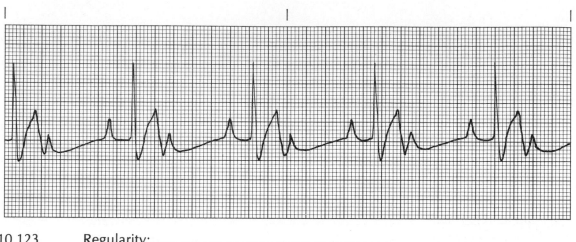

10.123   Regularity: _____
          Rate: _____
          P Waves: _____
          PRI: _____
          QRS: _____
          Interp: _____

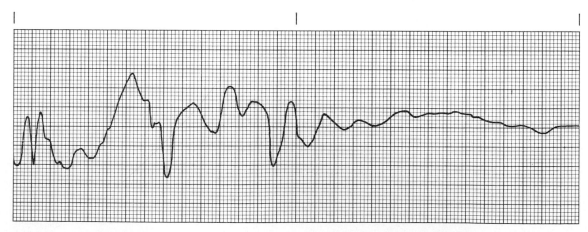

10.124   Regularity: _____
          Rate: _____
          P Waves: _____
          PRI: _____
          QRS: _____
          Interp: _____

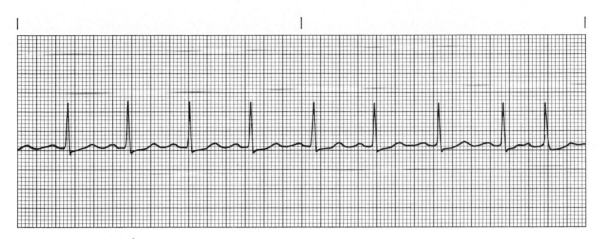

10.125   Regularity: _____
          Rate: _____
          P Waves: _____
          PRI: _____
          QRS: _____
          Interp: _____

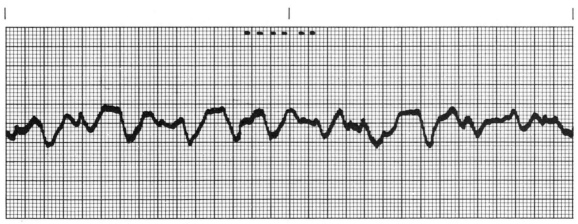

10.126   Regularity: _____
          Rate: _____
          P Waves: _____
          PRI: _____
          QRS: _____
          Interp: _____

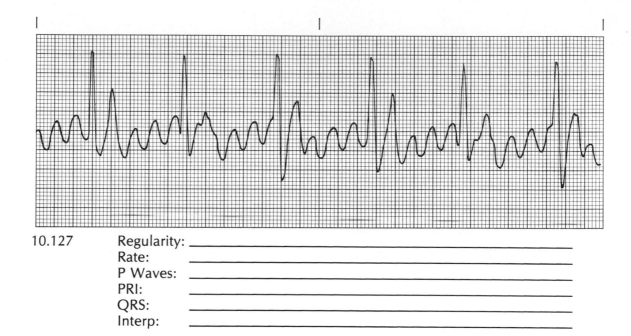

10.127   Regularity: _____
          Rate: _____
          P Waves: _____
          PRI: _____
          QRS: _____
          Interp: _____

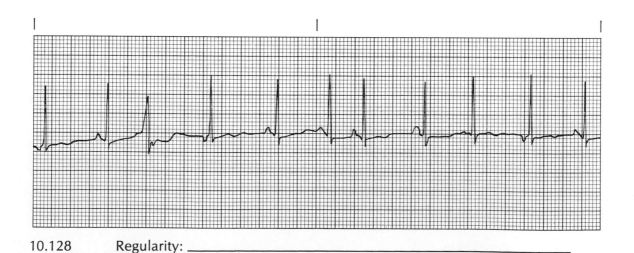

10.128   Regularity: _____
          Rate: _____
          P Waves: _____
          PRI: _____
          QRS: _____
          Interp: _____

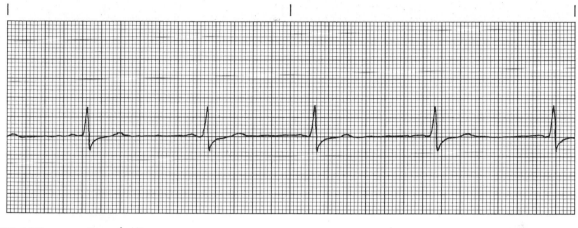

10.129   Regularity: _____
          Rate: _____
          P Waves: _____
          PRI: _____
          QRS: _____
          Interp: _____

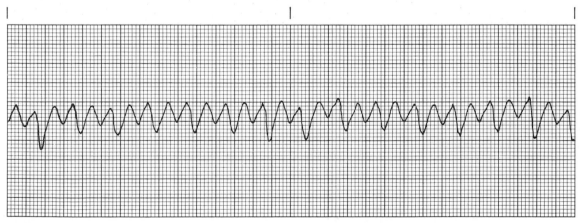

10.130   Regularity: _____
          Rate: _____
          P Waves: _____
          PRI: _____
          QRS: _____
          Interp: _____

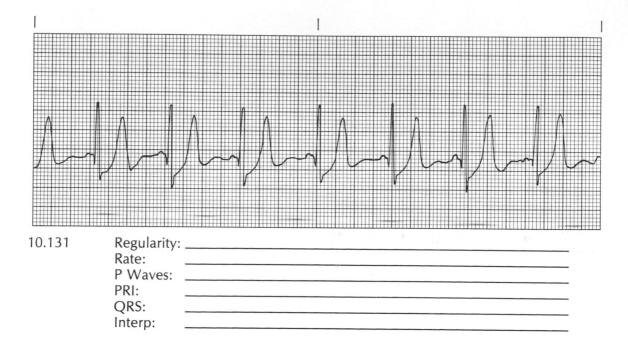

10.131   Regularity: _____
         Rate: _____
         P Waves: _____
         PRI: _____
         QRS: _____
         Interp: _____

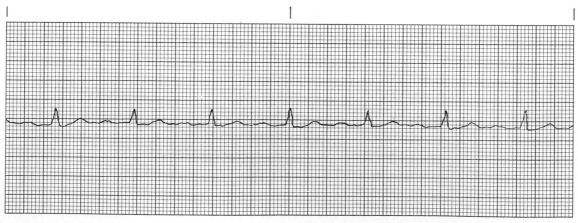

10.132   Regularity: _____
         Rate: _____
         P Waves: _____
         PRI: _____
         QRS: _____
         Interp: _____

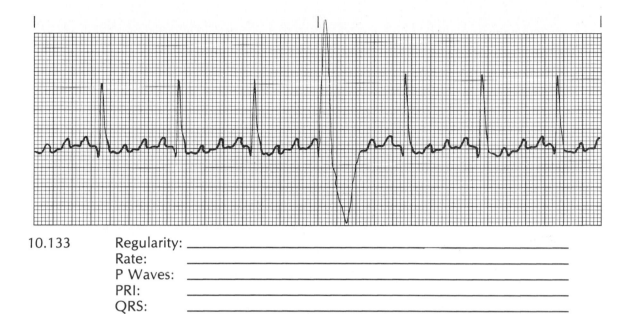

10.133   Regularity: _____
             Rate: _____
             P Waves: _____
             PRI: _____
             QRS: _____
             Interp: _____

10.134   Regularity: _____
             Rate: _____
             P Waves: _____
             PRI: _____
             QRS: _____
             Interp: _____

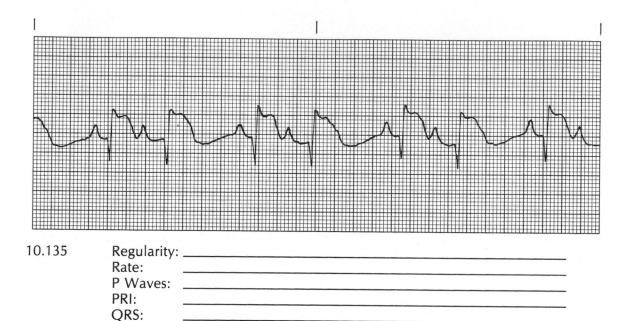

10.135   Regularity: _____

Rate: _____

P Waves: _____

PRI: _____

QRS: _____

Interp: _____

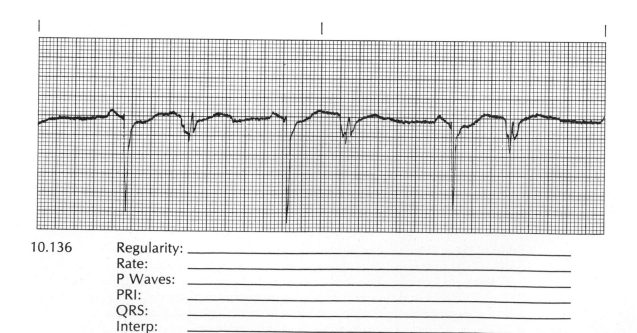

10.136   Regularity: _____

Rate: _____

P Waves: _____

PRI: _____

QRS: _____

Interp: _____

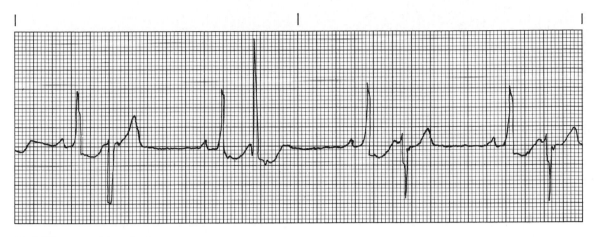

10.137   Regularity: _____
          Rate: _____
          P Waves: _____
          PRI: _____
          QRS: _____
          Interp: _____

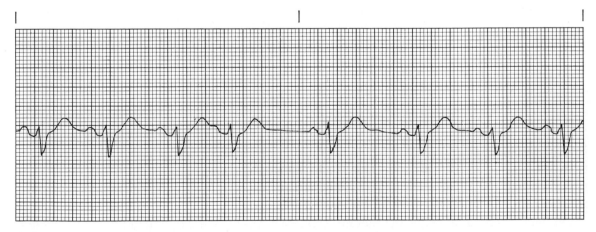

10.138   Regularity: _____
          Rate: _____
          P Waves: _____
          PRI: _____
          QRS: _____
          Interp: _____

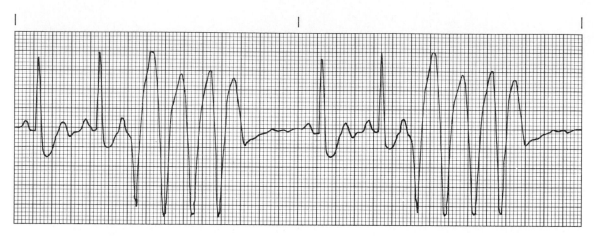

10.139   Regularity: _____
          Rate: _____
          P Waves: _____
          PRI: _____
          QRS: _____
          Interp: _____

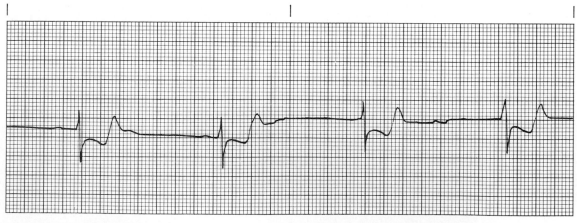

10.140   Regularity: _____
          Rate: _____
          P Waves: _____
          PRI: _____
          QRS: _____
          Interp: _____

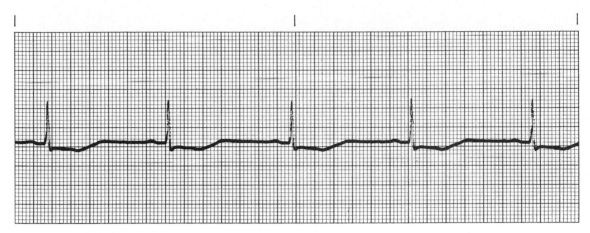

10.141   Regularity: _____
         Rate: _____
         P Waves: _____
         PRI: _____
         QRS: _____
         Interp: _____

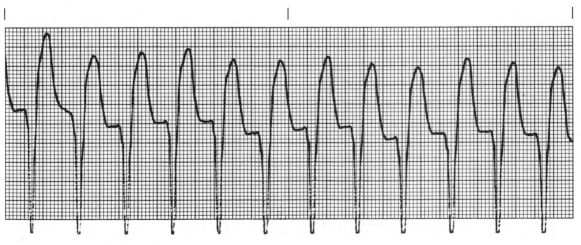

10.142   Regularity: _____
         Rate: _____
         P Waves: _____
         PRI: _____
         QRS: _____
         Interp: _____

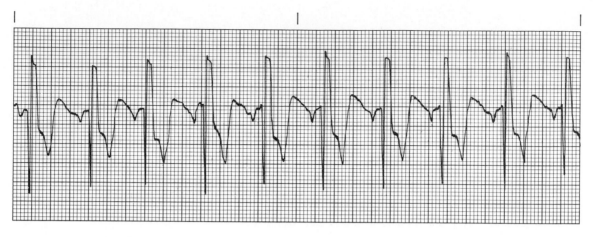

10.143   Regularity: _____
          Rate: _____
          P Waves: _____
          PRI: _____
          QRS: _____
          Interp: _____

10.144   Regularity: _____
          Rate: _____
          P Waves: _____
          PRI: _____
          QRS: _____
          Interp: _____

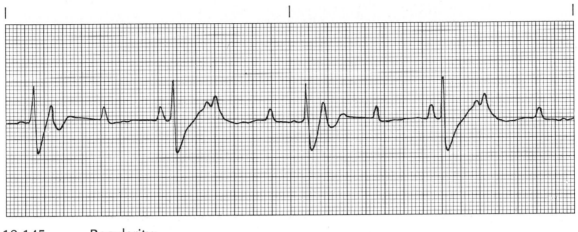

10.145   Regularity: _____
              Rate: _____
              P Waves: _____
              PRI: _____
              QRS: _____
              Interp: _____

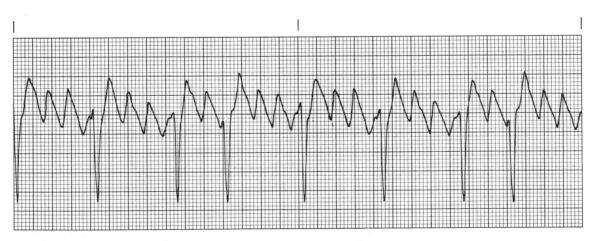

10.146   Regularity: _____
              Rate: _____
              P Waves: _____
              PRI: _____
              QRS: _____
              Interp: _____

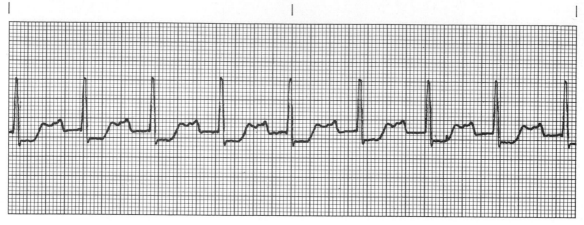

10.147   Regularity: _____
          Rate: _____
          P Waves: _____
          PRI: _____
          QRS: _____
          Interp: _____

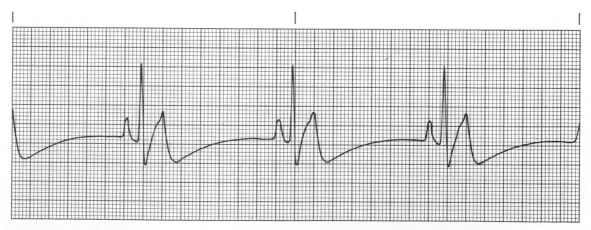

10.148   Regularity: _____
          Rate: _____
          P Waves: _____
          PRI: _____
          QRS: _____
          Interp: _____

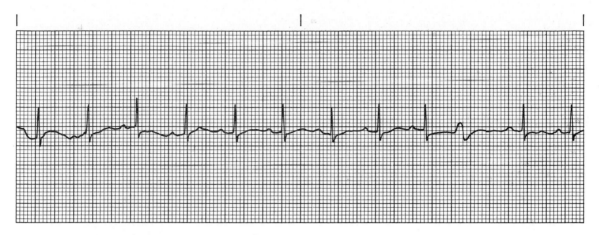

10.149   Regularity: _____
              Rate: _____
              P Waves: _____
              PRI: _____
              QRS: _____
              Interp: _____

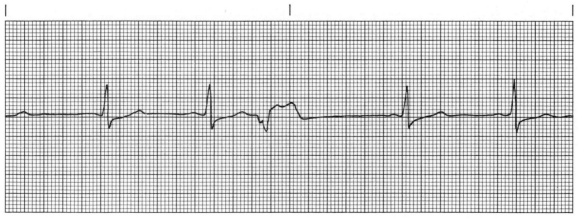

10.150   Regularity: _____
              Rate: _____
              P Waves: _____
              PRI: _____
              QRS: _____
              Interp: _____

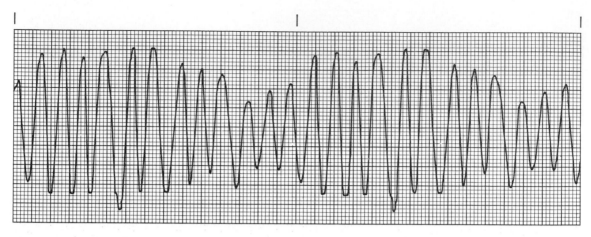

10.151   Regularity: _____
         Rate: _____
         P Waves: _____
         PRI: _____
         QRS: _____
         Interp: _____

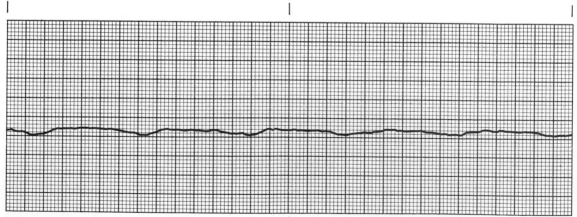

10.152   Regularity: _____
         Rate: _____
         P Waves: _____
         PRI: _____
         QRS: _____
         Interp: _____

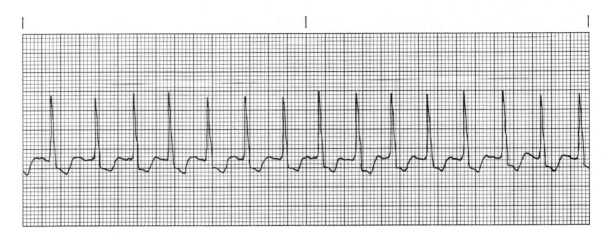

10.153   Regularity: _____
              Rate: _____
              P Waves: _____
              PRI: _____
              QRS: _____
              Interp: _____

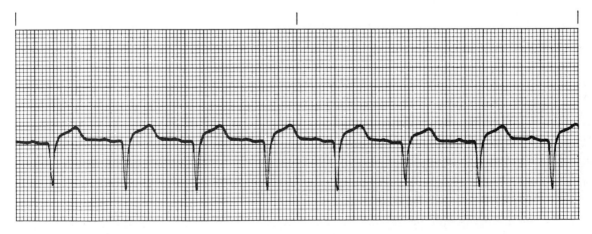

10.154   Regularity: _____
              Rate: _____
              P Waves: _____
              PRI: _____
              QRS: _____
              Interp: _____

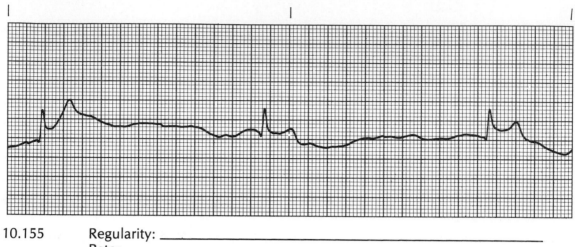

10.155   Regularity: _____
         Rate: _____
         P Waves: _____
         PRI: _____
         QRS: _____
         Interp: _____

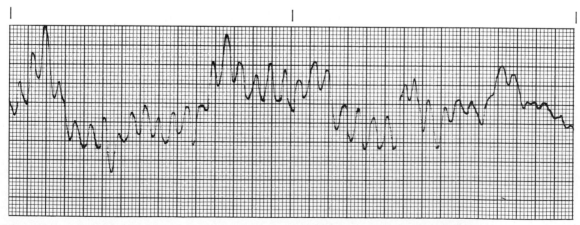

10.156   Regularity: _____
         Rate: _____
         P Waves: _____
         PRI: _____
         QRS: _____
         Interp: _____

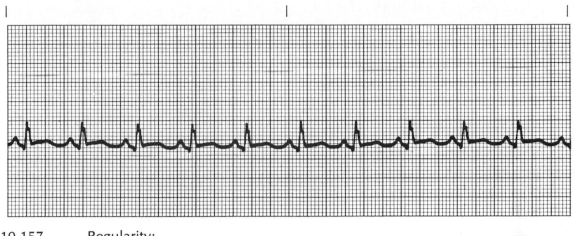

10.157   Regularity: _____
           Rate: _____
           P Waves: _____
           PRI: _____
           QRS: _____
           Interp: _____

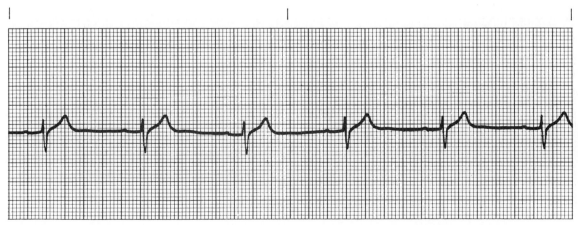

10.158   Regularity: _____
           Rate: _____
           P Waves: _____
           PRI: _____
           QRS: _____
           Interp: _____

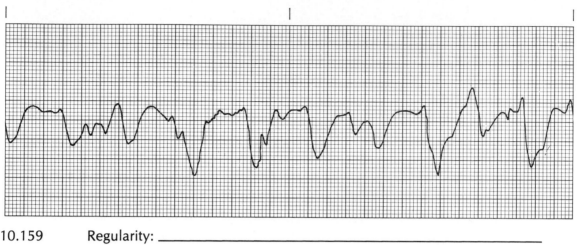

10.159   Regularity: _____
          Rate: _____
          P Waves: _____
          PRI: _____
          QRS: _____
          Interp: _____

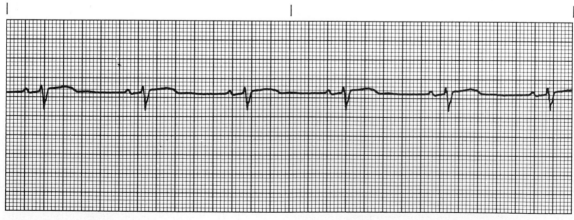

10.160   Regularity: _____
          Rate: _____
          P Waves: _____
          PRI: _____
          QRS: _____
          Interp: _____

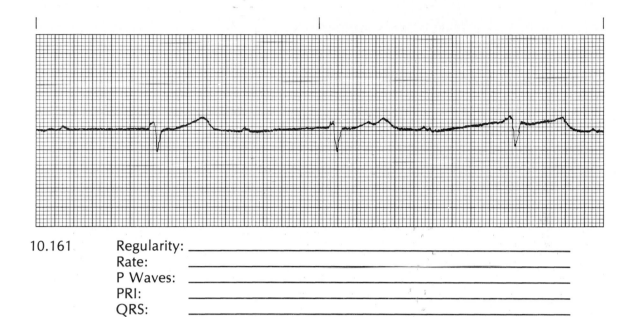

10.161   Regularity: _____
          Rate: _____
          P Waves: _____
          PRI: _____
          QRS: _____
          Interp: _____

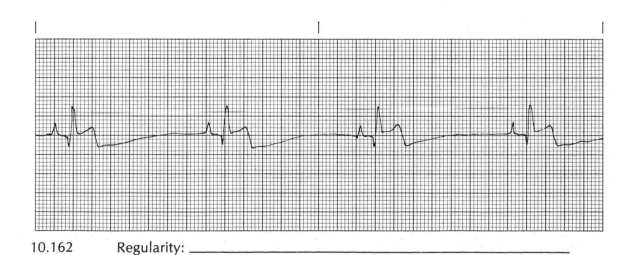

10.162   Regularity: _____
          Rate: _____
          P Waves: _____
          PRI: _____
          QRS: _____
          Interp: _____

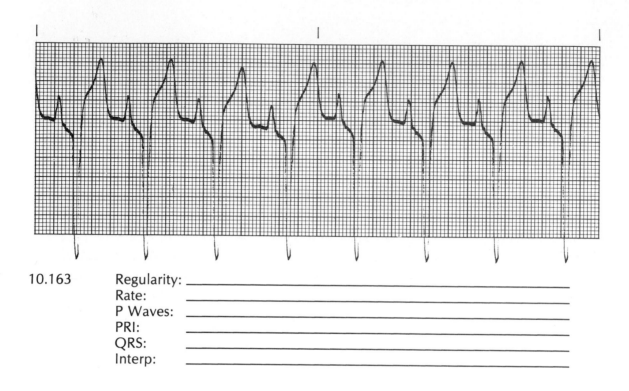

10.163   Regularity: _____
          Rate: _____
          P Waves: _____
          PRI: _____
          QRS: _____
          Interp: _____

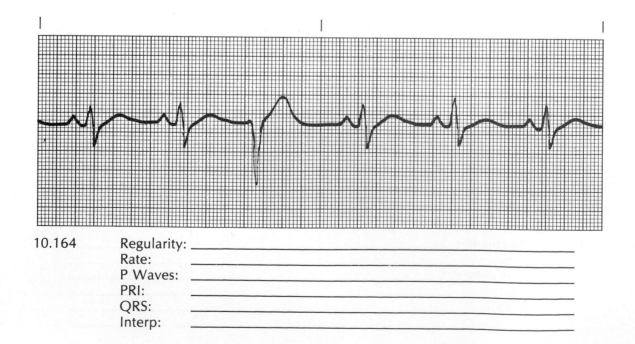

10.164   Regularity: _____
          Rate: _____
          P Waves: _____
          PRI: _____
          QRS: _____
          Interp: _____

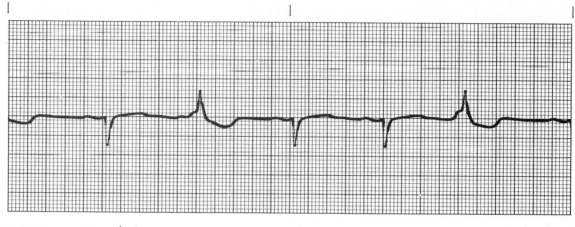

10.165   Regularity: _____
          Rate: _____
          P Waves: _____
          PRI: _____
          QRS: _____
          Interp: _____

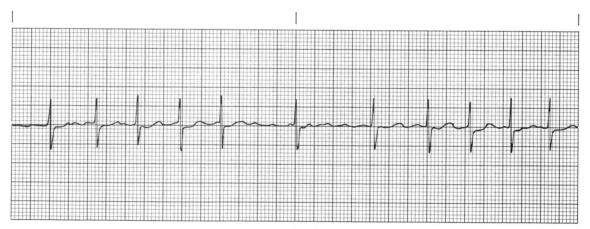

10.166   Regularity: _____
          Rate: _____
          P Waves: _____
          PRI: _____
          QRS: _____
          Interp: _____

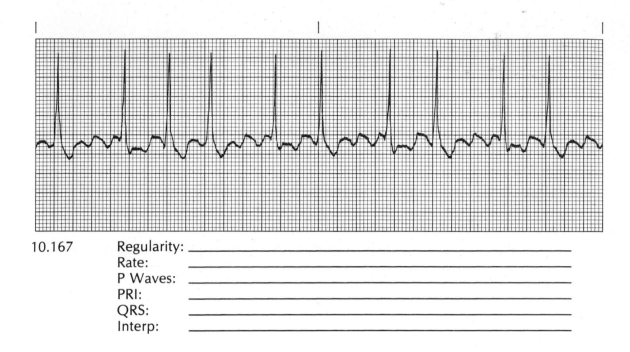

10.167   Regularity: _____
           Rate: _____
           P Waves: _____
           PRI: _____
           QRS: _____
           Interp: _____

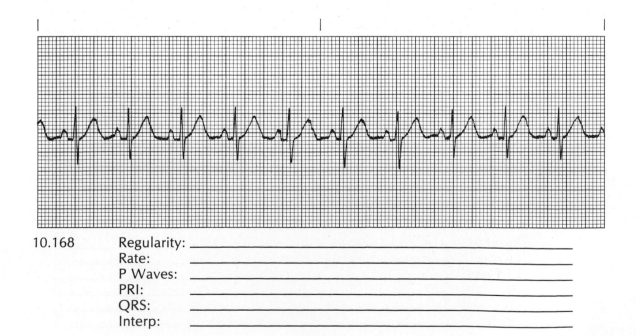

10.168   Regularity: _____
           Rate: _____
           P Waves: _____
           PRI: _____
           QRS: _____
           Interp: _____

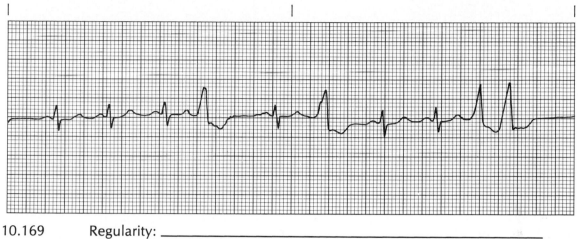

10.169   Regularity: _____
          Rate: _____
          P Waves: _____
          PRI: _____
          QRS: _____
          Interp: _____

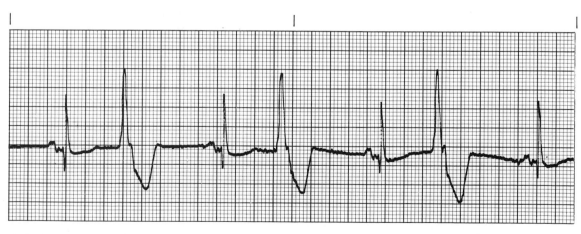

10.170   Regularity: _____
          Rate: _____
          P Waves: _____
          PRI: _____
          QRS: _____
          Interp: _____

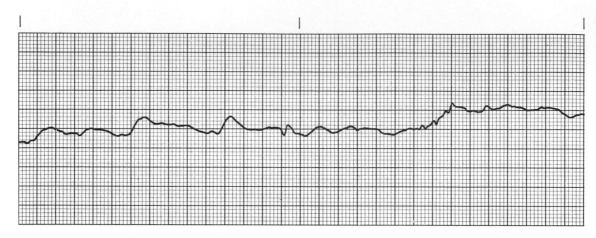

10.171   Regularity: _____
          Rate: _____
          P Waves: _____
          PRI: _____
          QRS: _____
          Interp: _____

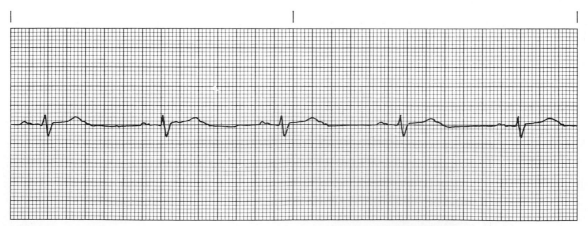

10.172   Regularity: _____
          Rate: _____
          P Waves: _____
          PRI: _____
          QRS: _____
          Interp: _____

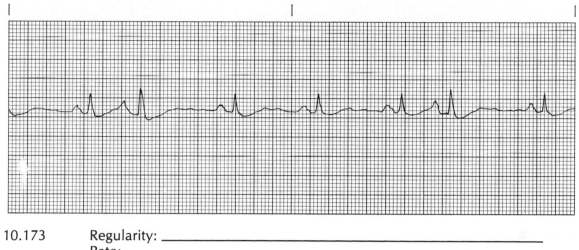

10.173   Regularity: _____
           Rate: _____
           P Waves: _____
           PRI: _____
           QRS: _____
           Interp: _____

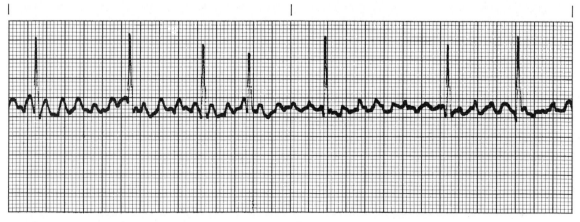

10.174   Regularity: _____
           Rate: _____
           P Waves: _____
           PRI: _____
           QRS: _____
           Interp: _____

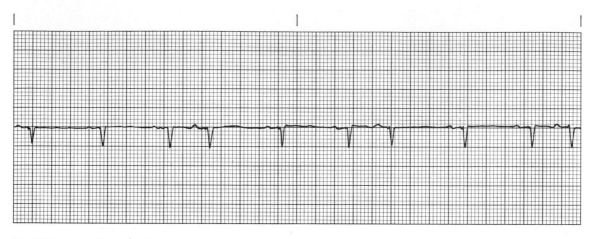

10.175   Regularity: _____
          Rate: _____
          P Waves: _____
          PRI: _____
          QRS: _____
          Interp: _____

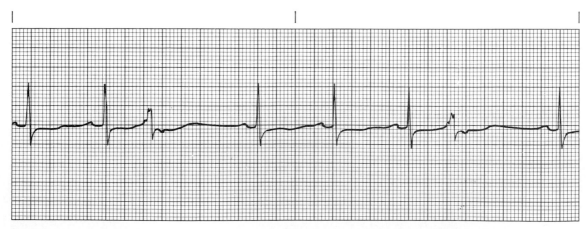

10.176   Regularity: _____
          Rate: _____
          P Waves: _____
          PRI: _____
          QRS: _____
          Interp: _____

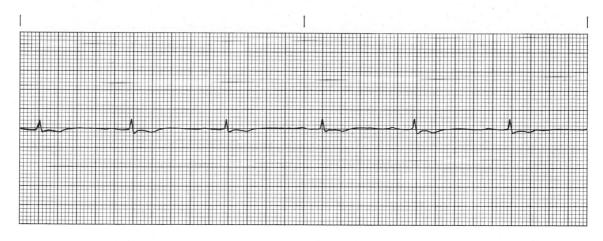

10.177   Regularity: _____
          Rate: _____
          P Waves: _____
          PRI: _____
          QRS: _____
          Interp: _____

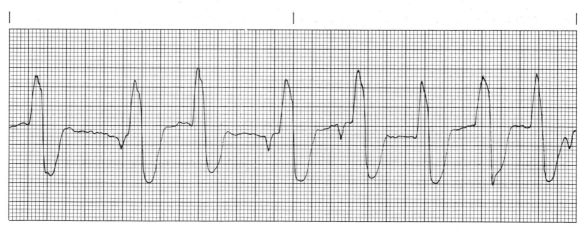

10.178   Regularity: _____
          Rate: _____
          P Waves: _____
          PRI: _____
          QRS: _____
          Interp: _____

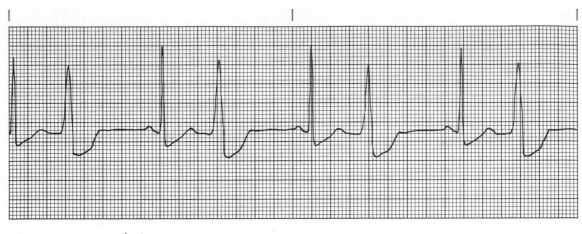

10.179   Regularity: _____
          Rate: _____
          P Waves: _____
          PRI: _____
          QRS: _____
          Interp: _____

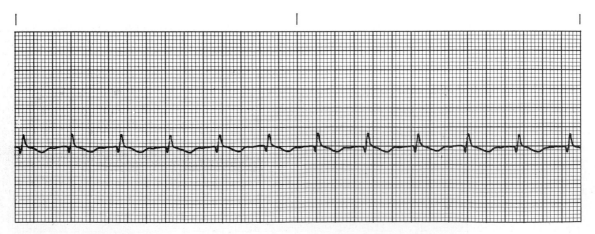

10.180   Regularity: _____
          Rate: _____
          P Waves: _____
          PRI: _____
          QRS: _____
          Interp: _____

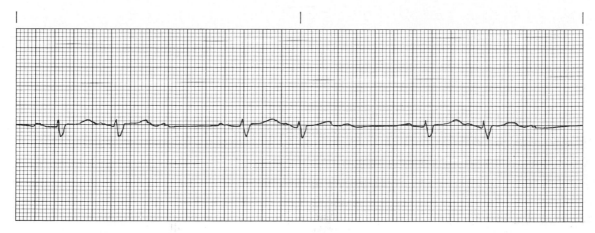

10.181   Regularity: _____
          Rate: _____
          P Waves: _____
          PRI: _____
          QRS: _____
          Interp: _____

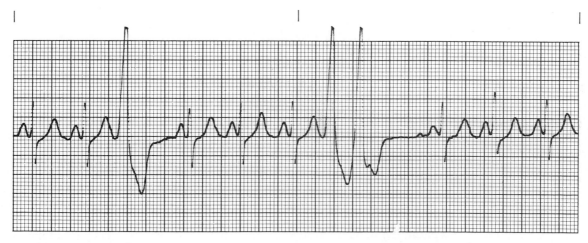

10.182   Regularity: _____
          Rate: _____
          P Waves: _____
          PRI: _____
          QRS: _____
          Interp: _____

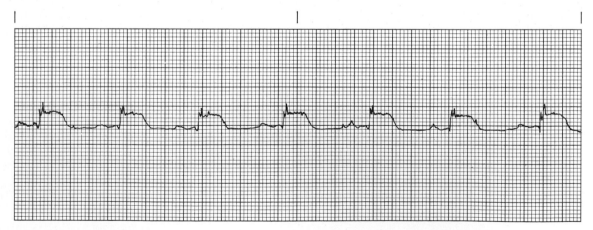

10.183   Regularity: _____

Rate: _____

P Waves: _____

PRI: _____

QRS: _____

Interp: _____

10.184   Regularity: _____

Rate: _____

P Waves: _____

PRI: _____

QRS: _____

Interp: _____

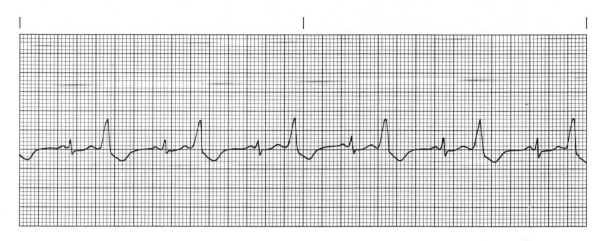

10.185   Regularity: _____
          Rate: _____
          P Waves: _____
          PRI: _____
          QRS: _____
          Interp: _____

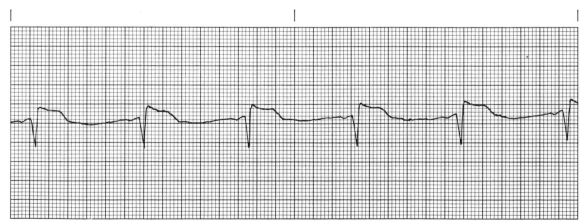

10.186   Regularity: _____
          Rate: _____
          P Waves: _____
          PRI: _____
          QRS: _____
          Interp: _____

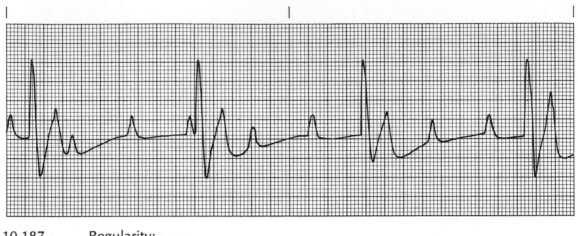

10.187   Regularity: _____
          Rate: _____
          P Waves: _____
          PRI: _____
          QRS: _____
          Interp: _____

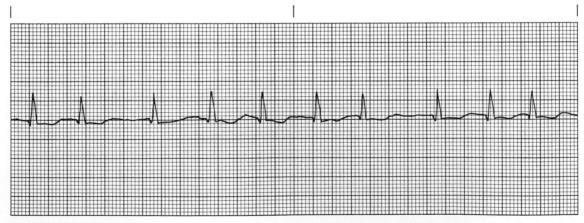

10.188   Regularity: _____
          Rate: _____
          P Waves: _____
          PRI: _____
          QRS: _____
          Interp: _____

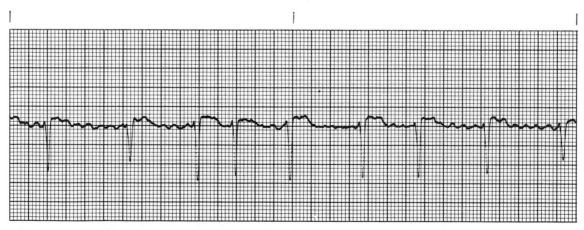

10.189   Regularity: _____
                Rate: _____
                P Waves: _____
                PRI: _____
                QRS: _____
                Interp: _____

10.190   Regularity: _____
                Rate: _____
                P Waves: _____
                PRI: _____
                QRS: _____
                Interp: _____

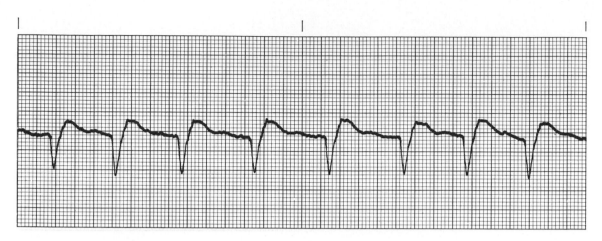

10.191   Regularity: _____
                    Rate: _____
                    P Waves: _____
                    PRI: _____
                    QRS: _____
                    Interp: _____

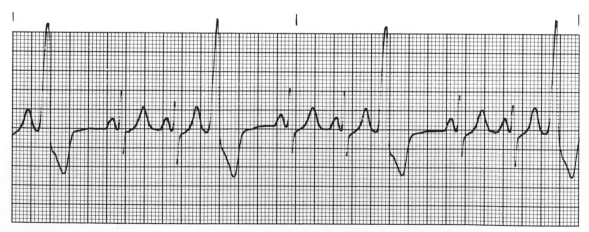

10.192   Regularity: _____
                    Rate: _____
                    P Waves: _____
                    PRI: _____
                    QRS: _____
                    Interp: _____

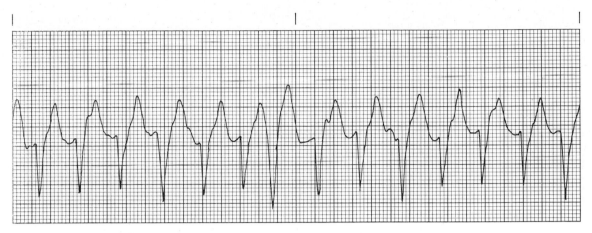

10.193   Regularity: _____
          Rate: _____
          P Waves: _____
          PRI: _____
          QRS: _____
          Interp: _____

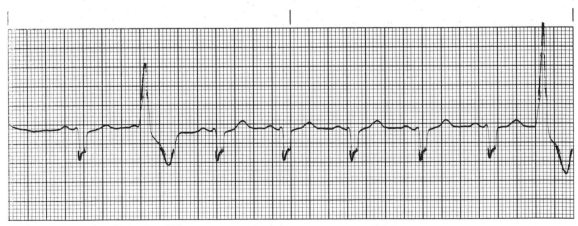

10.194   Regularity: _____
          Rate: _____
          P Waves: _____
          PRI: _____
          QRS: _____
          Interp: _____

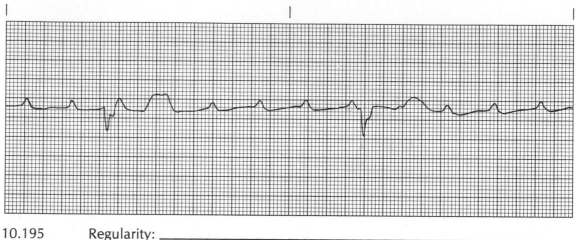

10.195   Regularity: _____
          Rate: _____
          P Waves: _____
          PRI: _____
          QRS: _____
          Interp: _____

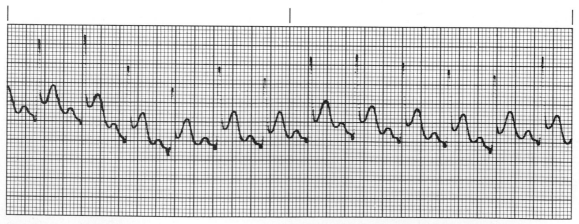

10.196   Regularity: _____
          Rate: _____
          P Waves: _____
          PRI: _____
          QRS: _____
          Interp: _____

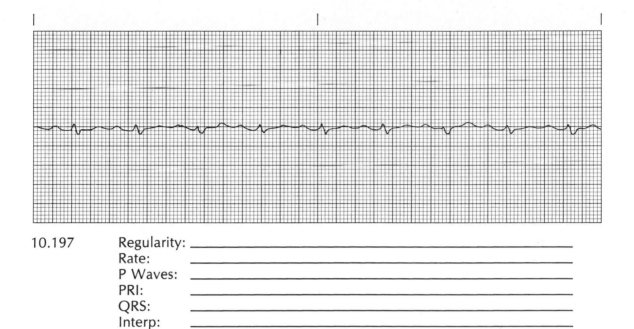

10.197   Regularity: _____
            Rate: _____
            P Waves: _____
            PRI: _____
            QRS: _____
            Interp: _____

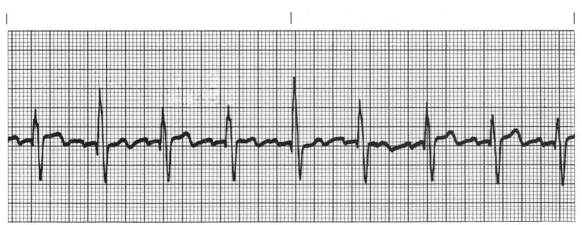

10.198   Regularity: _____
            Rate: _____
            P Waves: _____
            PRI: _____
            QRS: _____
            Interp: _____

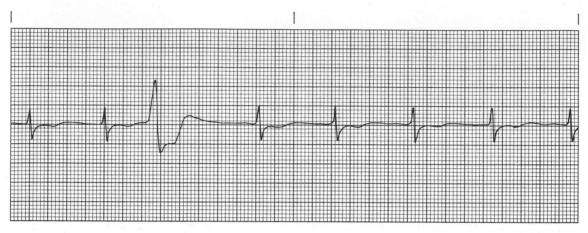

10.199   Regularity: _____
            Rate: _____
            P Waves: _____
            PRI: _____
            QRS: _____
            Interp: _____

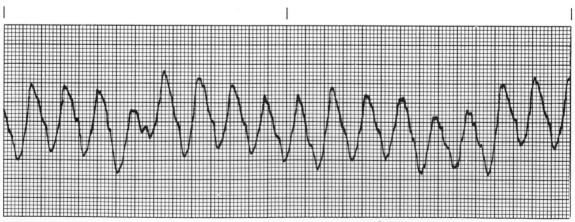

10.200   Regularity: _____
            Rate: _____
            P Waves: _____
            PRI: _____
            QRS: _____
            Interp: _____

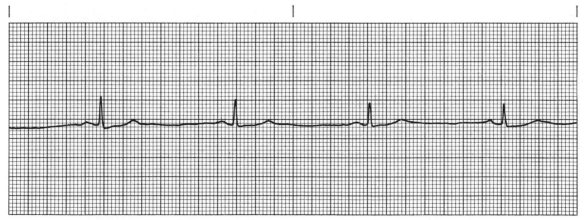

10.205   Regularity: _____
          Rate: _____
          P Waves: _____
          PRI: _____
          QRS: _____
          Interp: _____

10.206   Regularity: _____
          Rate: _____
          P Waves: _____
          PRI: _____
          QRS: _____
          Interp: _____

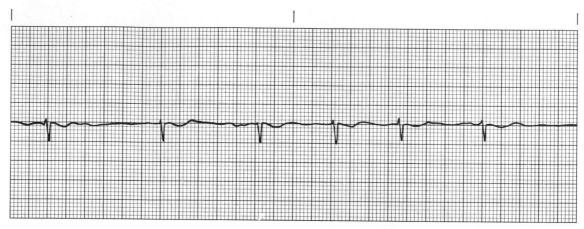

10.207   Regularity: _____
          Rate: _____
          P Waves: _____
          PRI: _____
          QRS: _____
          Interp: _____

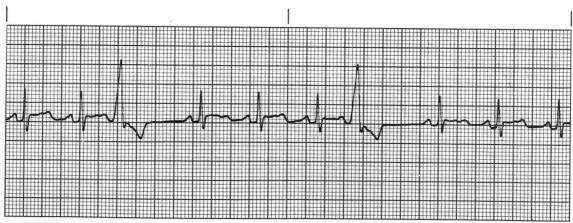

10.208   Regularity: _____
          Rate: _____
          P Waves: _____
          PRI: _____
          QRS: _____
          Interp: _____

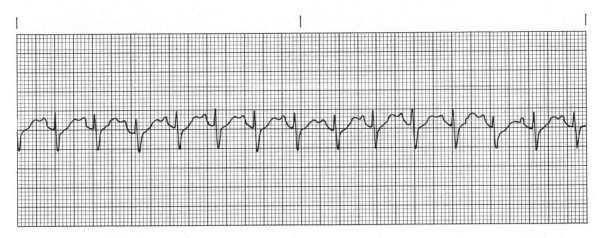

10.209   Regularity: _____
          Rate: _____
          P Waves: _____
          PRI: _____
          QRS: _____
          Interp: _____

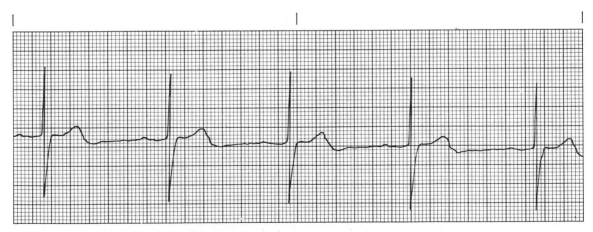

10.210   Regularity: _____
          Rate: _____
          P Waves: _____
          PRI: _____
          QRS: _____
          Interp: _____

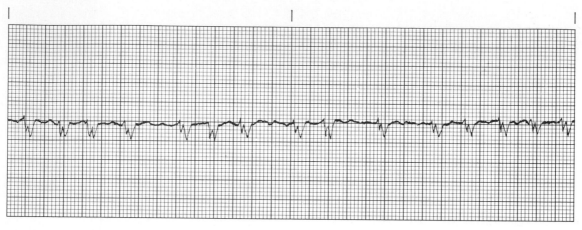

10.211   Regularity: _____
          Rate: _____
          P Waves: _____
          PRI: _____
          QRS: _____
          Interp: _____

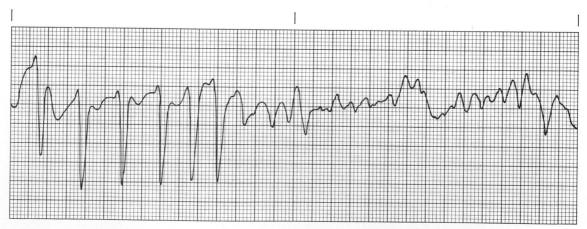

10.212   Regularity: _____
          Rate: _____
          P Waves: _____
          PRI: _____
          QRS: _____
          Interp: _____

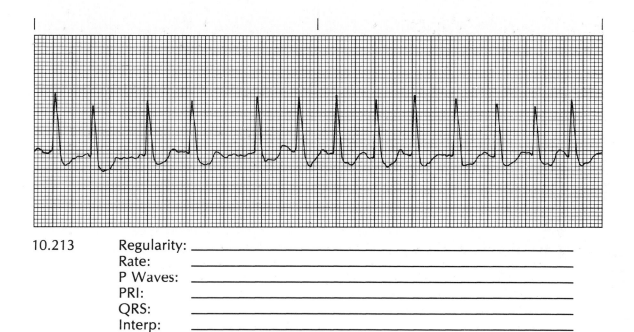

10.213   Regularity: _____
           Rate: _____
           P Waves: _____
           PRI: _____
           QRS: _____
           Interp: _____

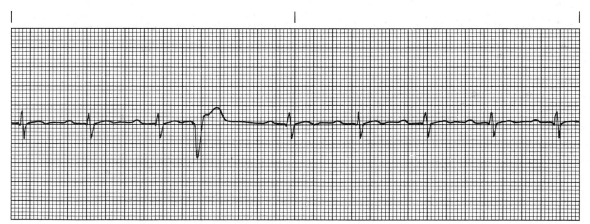

10.214   Regularity: _____
           Rate: _____
           P Waves: _____
           PRI: _____
           QRS: _____
           Interp: _____

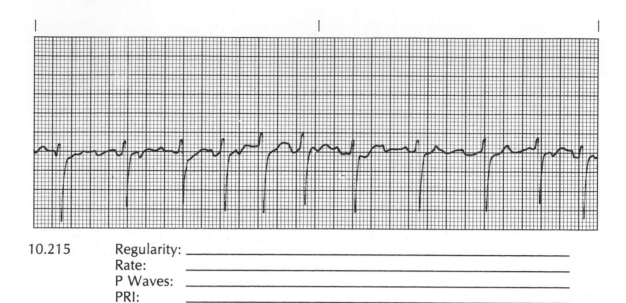

10.215   Regularity: _____
          Rate: _____
          P Waves: _____
          PRI: _____
          QRS: _____
          Interp: _____

10.216   Regularity: _____
          Rate: _____
          P Waves: _____
          PRI: _____
          QRS: _____
          Interp: _____

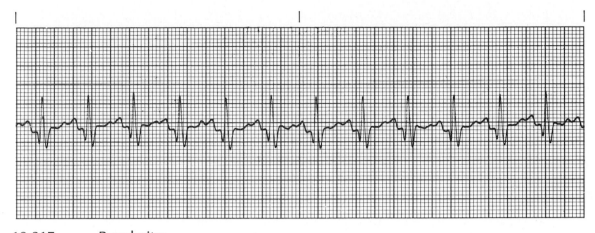

10.217　　　Regularity: _____
　　　　　　Rate: _____
　　　　　　P Waves: _____
　　　　　　PRI: _____
　　　　　　QRS: _____
　　　　　　Interp: _____

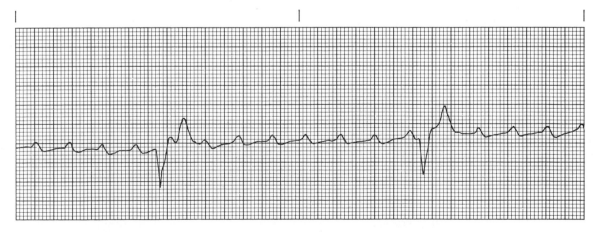

10.218　　　Regularity: _____
　　　　　　Rate: _____
　　　　　　P Waves: _____
　　　　　　PRI: _____
　　　　　　QRS: _____
　　　　　　Interp: _____

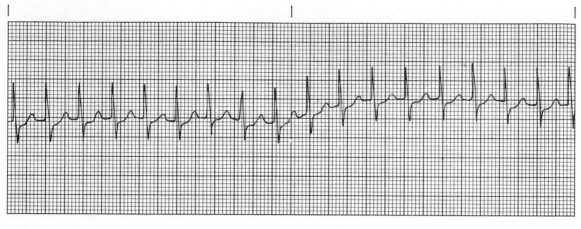

10.219
Regularity: _____
Rate: _____
P Waves: _____
PRI: _____
QRS: _____
Interp: _____

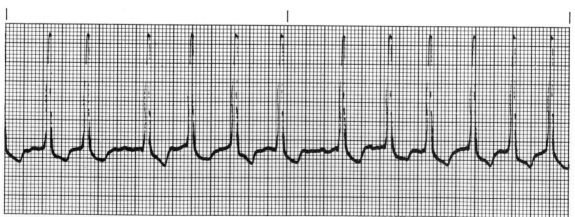

10.220
Regularity: _____
Rate: _____
P Waves: _____
PRI: _____
QRS: _____
Interp: _____

Answer Keys

The following pages contain the answers to all of the practice strips found in the preceding chapters. Before you begin comparing results, you should know something about how these answers were calculated.

Regularity: This will usually reflect the regularity of the underlying rhythm, but it may sometimes include the effect of any ectopics. A rhythm is considered regular if it is not off by more than one small square on faster rhythms, or more than two small squares on slower rhythms.

Rate: This measurement will always refer to the ventricular rate, unless the atrial and ventricular rates differ, in which case both will be given. The rates are all calculated by counting the number of small squares between two R waves (or the P waves if the atrial rate is being calculated) and dividing it into 1500. On irregular rhythms, the rate is calculated by counting the number of R waves in a six-second strip and multiplying it by 10. If ectopics are present in a regular arrhythmia, the rate is calculated by measuring the R–R interval in an uninterrupted section of the strip. In irregular arrhythmias with ectopics, the ectopics are included in the calculation of the rate unless they are PVCs, in which case they are *not* included. PVCs are not included in rate calculations because they frequently fail to produce a pulse. In calculating a rate on a bigeminy of PVCs, it is not possible to measure the R–R interval of the sinus beats, because the PVCs obscure them. In this rhythm, however, the sinus mechanism is healthy but is overridden by the irritable ectopics. We assume that sinus beats would continue if the PVCs were suppressed, and we assume that without the PVCs we would see twice as many sinus beats. Thus, in bigeminy of PVCs, the rate given is twice the rate of the visible R–R interval of the sinus beats.

P Waves: This is not an area of measurement, it is an area of observation. The primary task is to identify all of the P waves and see if they can be mapped out across the entire strip. You should also note the configuration of the P waves, and whether or not their shape changes from one beat to the next.

PR Intervals: All PRIs are measured from the beginning of the P wave to the beginning of the QRS complex. The P wave is considered to begin when it changes configuration from the preceding electrical activity. If no P waves are visible, the PRI is unknown. In cases of atrial fibrillation and atrial flutter, where it is impossible to tell which atrial depolarization was transmitted to the ventricles, the PRI is unknown. If there are no P waves, or if they are not related to the QRS complexes, there is no PRI. Your measurement should be within .04 seconds of the answer given in order to be considered correct.

QRS Complexes: The QRS complex is considered to begin when a deflection terminates the PR segment, whether that deflection is a Q wave or an R wave. The end-point of measurement is when the S wave changes at the juncture with the ST segment (sometimes called the J point). Your measurement should be within .04 seconds of the answer given in order to be considered correct.

As you compare your findings to those given, keep in mind what you learned in Chapter 3: the interpretation of an arrhythmia is a matter of collecting all the available data from the strip, and then comparing your findings to the rules for each arrhythmia. The arrhythmia that most closely parallels your findings is most probably the correct identification.

If your answer does not match exactly with the key, that does not necessarily mean that you are entirely wrong. But look to see how the answer given may have a closer parallel to the rules than yours does. If you have access to an instructor, this might be a good time to seek individual help and clear up any misunderstandings.

Practice Sheet 1:
Answers

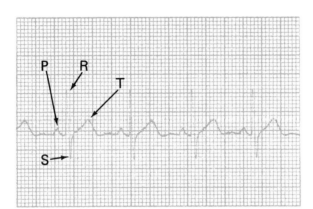

1.1

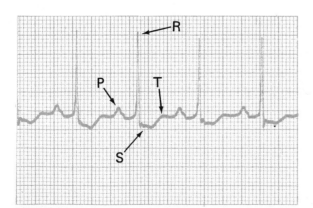

1.2

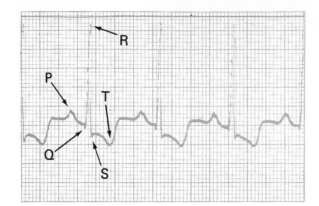

1.3

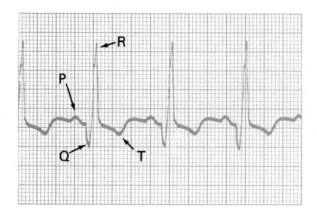

1.4

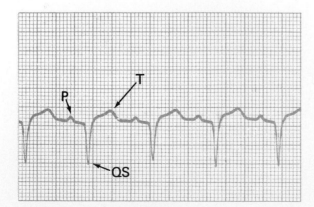

1.5

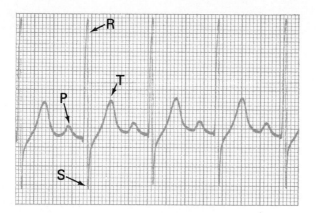

1.6

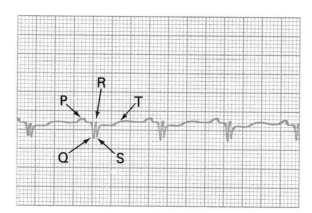

1.7

Practice Sheet 2:
Answers

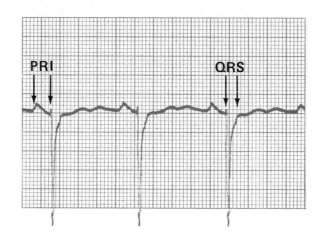

PRI: .18 seconds
QRS: .12 seconds

2.1

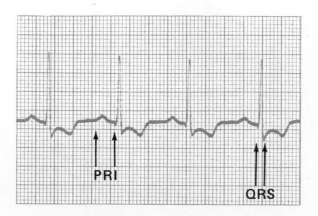

PRI: .20 seconds
QRS: .08 seconds

2.2

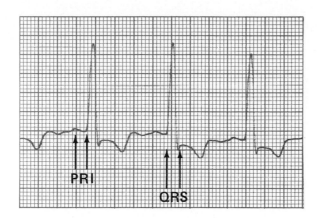

PRI: .16 seconds
QRS: .14 seconds

2.3

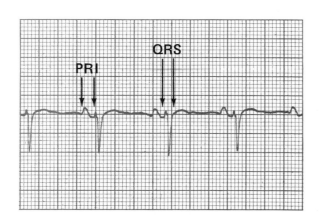

PRI: .12 seconds
QRS: .10 seconds

2.4

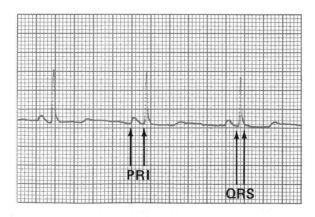

PRI: .14 seconds
QRS: .08 seconds

2.5

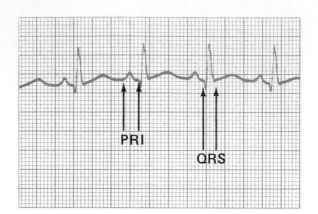

PRI: .16 seconds
QRS: .10 seconds

2.6

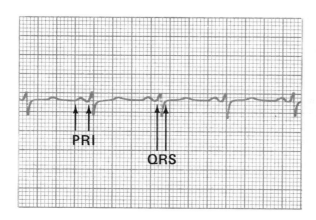

PRI: .14 seconds
QRS: .10 seconds

2.7

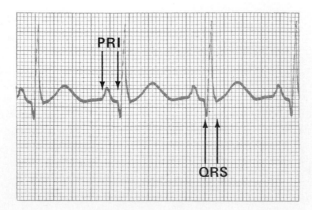

PRI: .16 seconds
QRS: .14 seconds

2.8

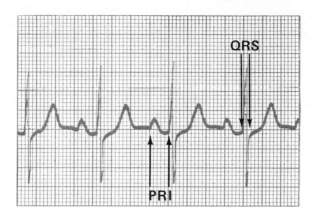

PRI: .20 seconds
QRS: .08 seconds

2.9

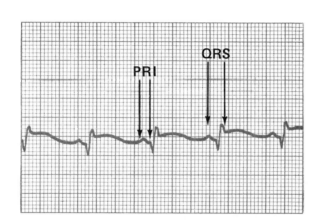

PRI: .12 seconds
QRS: .10 seconds

2.10

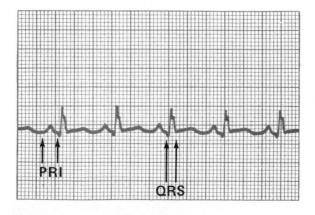

PRI: .16 seconds
QRS: .11 seconds

2.11

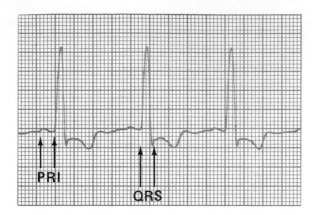

PRI: .16 seconds
QRS: .14 seconds

2.12

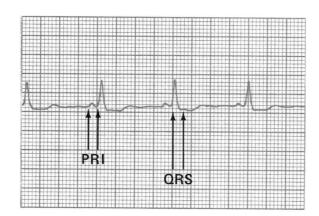

PRI: .10 seconds
QRS: .10 seconds

2.13

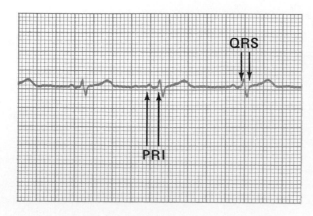

PRI: .12 seconds
QRS: .08 seconds

2.14

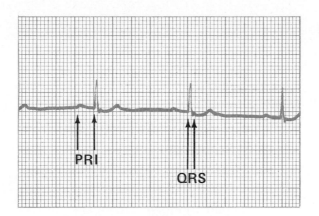

PRI: .18 seconds
QRS: .06 seconds

2.15

Practice Sheet 3:
Answers

3.1   Regularity: regular
          Rate: 79 beats per minute
          P Waves: regular P–P interval; uniform waves
          PRI: .16 seconds and constant
          QRS: .08 seconds

3.2   Regularity: irregular
          Rate: approximately 100 beats per minute
          P Waves: uniform; regular P–P interval
          PRI: .12 seconds and constant
          QRS: .08 seconds

3.3   Regularity: regular
          Rate: 63 beats per minute
          P Waves: uniform; regular P–P interval
          PRI: .16 seconds and constant
          QRS: .10 seconds

3.4   Regularity: regular
          Rate: 125 beats per minute
          P Waves: uniform, regular P–P interval
          PRI: .16 seconds and constant
          QRS: .08 seconds

3.5   Regularity: regular
          Rate: 81 beats per minute
          P Waves: uniform; regular P–P interval
          PRI: .16 seconds and constant
          QRS: .12 seconds

Practice Sheet 4:
Answers

4.1   Regularity: regular
             Rate: 107 beats per minute
             P Waves: uniform; regular P–P interval
             PRI: .20 seconds and constant
             QRS: .10 seconds

4.2   Regularity: regular
             Rate: 79 beats per minute
             P Waves: uniform; regular P–P intervals
             PRI: .10 seconds and constant
             QRS: .06 seconds

4.3   Regularity: regular
             Rate: 79 beats per minute
             P Waves: uniform; regular P–P interval
             PRI: .16 seconds and constant
             QRS: .10 seconds

4.4   Regularity: regular
             Rate: 83 beats per minute
             P Waves: uniform, regular P–P interval
             PRI: .20 seconds and constant
             QRS: .08 seconds

4.5   Regularity: irregular
             Rate: approximately 80 beats per minute
             P Waves: uniform; irregular P–P interval
             PRI: .16 seconds and constant
             QRS: .10 seconds

Practice Sheet 5:
Answers

5.1   Regularity: regular (slightly irregular)
        Rate: 48 beats per minute
        P Waves: uniform and upright; regular P–P interval
        PRI: .18 seconds and constant
        QRS: .12 seconds
        Interp: Sinus Bradycardia

5.2   Regularity: irregular
        Rate: approximately 80 beats per minute
        P Waves: uniform and upright; regular P–P interval
        PRI: .14 seconds and constant
        QRS: .06 seconds
        Interp: Sinus Arrhythmia

5.3   Regularity: regular
        Rate: 75 beats per minute
        P Waves: uniform and upright; regular P–P interval
        PRI: .16 seconds and constant
        QRS: .08 seconds
        Interp: Normal Sinus Rhythm

5.4   Regularity: regular
        Rate: 136 beats per minute
        P Waves: uniform and upright; regular P–P interval
        PRI: .16 seconds and constant
        QRS: .06 seconds
        Interp: Sinus Tachycardia

5.5   Regularity: irregular
        Rate: approximately 80 beats per minute
        P Waves: uniform P waves with an irregular P–P interval
        PRI: .16 seconds and constant
        QRS: .08 seconds
        Interp: Sinus Arrhythmia

5.6   Regularity: regular
        Rate: 107 beats per minute
        P Waves: uniform and upright; regular P–P interval
        PRI: .16 seconds and constant
        QRS: .12 seconds
        Interp: Sinus Tachycardia (with a wide QRS)

5.7   Regularity: regular
           Rate: 54 beats per minute
           P Waves: uniform and upright; regular P–P interval
           PRI: .16 seconds and constant
           QRS: .12 seconds
           Interp: Sinus Bradycardia (with a wide QRS)

5.8   Regularity: regular
           Rate: 71 beats per minute
           P Waves: uniform and upright; regular P–P interval
           PRI: .14 seconds and constant
           QRS: .08 seconds
           Interp: Normal Sinus Rhythm

5.9   Regularity: regular
           Rate: 94 beats per minute
           P Waves: uniform and upright; regular P–P interval
           PRI: .16 seconds and constant
           QRS: .12 seconds
           Interp: Normal Sinus Rhythm (with a wide QRS)

5.10   Regularity: slightly irregular
           Rate: approximately 30 beats per minute
           P Waves: uniform and upright; irregular P–P interval
           PRI: .18 seconds and constant
           QRS: .08 seconds
           Interp: Sinus Brady-Arrhythmia

5.11   Regularity: regular
           Rate: 77 beats per minute
           P Waves: uniform and upright; regular P–P interval
           PRI: .18 seconds and constant
           QRS: .06 seconds
           Interp: Normal Sinus Rhythm

5.12   Regularity: irregular
           Rate: 90 beats per minute
           P Waves: uniform and upright; irregular P–P interval
           PRI: .20 seconds and constant
           QRS: .06 seconds
           Interp: Sinus Arrhythmia

5.13   Regularity: regular
           Rate: 48 beats per minute
           P Waves: uniform and upright; regular P–P interval
           PRI: .20 seconds and constant
           QRS: .08 seconds
           Interp: Sinus Bradycardia

5.14

Regularity: irregular
Rate: approximately 70 beats per minute
P Waves: uniform and upright; regular P–P interval
PRI: .14 seconds and constant
QRS: .06 seconds
Interp: Sinus Arrhythmia

5.15

Regularity: regular
Rate: 79 beats per minute
P Waves: uniform and upright; regular P–P interval
PRI: .16 seconds and constant
QRS: .08 seconds
Interp: Normal Sinus Rhythm

5.16

Regularity: regular
Rate: 115 beats per minute
P Waves: uniform and upright; regular P–P interval
PRI: .14 seconds and constant
QRS: .16 seconds
Interp: Sinus Tachycardia

5.17

Regularity: regular
Rate: 65 beats per minute
P Waves: uniform and upright; regular P–P interval
PRI: .12 seconds and constant
QRS: .08 seconds
Interp: Normal Sinus Rhythm

5.18

Regularity: irregular
Rate: approximately 80 beats per minute
P Waves: uniform and upright; regular P–P interval
PRI: .12 seconds and constant
QRS: .08 seconds
Interp: Sinus Arrhythmia

5.19

Regularity: regular
Rate: 88 beats per minute
P Waves: uniform and upright; regular P–P interval
PRI: .16 seconds and constant
QRS: .08 seconds
Interp: Normal Sinus Rhythm

Practice Sheet 6:
Answers

6.1   Regularity: irregular
           Rate: approximately 100 beats per minute
           P Waves: not discernible; only undulations are present
           PRI: none
           QRS: .08 seconds
           Interp: uncontrolled Atrial Fibrillation

6.2   Regularity: regular
           Rate: atrial rate is 300 beats per minute; ventricular rate is 150
                       beats per minute
           P Waves: uniform; sawtooth appearance
           PRI: none
           QRS: .10 seconds (QRS is difficult to measure due to obscur-
                       ing by flutter waves)
           Interp: Atrial Flutter with 2:1 response

6.3   Regularity: regular underlying rhythm interrupted by an ectopic
           Rate: 71 beats per minute
           P Waves: uniform in underlying rhythm; one differently shaped
                       P wave before ectopic
           PRI: .16 seconds and constant
           QRS: .10 seconds
           Interp: Sinus Rhythm with one PAC

6.4   Regularity: irregular
           Rate: approximately 90 beats per minute
           P Waves: not discernible; undulations present
           PRI: none
           QRS: .12 seconds
           Interp: controlled Atrial Fibrillation (with wide QRS)

6.5   Regularity: regular
           Rate: atrial rate is 328 beats per minute; ventricular rate is
                       82 beats per minute
           P Waves: uniform; sawtooth appearance
           PRI: none
           QRS: .08 seconds
           Interp: Atrial Flutter with 4:1 response

6.6   Regularity: irregular
        Rate: approximately 50 beats per minute
        P Waves: not discernible; undulations present
        PRI: none
        QRS: .08 seconds (QRS complexes are sometimes obscured
                     by fibrillatory waves)
        Interp: controlled Atrial Fibrillation

6.7   Regularity: regular underlying rhythm interrupted by ectopics
        Rate: 115 beats per minute
        P Waves: uniform in the underlying rhythm; shape of P wave
                     changes before each ectopic
        PRI: .12 seconds
        QRS: .08 seconds; shape of QRS is uniform in both under-
                     lying beats and ectopics
        Interp: Sinus Tachycardia with three PACs

6.8   Regularity: irregular
        Rate: approximately 90 beats per minute
        P Waves: not discernible; undulations present
        PRI: none
        QRS: .08 seconds
        Interp: controlled Atrial Fibrillation

6.9   Regularity: irregular
        Rate: approximately 140 beats per minute
        P Waves: not discernible
        PRI: none
        QRS: .06 seconds
        Interp: uncontrolled Atrial Fibrillation

6.10   Regularity: regular underlying rhythm interrupted by an ectopic
        Rate: 65 beats per minute (rate changes after the ectopic be-
                     cause sinus firing mechanism resets itself)
        P Waves: uniform in underlying rhythm; shape differs in ectopic
        PRI: .16 seconds and constant; .20 seconds in ectopic
        QRS: .10 seconds
        Interp: Sinus Rhythm with one PAC

6.11   Regularity: irregular
        Rate: atrial rate 300 beats per minute; ventricular rate ap-
                     proximately 130 beats per minute
        P Waves: uniform; sawtooth appearance
        PRI: none
        QRS: .08 seconds
        Interp: Atrial Flutter with variable response

6.12

Regularity: irregular
Rate: approximately 80 beats per minute
P Waves: not discernible
PRI: none
QRS: .10 seconds
Interp: controlled Atrial Fibrillation

6.13

Regularity: regular
Rate: atrial rate is 332 beats per minute; ventricular rate is
            83 beats per minute
P Waves: uniform; sawtooth in appearance
PRI: none
QRS: .08 seconds
Interp: Atrial Flutter with 4:1 response

6.14

Regularity: regular
Rate: atrial rate is 300 beats per minute; ventricular rate is 75
            beats per minute
P Waves: uniform; there are four P waves for every QRS complex
PRI: none
QRS: .10 seconds
Interp: Atrial Flutter with 4:1 response

6.15

Regularity: irregular
Rate: approximately 40 beats per minute
P Waves: shape changes
PRI: varies from .12–.20 seconds; not constant
QRS: .08 seconds
Interp: Wandering Pacemaker

6.16

Regularity: irregular
Rate: approximately 80 beats per minute
P Waves: not visible; only undulations are present
PRI: none
QRS: .04 seconds
Interp: controlled Atrial Fibrillation

6.17

Regularity: regular
Rate: atrial rate is 334 beats per minute; ventricular rate is
            166 beats per minute
P Waves: uniform; sawtooth appearance; two P waves for every
            QRS complex
PRI: none
QRS: .10 seconds; slightly obscured by flutter waves
Interp: Atrial Flutter with 2:1 response

6.18   Regularity: irregular
            Rate: approximately 120 beats per minute
            P Waves: not discernible; only undulations are present
            PRI: none
            QRS: .08 seconds
            Interp: uncontrolled Atrial Fibrillation

6.19   Regularity: irregular
            Rate: approximately 70 beats per minute
            P Waves: not discernible; only fine undulations are present
            PRI: none
            QRS: .04 seconds
            Interp: controlled Atrial Fibrillation

6.20   Regularity: irregular
            Rate: approximately 110 beats per minute
            P Waves: what appear to be P waves do not map out; they are
                         actually coarse fibrillatory waves
            PRI: none
            QRS: .06 seconds; QRS complexes are obscured by fibrilla-
                         tory waves
            Interp: uncontrolled Atrial Fibrillation

6.21   Regularity: irregular
            Rate: approximately 150 beats per minute
            P Waves: unable to map out; undulations present
            PRI: none
            QRS: .06 seconds (QRS complexes are obscured by fibrilla-
                         tory waves)
            Interp: uncontrolled Atrial Fibrillation

6.22   Regularity: irregular
            Rate: approximately 40 beats per minute
            P Waves: shapes change; P–P interval is irregular
            PRI: varies (.12–.16 seconds)
            QRS: .08 seconds
            Interp: Wandering Pacemaker

Practice Sheet 7:
Answers

7.1   Regularity: regular underlying rhythm interrupted by an ectopic
               Rate: 107 beats per minute
               P Waves: uniform P waves except one missing before ectopic QRS
               PRI: .16 seconds and constant
               QRS: .08 seconds; QRS of ectopic beat is same size and shape as QRS of underlying rhythm
               Interp: Sinus Tachycardia with one PJC

7.2   Regularity: regular
               Rate: 83 beats per minute
               P Waves: no visible P waves
               PRI: none
               QRS: .08 seconds
               Interp: Accelerated Junctional Rhythm

7.3   Regularity: regular
               Rate: 100 beats per minute
               P Waves: all P waves are inverted
               PRI: .12 seconds and constant
               QRS: .06 seconds
               Interp: Junctional Tachycardia

7.4   Regularity: regular
               Rate: 43 beats per minute
               P Waves: no visible P waves
               PRI: none
               QRS: .08 seconds
               Interp: Junctional Escape Rhythm

7.5   Regularity: slightly irregular underlying rhythm interrupted by an ectopic
               Rate: 50 beats per minute
               P Waves: uniform, upright P waves; one inverted P wave before ectopic QRS
               PRI: .16 seconds and constant for underlying rhythm; .12 seconds for ectopic
               QRS: .08 seconds; QRS of ectopic is same shape and width as QRS of underlying rhythm
               Interp: Sinus Bradycardia with one PJC

7.6
Regularity: regular
Rate: 71 beats per minute
P Waves: no visible P waves
PRI: none
QRS: .10 seconds
Interp: Accelerated Junctional Rhythm

7.7
Regularity: regular
Rate: 167 beats per minute
P Waves: P waves are not visible
PRI: none
QRS: .06 seconds
Interp: Supraventricular Tachycardia

7.8
Regularity: regular
Rate: 79 beats per minute
P Waves: no visible P waves
PRI: none
QRS: .06 seconds
Interp: Accelerated Junctional Rhythm

7.9
Regularity: regular
Rate: 214 beats per minute
P Waves: P waves are not visible
PRI: none
QRS: .08 seconds
Interp: Supraventricular Tachycardia

7.10
Regularity: regular underlying rhythm interrupted by an ectopic
Rate: 81 beats per minute
P Waves: uniform and upright except for one inverted P wave in front of ectopic QRS
PRI: .16 seconds and constant for underlying rhythm; .12 seconds for ectopic
QRS: .08 seconds for both underlying rhythm and ectopic
Interp: Sinus Rhythm with one PJC

7.11
Regularity: regular
Rate: 150 beats per minute
P Waves: P waves are not visible
PRI: none
QRS: .10 seconds
Interp: Supraventricular Tachycardia

7.12   Regularity: regular
              Rate: 43 beats per minute
              P Waves: P waves are not visible
              PRI: none
              QRS: .10 seconds
              Interp: Junctional Escape Rhythm

7.13   Regularity: regular
              Rate: 88 beats per minute
              P Waves: inverted and uniform P waves
              PRI: .12 seconds and constant
              QRS: .10 seconds
              Interp: Accelerated Junctional Rhythm

Practice Sheet 8:
Answers

8.1
Regularity: regular
Rate: 51 beats per minute
P Waves: uniform and upright; regular P–P interval
PRI: .24 seconds and constant
QRS: .10 seconds
Interp: Sinus Bradycardia with First Degree Heart Block

8.2
Regularity: irregular with a pattern of grouped beating
Rate: atrial rate 115 beats per minute; ventricular rate approximately 90 beats per minute
P Waves: uniform; regular P–P intervals; more P waves than QRS complexes
PRI: changes; progressively lengthens from .20 seconds to .32 seconds
QRS: .08 seconds
Interp: Wenckebach (Second Degree Heart Block Mobitz I)

8.3
Regularity: regular
Rate: atrial rate 157 beats per minute; ventricular rate 33 beats per minute
P Waves: uniform; regular P–P intervals; more P waves than QRS complexes
PRI: P waves are not associated with QRS complexes
QRS: .12 seconds
Interp: Third Degree Heart Block (CHB) with ventricular escape focus

8.4
Regularity: regular
Rate: 73 beats per minute
P Waves: non-conducted P waves are more apparent after mapping the P–P interval, since some P waves are hidden within the QRS complexes and T waves
PRI: P waves are not associated with QRS complexes
QRS: .08 seconds
Interp: Third Degree Heart Block (CHB) with junctional escape focus

8.5
Regularity: regular
Rate: 88 beats per minute
P Waves: uniform and upright; regular P–P interval
PRI: .26 seconds and constant
QRS: .12 seconds
Interp: Sinus Rhythm with First Degree Heart Block (with wide QRS)

8.6   Regularity: irregular with a pattern of grouped beating
       Rate: atrial rate 100 beats per minute; ventricular rate 80
                   beats per minute
       P Waves: uniform; regular P–P interval
       PRI: changing; progressively lengthen from .16 seconds to
                   .24 seconds
       QRS: .08 seconds
       Interp: Wenckebach (Second Degree Heart Block Mobitz I)

8.7   Regularity: irregular with a pattern of grouped beating
       Rate: atrial rate 75 beats per minute; ventricular rate approx-
                   imately 60 beats per minute
       P Waves: uniform; regular P–P interval; more P waves than QRS
                   complexes
       PRI: changing; progressively lengthens from .20 seconds to
                   .30 seconds
       QRS: .06 seconds
       Interp: Wenckebach (Second Degree Heart Block Mobitz I)

8.8   Regularity: regular
       Rate: atrial rate 120 beats per minute; ventricular rate 60
                   beats per minute
       P Waves: uniform and upright; regular P–P interval; consistently
                   two P waves for every QRS complex
       PRI: .38 seconds and constant
       QRS: .10 seconds
       Interp: Classical Second Degree Heart Block (Mobitz II) with
                   2:1 conduction

8.9   Regularity: irregular with a pattern of grouped beating
       Rate: atrial rate 125 beats per minute; ventricular rate ap-
                   proximately 80 beats per minute
       P Waves: uniform; regular P–P interval; more P waves than QRS
                   complexes
       PRI: changing; progressively lengthens from .20 seconds to
                   .28 seconds
       QRS: .12 seconds
       Interp: Wenckebach (Second Degree Heart Block Mobitz I)
                   (with wide QRS)

8.10   Regularity: irregular (see note)
       Rate: approximately 25 beats per minute
       P Waves: uniform; regular P–P intervals; more P waves than QRS
                   complexes
       PRI: the P waves are not associated to the QRS complexes
       QRS: .20 seconds

Interp: Third Degree Heart Block (CHB) with ventricular es-
            cape focus
Note: The ventricular pacemaker site usually has a regular fir-
            ing mechanism; but if a dangerous ventricular rhythm
            is allowed to continue untreated, its serious effects on
            the myocardium will ultimately cause the firing site to
            slow or die out. In this strip, the change in ventricular
            rate demonstrates this slowing phenomenon.

8.11   Regularity: regular
        Rate: 75 beats per minute
        P Waves: uniform; regular P–P interval
        PRI: .30 seconds and constant
        QRS: .14 seconds
        Interp: Sinus Rhythm with First Degree Heart Block (with wide
                     QRS)

8.12   Regularity: regular
        Rate: atrial rate 74 beats per minute; ventricular rate 37 beats
                     per minute
        P Waves: uniform; regular P–P interval; consistently two P waves
                     for every QRS complex
        PRI: .26 seconds and constant
        QRS: .12 seconds
        Interp: Classical Second Degree Heart Block (Mobitz II) with
                     2:1 conduction

8.13   Regularity: irregular with a pattern of grouped beating
        Rate: approximately 60 beats per minute
        P Waves: uniform; regular P–P interval
        PRI: changes; progressively lengthens from .28 seconds to
                     .48 seconds
        QRS: .06 seconds
        Interp: Wenckebach (Second Degree Heart Block Mobitz I)

8.14   Regularity: regular
        Rate: atrial rate 100 beats per minute; ventricular rate 35
                     beats per minute
        P Waves: uniform; regular P–P interval; more P waves than QRS
                     complexes
        PRI: the P waves are not associated with the QRS complexes
        QRS: .12 seconds
        Interp: Third Degree Heart Block (CHB) with ventricular es-
                     cape focus

8.15   Regularity: regular
            Rate: 65 beats per minute
            P Waves: Uniform and upright; regular P–P interval
            PRI: .26 seconds and constant
            QRS: .10 seconds
            Interp: Sinus Rhythm with First Degree Heart Block

8.16   Regularity: slightly irregular
            Rate: atrial rate 64 beats per minute; ventricular rate 32 beats
                        per minute
            P Waves: uniform; slight irregularity of the P–P interval (see
                        note); consistently two P waves for every QRS complex
            PRI: .20 seconds
            QRS: .12 seconds
            Interp: Classical Second Degree Heart Block (Mobitz II) with
                        2:1 conduction
            Note: A rhythm with a consistent 2:1 conduction ratio usu-
                        ally produces a regular rhythm. In this strip, however,
                        the presence of an underlying sinus arrhythmia results
                        in an irregular P–P, with an ultimate irregularity of the
                        ventricular response.

8.17   Regularity: regular
            Rate: atrial rate 100 beats per minute; ventricular rate 24
                        beats per minute
            P Waves: uniform; regular P–P interval; more P waves than QRS
                        complexes
            PRI: the P waves are not associated with the QRS complexes
            QRS: .08 seconds
            Interp: Third Degree Heart Block (CHB) with a junctional es-
                        cape focus
            Note: The ventricular rate in this strip is slower than the usual
                        junctional rate, but the QRS measurement of .10 sec-
                        onds could not have been produced by a ventricular
                        pacemaker; thus, the escape focus must have been
                        junctional.

8.18   Regularity: irregular with a pattern of grouped beating
            Rate: atrial rate 107 beats per minute; ventricular rate ap-
                        proximately 90 beats per minute
            P Waves: uniform; regular P–P interval; more P waves than QRS
                        complexes
            PRI: changes; progressively lengthens from .20 seconds to
                        .36 seconds
            QRS: .10 seconds
            Interp: Wenckebach (Second Degree Heart Block Mobitz I)

Practice Sheet 9:
Answers

9.1   Regularity: regular underlying rhythm interrupted by ectopics
         Rate: 75 beats per minute
         P Waves: uniform; regular P–P interval
         PRI: .18 seconds
         QRS: .12 seconds in underlying complex:
                     .12 seconds in ectopics
                     ectopics have bizarre configuration
         Interp: Sinus Rhythm (with wide QRS) with two PVCs

9.2   Regularity: regular underlying rhythm interrupted by ectopics in a
                     pattern of grouped beating
         Rate: 39 beats per minute according to visible P waves; true
                     sinus rate is probably 78 beats per minute
         P Waves: uniform; regular P–P interval
         PRI: .18 seconds
         QRS: .08 seconds in underlying rhythm: .14 seconds in ectopic
         Interp: Sinus Rhythm with bigeminy of PVCs

9.3   Regularity: regular underlying rhythm interrupted by an ectopic
         Rate: 60 beats per minute
         P Waves: uniform; regular P–P interval
         PRI: .20 seconds
         QRS: .10 seconds in underlying rhythm;
                     .18 seconds in ectopic;
                     ectopic has bizarre configuration
         Interp: Sinus Rhythm (borderline bradycardia) with one PVC

9.4   Regularity: slightly irregular
         Rate: approximately 170 beats per minute
         P Waves: not visible
         PRI: none
         QRS: .12 seconds; configuration is bizarre
         Interp: Ventricular Tachycardia

9.5   Regularity: regular underlying rhythm interrupted by ectopics
         Rate: 79 beats per minute (underlying rhythm)
         P Waves: uniform; regular P–P interval
         PRI: .16 seconds
         QRS: .06 seconds in underlying rhythm;
                     .20 seconds in ectopics;
                     ectopics have bizarre configuration
         Interp: Sinus Rhythm with three unifocal PVCs (possibly tri-
                     geminy)

9.6
Regularity: totally chaotic baseline
Rate: cannot be determined
P Waves: none
PRI: none
QRS: none
Interp: Ventricular Fibrillation

9.7
Regularity: regular underlying rhythm interrupted by ectopics
Rate: 107 beats per minute (underlying rhythm)
P Waves: uniform; regular P–P interval interrupted by ectopics
PRI: .14 seconds
QRS: .10 seconds in underlying rhythm;
.14 seconds in ectopics;
ectopics have bizarre configuration
Interp: Sinus Rhythm with two unifocal PVCs and a short burst of Ventricular Tachycardia

9.8
Regularity: regular
Rate: 167 beats per minute
P Waves: not visible
PRI: none
QRS: .16 seconds; bizarre configuration
Interp: Ventricular Tachycardia

9.9
Regularity: regular underlying rhythm interrupted by ectopics
Rate: 83 beats per minute
P Waves: uniform; regular P–P interval
PRI: .16 seconds
QRS: .14 seconds in underlying rhythm;
.16 seconds in ectopics;
ectopics have bizarre configuration
Interp: Sinus Rhythm (with wide QRS) with two multifocal PVCs

9.10
Regularity: regular
Rate: 150 beats per minute
P Waves: not visible
PRI: none
QRS: .20 seconds; bizarre configuration
Interp: Ventricular Tachycardia

9.11
Regularity: regular underlying rhythm interrupted by ectopics
Rate: 100 beats per minute
P Waves: uniform; regular P–P interval
PRI: .14 seconds
QRS: .06 seconds in underlying rhythm;
.12 seconds in ectopics;
ectopics have bizarre configuration
Interp: Sinus Tachycardia with three unifocal PVCs

9.12   Regularity: regular
                       Rate: 167 beats per minute
                       P Waves: not visible
                       PRI: none
                       QRS: .16 seconds; bizarre configuration
                       Interp: Ventricular Tachycardia

9.13   Regularity: regular underlying rhythm interrupted by ectopics in a pattern of grouped beating
                       Rate: 38 beats per minute according to visible P waves; true sinus rate is probably 76 beats per minute
                       P Waves: uniform; regular P–P interval
                       PRI: .20 seconds
                       QRS: .10 seconds in underlying rhythm; .14 seconds in ectopics; ectopics have bizarre configuration
                       Interp: Sinus Rhythm with bigeminy of PVCs

9.14   Regularity: totally chaotic baseline
                       Rate: cannot be determined
                       P Waves: none
                       PRI: none
                       QRS: none
                       Interp: Ventricular Fibrillation

9.15   Regularity: regular
                       Rate: 40 beats per minute
                       P Waves: none
                       PRI: none
                       QRS: .20 seconds; bizarre configuration
                       Interp: Idioventricular Rhythm

9.16   Regularity: regular underlying rhythm interrupted by ectopics
                       Rate: 94 beats per minute
                       P Waves: uniform; regular P–P interval
                       PRI: .12 seconds
                       QRS: .10 seconds in underlying rhythm; .16 seconds in ectopics ectopics have bizarre configuration; ectopics occur consecutively
                       Interp: Sinus Rhythm with a run of PVCs

9.17   Regularity: regular
                       Rate: 150 beats per minute
                       P Waves: are visible through QRS complexes, but do not appear related to QRS complexes

PRI:	none
QRS:	.28 seconds; bizarre configuration
Interp:	Ventricular Tachycardia

9.18
Regularity: totally chaotic baseline
Rate: cannot be determined
P Waves: none
PRI: none
QRS: none
Interp: Ventricular Fibrillation

9.19
Regularity: regular underlying rhythm interrupted by an ectopic
Rate: 79 beats per minute
P Waves: uniform; regular P–P interval
PRI: .16 seconds
QRS: .08 seconds
Interp: Sinus Rhythm with one PVC

9.20
Regularity: totally chaotic baseline
Rate: cannot be determined
P Waves: none
PRI: none
QRS: none
Interp: Ventricular Fibrillation

9.21
Regularity: first part of rhythm is regular, but then changes into a totally chaotic pattern
Rate: 167 beats per minute (first part of strip)
P Waves: not visible
PRI: none
QRS: .20 seconds in first part of strip; cannot be identified in latter part of strip
Interp: Ventricular Tachycardia changing into Ventricular Fibrillation

9.22
Regularity: regular underlying rhythm interrupted by ectopics
Rate: 79 beats per minute
P Waves: uniform; regular P–P interval
PRI: .20 seconds
QRS: .10 seconds in underlying rhythm; .14 seconds in ectopics; ectopics have bizarre configuration
Interp: Sinus Rhythm with two unifocal PVCs

9.23
Regularity: regular
Rate: 42 beats per minute
P Waves: none

	PRI:	none
	QRS:	.12 seconds; bizarre configuration
	Interp:	Idioventricular Rhythm

9.24   Regularity: slightly irregular rhythm interrupted by ectopics
        Rate: approximately 65 beats per minute
        P Waves: uniform; slightly irregular P–P interval
        PRI: .18 seconds and constant
        QRS: .14 seconds in underlying rhythm;
                    .16 seconds in ectopics;
                    ectopics have bizarre configuration
        Interp: Sinus Arrhythmia (with wide QRS) with two unifocal
                    PVCs

9.25   Regularity: totally chaotic baseline
        Rate: cannot be determined
        P Waves: none
        PRI: none
        QRS: none
        Interp: Ventricular Fibrillation

9.26   Regularity: regular underlying rhythm interrupted by ectopics
        Rate: 83 beats per minute
        P Waves: uniform; regular P–P interval
        PRI: .14 seconds
        QRS: .12 seconds in underlying rhythm;
                    .16 seconds in ectopics;
                    ectopics have bizarre configuration
        Interp: Sinus Rhythm (with wide QRS) with two unifocal PVCs

9.27   Regularity: regular
        Rate: 37 beats per minute
        P Waves: none
        PRI: none
        QRS: .20 seconds; bizarre configuration
        Interp: Idioventricular Rhythm

9.28   Regularity: totally chaotic baseline
        Rate: cannot be determined
        P Waves: none
        PRI: none
        QRS: none
        Interp: Ventricular Fibrillation

9.29   Regularity: irregular underlying rhythm interrupted by an ectopic
        Rate: approximately 60 beats per minute (underlying rhythm)
        P Waves: uniform; regular P–P interval
        PRI: .16 seconds and constant

QRS:	.10 seconds in underlying rhythm; .12 seconds in ectopic; ectopic has bizarre configuration
Interp:	Sinus Rhythm with one PVC

9.30

Regularity:	regular
Rate:	188 beats per minute
P Waves:	none
PRI:	none
QRS:	.20 seconds; bizarre configuration
Interp:	Ventricular Tachycardia

9.31

Regularity:	regular underlying rhythm interrupted by ectopics
Rate:	94 beats per minute (underlying rhythm)
P Waves:	uniform; regular P–P interval
PRI:	.24 seconds and constant
QRS:	.10 seconds in underlying rhythm; .12–.20 seconds in ectopics; ectopics occur consecutively; ectopics have bizarre configuration
Interp:	Sinus Rhythm with First Degree Heart Block, with one PVC and run of PVCs

9.32

Regularity:	regular
Rate:	167 beats per minute
P Waves:	not visible
PRI:	none
QRS:	.14 seconds; bizarre configuration
Interp:	Ventricular Tachycardia

9.33

Regularity:	regular underlying rhythm interrupted by ectopics
Rate:	83 beats per minute (underlying rhythm)
P Waves:	uniform; regular P–P interval
PRI:	.16 seconds
QRS:	.10 seconds in underlying rhythm; .16 seconds in ectopics; ectopics have bizarre configuration
Interp:	Sinus Rhythm with two unifocal PVCs

9.34

Regularity:	irregular underlying rhythm interrupted by ectopics in pattern of grouped beating
Rate:	approximately 30 beats per minute (underlying rhythm)
P Waves:	not discernible; undulations present
PRI:	none
QRS:	.10 seconds in underlying rhythm; .14 seconds in ectopics; ectopics have bizarre configuration
Interp:	Atrial Fibrillation with bigeminy of unifocal PVCs

Practice Sheet 10:
Answers

10.1   Regularity: regular
        Rate: 60 beats per minute
        P Waves: uniform; regular P–P interval
        PRI: .28 seconds and constant
        QRS: .14 seconds
        Interp: Sinus Rhythm (borderline bradycardia) with First De-
                    gree Heart Block (with wide QRS)

10.2   Regularity: irregular
        Rate: approximately 50 beats per minute
        P Waves: not discernible; undulations present
        PRI: none
        QRS: .10 seconds
        Interp: controlled Atrial Fibrillation (bradycardia)

10.3   Regularity: regular underlying rhythm interrupted by ectopics
        Rate: 79 beats per minute
        P Waves: uniform; regular P–P interval
        PRI: .20 seconds and constant
        QRS: .08 seconds in underlying rhythm;
                    .12 seconds in ectopic beats; ectopic complexes differ
                    from normal complexes
        Interp: Sinus Rhythm with two unifocal PVCs

10.4   Regularity: regular underlying rhythm interrupted by ectopics in a
                    pattern of grouped beating
        Rate: 50 beats per minute according to visible P waves; true
                    sinus rate is probably 100 beats per minute
        P Waves: uniform; regular P–P interval
        PRI: .20 seconds and constant
        QRS: .14 seconds in underlying rhythm;
                    .14 seconds in ectopic beats; ectopic QRSs have a dif-
                    ferent configuration than normal QRSs
        Interp: Sinus Rhythm (with a wide QRS) with bigeminy of PVCs

10.5   Regularity: irregular R–R interval; regular P–P interval
        Rate: atrial rate 300 beats per minute
                    ventricular rate approximately 90 beats per minute
        P Waves: uniform; sawtooth appearance; regular P–P interval;
                    more P waves than QRS complexes
        PRI: none
        QRS: .08 seconds
        Interp: Atrial Flutter with variable block

10.6
Regularity:	regular underlying rhythm interrupted by ectopics
Rate:	60 beats per minute
P Waves:	uniform; regular P–P interval
PRI:	.22 seconds and constant
QRS:	.08 seconds in underlying rhythm;
	.12 seconds in ectopic beats; ectopic QRSs are bizarre
Interp:	Sinus Rhythm (borderline bradycardia) with First Degree Heart Block and two unifocal PVCs

10.7
Regularity:	regular
Rate:	48 beats per minute
P Waves:	uniform and upright; regular P–P interval
PRI:	.16 seconds and constant
QRS:	.10 seconds
Interp:	Sinus Bradycardia

10.8
Regularity:	regular underlying rhythm interrupted by ectopics in a pattern of grouped beating
Rate:	atrial rate 300 beats per minute;
	ventricular rate 40 beats per minute
P Waves:	uniform; sawtooth appearance; regular P–P interval; more P waves than QRS complexes
PRI:	none
QRS:	.06 seconds in underlying rhythm;
	.12 seconds in ectopics;
	ectopics have bizarre configuration
Interp:	Atrial Flutter with bigeminy of PVCs

10.9
Regularity:	irregular underlying rhythm interrupted by ectopics in a pattern of grouped beating
Rate:	approximately 40 beats per minute (excluding ectopics)
P Waves:	not discernible; undulations present
PRI:	none
QRS:	.10 seconds in underlying rhythm;
	.14 seconds in ectopics;
	ectopics have bizarre configuration
Interp:	Atrial Fibrillation with bigeminy of PVCs

10.10
Regularity:	irregular
Rate:	approximately 120 beats per minute
P Waves:	not discernible; undulations present
PRI:	none
QRS:	.10 seconds
Interp:	uncontrolled Atrial Fibrillation

10.11
Regularity:	totally chaotic baseline
Rate:	cannot determine

	P Waves:	none
	PRI:	none
	QRS:	none
	Interp:	Ventricular Fibrillation

10.12   Regularity: regular
Rate: atrial rate 300 beats per minute;
                 ventricular rate 75 beats per minute
P Waves: uniform, sawtooth appearance; regular P–P interval;
                 more P waves than QRS complexes
PRI: none
QRS: .10 seconds
Interp: Atrial Flutter with 4:1 response

10.13   Regularity: regular
Rate: 150 beats per minute
P Waves: not visible
PRI: none
QRS: .16 seconds; bizarre configuration
Interp: Ventricular Tachycardia

10.14   Regularity: slightly irregular
Rate: approximately 58 beats per minute
P Waves: uniform; irregular P–P interval
PRI: .16 seconds and constant
QRS: .16 seconds
Interp: Sinus Bradycardia (with a slight sinus arrhythmia)

10.15   Regularity: totally chaotic baseline
Rate: cannot determine
P Waves: none
PRI: none
QRS: none
Interp: Ventricular Fibrillation

10.16   Regularity: regular underlying rhythm interrupted by ectopics
Rate: 100 beats per minute
P Waves: uniform P waves; regular P–P interval
PRI: .22 seconds and constant
QRS: .12 seconds in underlying rhythm;
                 .20 seconds in ectopics;
                 ectopics have bizarre configuration
Interp: Sinus Rhythm (with wide QRS) with First Degree Heart
              Block and three unifocal PVCs (possibly quadrigeminy)

10.17   Regularity: irregular
Rate: approximately 170 beats per minute
P Waves: not discernible; undulations present
PRI: none
QRS: .08 seconds
Interp: uncontrolled Atrial Fibrillation

10.18   Regularity: regular underlying rhythm interrupted by ectopics
Rate: 107 beats per minute
P Waves: uniform P waves in underlying rhythm; shape of P waves changes in ectopic beats
PRI: .14 seconds
QRS: .08 seconds in both underlying rhythm and ectopics
Interp: Sinus Tachycardia with two PACs

10.19   Regularity: regular underlying rhythm interrupted by ectopics
Rate: 83 beats per minute
P Waves: uniform; regular P–P interval
PRI: .20 seconds
QRS: .08 seconds in underlying beats;
             .16 seconds in ectopics
Interp: Sinus Rhythm with three unifocal PVCs (possibly trigeminy)

10.20   Regularity: regular
Rate: 68 beats per minute
P Waves: uniform; regular P–P interval
PRI: .44 seconds and constant
QRS: .12 seconds
Interp: Sinus Rhythm with First Degree Heart Block (with wide QRS)

10.21   Regularity: regular underlying rhythm interrupted by ectopics
Rate: 83 beats per minute
P Waves: uniform; regular P–P interval
PRI: .12 seconds
QRS: .12 seconds in underlying rhythm;
             .12 seconds in ectopics;
             ectopics have bizarre configuration
Interp: Sinus Rhythm with multifocal PVCs

10.22   Regularity: regular
Rate: atrial rate 96 beats per minute; ventricular rate 48 beats per minute
P Waves: upright and uniform; regular P–P interval
PRI: .20 seconds
QRS: .16 seconds
Interp: Classical Second Degree Heart Block (2:1); Mobitz II

10.23   Regularity: regular underlying rhythm interrupted by ectopics in a
                      pattern of grouped beating
          Rate: 56 beats per minute according to visible P waves; true
                      sinus rate is probably 112 beats per minute
          P Waves: uniform; regular P–P interval
          PRI: .12 seconds
          QRS: .08 seconds in underlying rhythm;
                      .12 seconds in ectopics;
                      ectopics have bizarre configuration
          Interp: Sinus Rhythm with bigeminy of PVCs

10.24   Regularity: irregular
          Rate: approximately 60 beats per minute
          P Waves: not discernible; undulations present
          PRI: none
          QRS: .12 seconds
          Interp: controlled Atrial Fibrillation (with wide QRS)

10.25   Regularity: regular
          Rate: 94 beats per minute
          P Waves: uniform and upright; regular P–P interval
          PRI: .20 seconds and constant
          QRS: .10 seconds
          Interp: Normal Sinus Rhythm

10.26   Regularity: irregular rhythm interrupted by ectopics
          Rate: approximately 60 beats per minute; if ectopics are in-
                      cluded, the rate is 90 beats per minute
          P Waves: not discernible; undulations present
          PRI: none
          QRS: .08 seconds in underlying rhythm;
                      .14 seconds in ectopics;
                      ectopics have bizarre configuration
          Interp: Atrial Fibrillation with three unifocal PVCs

10.27   Regularity: regular underlying rhythm interrupted by ectopics
          Rate: 103 beats per minute
          P Waves: uniform in underlying rhythm; shape changes in ec-
                      topic beats
          PRI: .16 seconds
          QRS: .10 seconds in both underlying rhythm and ectopics;
                      shape does not change in ectopics
          Interp: Sinus Tachycardia with two PACs

10.28   Regularity: regular underlying rhythm interrupted by ectopics in a
                      pattern of grouped beating
          Rate: 54 beats per minute according to visible P waves; true
                      sinus rate is probably 108 beats per minute

P Waves:	uniform; regular P–P interval
PRI:	.16 seconds and constant
QRS:	.12 seconds in both underlying rhythm and ectopics; ectopics have bizarre configuration
Interp:	Sinus Rhythm (with a wide QRS) with bigeminy of PVCs

10.29

Regularity:	regular
Rate:	79 beats per minute
P Waves:	upright and uniform; regular P–P interval
PRI:	.20 seconds and constant
QRS:	.08 seconds
Interp:	Normal Sinus Rhythm

10.30

Regularity:	irregular underlying rhythm interrupted by ectopics
Rate:	approximately 70 beats per minute; if ectopics are included rate is 110 beats per minute
P Waves:	not discernible; undulations present
PRI:	none
QRS:	.12 seconds in underlying rhythm; .14 seconds in ectopics; ectopics have bizarre configurations
Interp:	Atrial Fibrillation (with wide QRS) with multifocal PVCs and one PVC couplet

10.31

Regularity:	irregular
Rate:	approximately 60 beats per minute
P Waves:	not discernible; undulations present
PRI:	none
QRS:	.08 seconds
Interp:	controlled Atrial Fibrillation

10.32

Regularity:	irregular
Rate:	atrial rate 300 beats per minute; ventricular rate 80 beats per minute
P Waves:	uniform; sawtooth appearance; regular P–P interval; more P waves than QRS complexes
PRI:	none
QRS:	.08 seconds
Interp:	Atrial Flutter with variable block

10.33

Regularity:	irregular
Rate:	atrial rate 94 beats per minute; ventricular rate 60 beats per minute
P Waves:	uniform; regular P–P interval; occasional nonconducted P waves
PRI:	changing; progressive lengthening from .20 seconds to .26 seconds

	QRS:	.08 seconds
	Interp:	Wenckebach (second degree Mobitz I)

10.34	Regularity:	regular
	Rate:	136 beats per minute
	P Waves:	uniform and upright; regular P–P interval
	PRI:	.12 seconds and constant
	QRS:	.06 seconds
	Interp:	Sinus Tachycardia

10.35	Regularity:	regular
	Rate:	83 beats per minute
	P Waves:	uniform and upright; regular P–P interval
	PRI:	.28 seconds and constant
	QRS:	.08 seconds
	Interp:	Sinus Rhythm with First Degree Heart Block

10.36	Regularity:	regular
	Rate:	136 beats per minute
	P Waves:	uniform; regular P–P interval
	PRI:	.14 seconds (partially obscured by T wave)
	QRS:	.10 seconds
	Interp:	Sinus Tachycardia

10.37	Regularity:	regular underlying rhythm interrupted by ectopics
	Rate:	atrial rate 284 beats per minute; ventricular rate 71 beats per minute
	P Waves:	uniform; sawtooth appearance; regular P–P interval; consistently four P waves for every QRS complex
	PRI:	none
	QRS:	.10 seconds in underlying rhythm; .16 seconds in ectopics; ectopics have bizarre configuration
	Interp:	Atrial Flutter with 4:1 response and two unifocal PVCs

10.38	Regularity:	regular underlying rhythm interrupted by ectopics
	Rate:	100 beats per minute
	P Waves:	uniform; regular P–P interval
	PRI:	.20 seconds and constant
	QRS:	.12 seconds in underlying rhythm and in ectopics; ectopics have bizarre configuration
	Interp:	Sinus Tachycardia (with a wide QRS) with two unifocal PVCs

10.39
Regularity:	regular
Rate:	71 beats per minute
P Waves:	uniform; regular P–P interval
PRI:	.14 seconds and constant
QRS:	.10 seconds
Interp:	Normal Sinus Rhythm

10.40
Regularity:	regular
Rate:	300 beats per minute
P Waves:	not visible
PRI:	none
QRS:	.16 seconds; bizarre configuration
Interp:	Ventricular Tachycardia (Ventricular Flutter)

10.41
Regularity:	irregular
Rate:	approximately 70 beats per minute
P Waves:	not discernible; undulations present
PRI:	none
QRS:	.08 seconds
Interp:	controlled Atrial Fibrillation

10.42
Regularity:	regular underlying rhythm interrupted by ectopic (rate changes following ectopic)
Rate:	approximately 80 beats per minute
P Waves:	uniform in underlying rhythm; configuration changes in ectopic beat
PRI:	.16 seconds
QRS:	.12 seconds
Interp:	Sinus Rhythm (with wide QRS) with one PAC

10.43
Regularity:	regular
Rate:	107 beats per minute
P Waves:	uniform; regular P–P interval
PRI:	.14 seconds
QRS:	.16 seconds
Interp:	Sinus Tachycardia (with wide QRS)

10.44
Regularity:	irregular
Rate:	approximately 110 beats per minute
P Waves:	not discernible; undulations present
PRI:	none
QRS:	.06 seconds
Interp:	uncontrolled Atrial Fibrillation

10.45
Regularity:	regular underlying rhythm interrupted by ectopics
Rate:	88 beats per minute
P Waves:	uniform; regular P–P interval

	PRI:	.20 seconds
	QRS:	.10 seconds in underlying rhythm; .14 seconds in ectopic; ectopic has bizarre configuration
	Interp:	Sinus Rhythm with one PVC

10.46   Regularity: regular
        Rate: 125 beats per minute
        P Waves: uniform; regular P–P interval
        PRI: .16 seconds
        QRS: .10 seconds
        Interp: Sinus Tachycardia

10.47   Regularity: irregular
        Rate: approximately 70 beats per minute
        P Waves: not discernible; undulations present
        PRI: none
        QRS: .10 seconds
        Interp: controlled Atrial Fibrillation

10.48   Regularity: regular
        Rate: 52 beats per minute
        P Waves: uniform; regular P–P interval
        PRI: .20 seconds and constant
        QRS: .08 seconds
        Interp: Sinus Bradycardia

10.49   Regularity: irregular
        Rate: atrial rate 375 beats per minute; ventricular rate approximately 100 beats per minute
        P Waves: uniform; sawtooth appearance; regular P–P interval; more P waves than QRS complexes
        PRI: none
        QRS: .08 seconds; complexes partially obscured by flutter waves
        Interp: Atrial Flutter with variable response

10.50   Regularity: regular
        Rate: 115 beats per minute
        P Waves: none visible
        PRI: none
        QRS: .08 seconds
        Interp: Junctional Tachycardia

10.51   Regularity: regular
        Rate: 107 beats per minute
        P Waves: uniform; regular P–P interval

PRI: .12 seconds and constant
QRS: .12 seconds
Interp: Sinus Tachycardia (with wide QRS)

10.52   Regularity: irregular
           Rate: atrial rate 300 beats per minute; ventricular rate 80
                       beats per minute
           P Waves: uniform; sawtooth appearance; regular P–P interval;
                       more P waves than QRS complexes
           PRI: none
           QRS: .08 seconds (complexes partially obscured by flutter
                       waves)
           Interp: Atrial Flutter with variable response

10.53   Regularity: regular underlying rhythm interrupted by ectopics
           Rate: 103 beats per minute (underlying rhythm)
           P Waves: uniform; regular P–P interval
           PRI: .14 seconds
           QRS: .06 seconds in underlying rhythm;
                       .12 seconds in ectopics;
                       ectopics have bizarre configuration
           Interp: Sinus Tachycardia with trigeminy of PVCs

10.54   Regularity: irregular
           Rate: approximately 80 beats per minute
           P Waves: not discernible; undulations present
           PRI: none
           QRS: .08 seconds
           Interp: controlled Atrial Fibrillation

10.55   Regularity: regular
           Rate: 167 beats per minute
           P Waves: not visible
           PRI: none
           QRS: .20 seconds; bizarre configuration
           Interp: Ventricular Tachycardia

10.56   Regularity: irregular
           Rate: atrial rate 300 beats per minute; ventricular rate ap-
                       proximately 140 beats per minute
           P Waves: uniform; sawtooth configuration; regular P–P interval;
                       more P waves than QRS complexes.
           PRI: none
           QRS: .08 seconds (complexes partially obscured by flutter
                       waves)
           Interp: Atrial Flutter with variable response

10.57   Regularity: totally chaotic baseline
         Rate: unable to determine
         P Waves: none
         PRI: none
         QRS: none
         Interp: Ventricular Fibrillation

10.58   Regularity: irregular
         Rate: approximately 110 beats per minute
         P Waves: not discernible; undulations present
         PRI: none
         QRS: .08 seconds
         Interp: uncontrolled Atrial Fibrillation

10.59   Regularity: regular
         Rate: 107 beats per minute
         P Waves: uniform; regular P–P interval
         PRI: .20 seconds
         QRS: .12 seconds
         Interp: Sinus Tachycardia (with wide QRS)

10.60   Regularity: irregular rhythm is interrupted by an ectopic
         Rate: approximately 70 beats per minute
         P Waves: uniform; irregular P–P interval; shape of P wave
                     changes in ectopic beat
         PRI: .14 seconds
         QRS: .12 seconds in both underlying beat and ectopic;
                     shape of complexes consistent
         Interp: Sinus Arrhythmia with one PAC

10.61   Regularity: irregular
         Rate: approximately 170 beats per minute
         P Waves: not discernible
         PRI: none
         QRS: .10 seconds
         Interp: uncontrolled Atrial Fibrillation

10.62   Regularity: regular underlying rhythm interrupted by ectopics
         Rate: 75 beats per minute
         P Waves: uniform in underlying rhythm; regular P–P interval
         PRI: .20 seconds
         QRS: .14 seconds in underlying complexes;
                     .16 seconds in ectopics;
                     ectopics differ in configuration from underlying com-
                     plexes
         Interp: Sinus Rhythm (with wide QRS) with two unifocal PVCs

10.63   Regularity: irregular
           Rate: approximately 130 beats per minute
           P Waves: not discernible; undulations present
           PRI: none
           QRS: .10 seconds
           Interp: uncontrolled Atrial Fibrillation

10.64   Regularity: regular
           Rate: atrial rate 300 beats per minute;
                       ventricular rate 75 beats per minute
           P Waves: uniform; sawtooth appearance; regular P–P interval;
                       consistently four P waves for every QRS complex
           PRI: none
           QRS: .08 seconds
           Interp: Atrial Flutter with 4:1 response

10.65   Regularity: regular
           Rate: 71 beats per minute
           P Waves: uniform; regular P–P interval
           PRI: .24 seconds and constant
           QRS: .10 seconds
           Interp: Sinus Rhythm with first Degree Heart Block

10.66   Regularity: regular
           Rate: 111 beats per minute
           P Waves: uniform; regular P–P interval
           PRI: .12 seconds
           QRS: .08 seconds
           Interp: Sinus Tachycardia

10.67   Regularity: irregular
           Rate: approximately 90 beats per minute
           P Waves: not discernible; undulations present
           PRI: none
           QRS: .08 seconds
           Interp: controlled Atrial Fibrillation

10.68   Regularity: irregular
           Rate: approximately 70 beats per minute
           P Waves: uniform; irregular P–P interval
           PRI: .12 seconds
           QRS: .08 seconds
           Interp: Sinus Arrhythmia

10.69   Regularity: irregular underlying rhythm interrupted by ectopics
           Rate: approximately 90 beats per minute
           P Waves: not discernible; undulations present

PRI: none
QRS: .12 seconds in underlying complexes;
            .14 seconds in ectopics;
            ectopics have bizarre configuration
Interp: Atrial Fibrillation (with wide QRS) with runs of PVCs

10.70   Regularity: totally chaotic baseline
            Rate: cannot be determined
            P Waves: none
            PRI: none
            QRS: none
            Interp: Ventricular Fibrillation

10.71   Regularity: regular underlying rhythm interrupted by ectopics
            Rate: 88 beats per minute
            P Waves: uniform in underlying rhythm; regular P–P interval;
                        shape changes in ectopic beats
            PRI: .16 seconds
            QRS: .14 seconds
            Interp: Sinus Rhythm (with wide QRS) with one PAC

10.72   Regularity: regular
            Rate: 91 beats per minute
            P Waves: uniform; regular P–P interval
            PRI: .28 seconds and constant
            QRS: .08 seconds
            Interp: Sinus Rhythm with First Degree Heart Block

10.73   Regularity: regular
            Rate: 150 beats per minute
            P Waves: not discernible
            PRI: none
            QRS: .08 seconds
            Interp: Supraventricular Tachycardia

10.74   Regularity: totally chaotic baseline
            Rate: cannot be determined
            P Waves: none
            PRI: none
            QRS: none
            Interp: Ventricular Fibrillation

10.75   Regularity: irregular
            Rate: approximately 110 beats per minute
            P Waves: not discernible; undulations present
            PRI: none
            QRS: .12 seconds
            Interp: uncontrolled Atrial Fibrillation (with wide QRS)

10.76

Regularity: regular
Rate: 56 beats per minute
P Waves: not visible
PRI: none
QRS: .16 seconds; configuration is bizarre
Interp: accelerated Idioventricular Rhythm
Note: This rhythm fits all of the rules for Idioventricular Rhythm except that the rate is faster than you would expect it to be, but not as fast as you would think a Ventricular Tachycardia would be. This patient may have been in an Idioventricular Rhythm at a slower rate, and then received a drug to make the rate increase and improve his/her condition.

10.77

Regularity: regular
Rate: atrial rate 260 beats per minute; ventricular rate 65 beats per minute
P Waves: uniform; sawtooth appearance; regular P–P interval; consistently four P waves for every QRS complex
PRI: none
QRS: .10 seconds
Interp: Atrial Flutter with 4:1 block

10.78

Regularity: irregular underlying rhythm interrupted by ectopics
Rate: approximately 60 beats per minute
P Waves: not discernible; undulations present
PRI: none
QRS: .10 seconds in underlying rhythm; .14 seconds in ectopic; ectopic has bizarre configuration
Interp: controlled Atrial Fibrillation with one PVC

10.79

Regularity: regular underlying rhythm interrupted by ectopics
Rate: 81 beats per minute
P Waves: uniform; regular P–P interval
PRI: .14 seconds
QRS: .12 seconds in underlying rhythm; .14 seconds in ectopic; ectopic has bizarre configuration
Interp: Sinus Rhythm with one PVC

10.80

Regularity: irregular
Rate: atrial rate 300 beats per minute; ventricular rate approximately 80 beats per minute
P Waves: uniform; sawtooth appearance; regular P–P interval; more P waves than QRS complexes
PRI: none
QRS: .10 seconds
Interp: Atrial Flutter with variable block

10.81   Regularity: totally chaotic baseline
         Rate: cannot be determined
         P Waves: none
         PRI: none
         QRS: none
         Interp: Ventricular Fibrillation

10.82   Regularity: irregular
         Rate: atrial rate 56 beats per minute;
                     ventricular rate 50 beats per minute
         P Waves: uniform; regular P–P interval; occasional nonconducted P waves
         PRI: changing PRI; progressively lengthens from .28 seconds to .40 seconds
         QRS: .08 seconds
         Interp: Wenckebach (Second Degree Heart Block Mobitz I)

10.83   Regularity: irregular rhythm interrupted by ectopics
         Rate: approximately 60 beats per minute;
                     (underlying rhythm)
         P Waves: uniform; irregular P–P interval
         PRI: .20 seconds
         QRS: .04 seconds in underlying rhythm;
                     .16 seconds in ectopics;
                     ectopics have bizarre configuration;
                     ectopics have different shapes than each other
         Interp: Sinus Arrhythmia with multifocal PVCs

10.84   Regularity: regular
         Rate: atrial rate 65 beats per minute
                     ventricular rate 29 beats per minute
         P Waves: uniform; regular P–P interval; more P waves than QRS complexes
         PRI: P waves are not associated with QRS complexes
         QRS: .20 seconds; bizarre configuration
         Interp: Third Degree Heart Block (CHB) with ventricular escape focus

10.85   Regularity: irregular
         Rate: approximately 90 beats per minute
         P Waves: not discernible; undulations present
         PRI: none
         QRS: .14 seconds
         Interp: controlled Atrial Fibrillation (with wide QRS)

10.86   Regularity: irregular
         Rate: approximately 120 beats per minute

	P Waves:	not discernible; undulations present
	PRI:	none
	QRS:	.10 seconds
	Interp:	uncontrolled Atrial Fibrillation

10.87
Regularity: regular
Rate: 75 beats per minute
P Waves: uniform and upright; regular P–P interval
PRI: .16 seconds and constant
QRS: .06 seconds
Interp: Normal Sinus Rhythm

10.88
Regularity: regular underlying rhythm interrupted by ectopics
Rate: 88 beats per minute
P Waves: uniform in underlying rhythm; form changes in ectopics
PRI: .12 seconds
QRS: .10 seconds in both underlying rhythm and ectopics; form does not change in ectopics
Interp: Sinus Rhythm with three PACs

10.89
Regularity: regular
Rate: 214 beats per minute
P Waves: not visible
PRI: none
QRS: .06 seconds
Interp: Supraventricular Tachycardia—probably Atrial Tachycardia
Note: Of all the supraventricular tachycardias, Atrial Tachycardia is the only one that can produce this ventricular rate with 1:1 conduction.

10.90
Regularity: regular
Rate: atrial rate 100 beats per minute; ventricular rate 44 beats per minute
P Waves: uniform; regular P–P interval; more P waves than QRS complexes
PRI: P waves are not associated with QRS complexes
QRS: .08 seconds
Interp: Third Degree Heart Block (CHB) with junctional escape focus

10.91
Regularity: regular, interrupted by ectopic
Rate: 83 beats per minute
P Waves: uniform; regular P–P interval
PRI: .24 seconds and constant in underlying rhythm; .12 seconds in ectopic
QRS: .14 seconds in underlying rhythm;

.14 seconds in ectopic

Interp: Sinus Rhythm (with wide QRS) with First Degree Heart Block and one PJC

10.92   Regularity: regular
Rate: 188 beats per minute
P Waves: none visible
PRI: not discernible
QRS: .10 seconds
Interp: Supraventricular Tachycardia

10.93   Regularity: slightly irregular
Rate: atrial rate 88 beats per minute; ventricular rate approximately 33 beats per minute
P Waves: uniform; regular P–P interval; more P waves than QRS complexes
PRI: none
QRS: .12 seconds
Interp: Third Degree Heart Block (CHB)

10.94   Regularity: totally chaotic baseline
Rate: unable to determine
P Waves: none visible
PRI: unable to determine
QRS: none visible
Interp: Ventricular Fibrillation (agonal rhythm)

10.95   Regularity: regular
Rate: 50 beats per minute
P Waves: uniform; regular P–P interval
PRI: .16 seconds and constant
QRS: .14 seconds
Interp: Sinus Bradycardia (with wide QRS)

10.96   Regularity: slightly irregular underlying rhythm interrupted by ectopics
Rate: approximately 107 beats per minute (underlying rhythm)
P Waves: not discernible (see note); ectopics not preceded by P waves
PRI: none
QRS: .08 seconds in underlying rhythm; .12 seconds and .16 seconds in ectopics
Interp: controlled Atrial Fibrillation with two multifocal PVCs
Note: small waves precede some QRS complexes, but by too short a distance to have been conducted; furthermore, these waves do not map out across the strip

10.97   Regularity: slightly irregular
       Rate: approximately 37 beats per minute
       P Waves: uniform; regular P–P interval
       PRI: .20 seconds and constant
       QRS: .08 seconds
       Interp: Sinus Bradycardia (with slight sinus arrhythmia)

10.98   Regularity: regular
       Rate: 125 beats per minute
       P Waves: uniform; regular P–P interval
       PRI: .16 seconds and constant (obscured slightly by T waves)
       QRS: .08 seconds
       Interp: Sinus Tachycardia

10.99   Regularity: slightly irregular
       Rate: approximately 110 beats per minute
       P Waves: shape changes from beat to beat
       PRI: approximately .16 seconds; varies slightly
       QRS: .12 seconds
       Interp: Wandering Pacemaker (with a wide QRS)

10.100 Regularity: slightly irregular
       Rate: approximately 170 beats per minute
       P Waves: none visible
       PRI: none
       QRS: .24 seconds
       Interp: Ventricular Tachycardia

10.101 Regularity: irregular
       Rate: approximately 130 beats per minute
       P Waves: none visible, undulations present
       PRI: none
       QRS: .06 seconds
       Interp: uncontrolled Atrial Fibrillation

10.102 Regularity: totally chaotic baseline
       Rate: not discernible
       P Waves: none visible
       PRI: none
       QRS: none visible
       Interp: Ventricular Fibrillation

10.103 Regularity: Regular underlying rhythm interrupted by ectopics in a
             pattern of grouped beating
       Rate: 68 beats per minute
       P Waves: uniform; regular P–P interval in underlying rhythm; no
             P waves preceding ectopics
       PRI: .16 seconds and constant

	QRS:	.08 seconds in underlying rhythm;
		.14 seconds in ectopics
	Interp:	Sinus Rhythm with bigeminy of PVCs

10.104

Regularity:	regular underlying rhythm interrupted by ectopics
Rate:	100 beats per minute
P Waves:	uniform; regular P–P interval;
	no P waves preceding ectopics
PRI:	.14 seconds and constant
QRS:	.12 seconds
Interp:	Sinus Tachycardia (with a wide QRS) and two PJCs

10.105

Regularity:	regular (very slightly irregular)
Rate:	approximately 70 beats per minute
P Waves:	uniform; regular P–P interval
PRI:	.30 seconds and constant
QRS:	.08 seconds
Interp:	Sinus Rhythm with First Degree Heart Block

10.106

Regularity:	totally chaotic baseline
Rate:	unable to determine
P Waves:	none visible
PRI:	none
QRS:	none visible
Interp:	Ventricular Fibrillation

10.107

Regularity:	slight irregular underlying rhythm interrupted by ectopics
Rate:	approximately 50 beats per minute
P Waves:	uniform and upright
PRI:	.08 seconds and constant
QRS:	.08 seconds in underlying rhythm;
	.20 seconds in ectopic
Interp:	Sinus Bradycardia with one PVC

10.108

Regularity:	irregular
Rate:	atrial rate 214 beats per minute; ventricular rate approximately 100 beats per minute
P Waves:	characteristic sawtooth pattern
PRI:	unable to determine
QRS:	.10 seconds
Interp:	Atrial Flutter with variable response

10.109

Regularity:	regular
Rate:	75 beats per minute
P Waves:	uniform; regular P–P interval
PRI:	.24 seconds and constant

| QRS: | .08 seconds |
| Interp: | Sinus Rhythm with First Degree Heart Block |

10.110
Regularity:	slightly irregular
Rate:	approximately 150 beats per minute
P Waves:	none visible
PRI:	none
QRS:	.12 seconds
Interp:	Ventricular Tachycardia

10.111
Regularity:	irregular
Rate:	approximately 70 beats per minute
P Waves:	none visible; undulations present
PRI:	none
QRS:	.14 seconds
Interp:	controlled Atrial Fibrillation (with wide QRS)

10.112
Regularity:	regular
Rate:	63 beats per minute
P Waves:	inverted before every QRS complex
PRI:	.12 seconds and constant
QRS:	.08 seconds
Interp:	Junctional Escape Rhythm

10.113
Regularity:	irregular
Rate:	approximately 150 beats per minute initially; then 0
P Waves:	none
PRI:	none
QRS:	approximately .20 seconds
Interp:	Ventricular Tachycardia into Asystole

10.114
Regularity:	irregular underlying rhythm with a pattern of grouped beating
Rate:	approximately 80 beats per minute
P Waves:	uniform; regular P–P interval
PRI:	varies; progressively lengthens until one P wave is not conducted
QRS:	.12 seconds
Interp:	Wenckebach (with wide QRS)

10.115
Regularity:	slightly irregular
Rate:	approximately 150 beats per minute
P Waves:	none visible
PRI:	none
QRS:	approximately .24 seconds
Interp:	Ventricular Tachycardia

10.116   Regularity: regular underlying rhythm interrupted by ectopic
          Rate: 63 beats per minute
          P Waves: uniform; regular P–P interval
          PRI: .20 seconds and constant
          QRS: .08 seconds in underlying rhythm;
                       .14 seconds in ectopic
          Interp: Sinus Rhythm with PVC

10.117   Regularity: regular underlying rhythm interrupted by ectopics in a
                       pattern of grouped beating
          Rate: 79 beats per minute
          P Waves: uniform; regular P–P interval; no P waves preceding
                       ectopics
          PRI: .22 seconds and constant
          QRS: .10 seconds in underlying rhythm;
                       .16 seconds in ectopics
          Interp: Sinus Rhythm with First Degree Heart Block with tri-
                       geminy of PVCs

10.118   Regularity: regular
          Rate: 150 beats per minute
          P Waves: none visible
          PRI: none
          QRS: .14 seconds
          Interp: Ventricular Tachycardia

10.119   Regularity: regular, interrupted by ectopics
          Rate: 79 beats per minute
          P Waves: uniform; regular P–P interval
          PRI: .20 seconds and constant
          QRS: .08 seconds in underlying rhythm;
                       .12 seconds in ectopics
          Interp: NSR with two PVCs

10.120   Regularity: slightly irregular
          Rate: approximately 107 beats per minute
          P Waves: none visible
          PRI: none
          QRS: .22 seconds
          Interp: slow Ventricular Tachycardia

10.121   Regularity: regular underlying rhythm interrupted by ectopic
          Rate: 83 beats per minute
          P Waves: uniform; regular P–P interval;
                       no P wave preceding ectopic
          PRI: .14 seconds and constant

QRS:	.08 seconds in underlying rhythm; .16 seconds in ectopic	
Interp:	Normal Sinus Rhythm with PVC	

10.122
Regularity:	regular underlying rhythm interrupted by ectopic
Rate:	77 beats per minute
P Waves:	uniform; regular P–P interval; no P wave preceding ectopic
PRI:	.26 seconds and constant
QRS:	.08 seconds in underlying rhythm; .12 seconds in ectopic
Interp:	Sinus Rhythm with First Degree Heart Block and one PVC

10.123
Regularity:	regular
Rate:	atrial rate 94 beats per minute; ventricular rate 47 beats per minute
P Waves:	uniform; regular P–P interval; three P waves for every QRS complex
PRI:	.28 seconds and constant
QRS:	.12 seconds
Interp:	Classical Second Degree Heart Block with 2:1 conduction (with wide QRS)

10.124
Regularity:	totally chaotic baseline
Rate:	unable to determine
P Waves:	none visible
PRI:	none
QRS:	none visible
Interp:	Ventricular Fibrillation into Asystole

10.125
Regularity:	regular underlying rhythm interrupted by ectopic
Rate:	88 beats per minute
P Waves:	uniform; regular P–P interval; ectopic is preceded by upright P wave
PRI:	.20 seconds and constant
QRS:	.08 seconds
Interp:	Normal Sinus Rhythm with one PAC

10.126
Regularity:	totally chaotic baseline
Rate:	unable to determine
P Waves:	none visible
PRI:	none
QRS:	none visible
Interp:	Ventricular Fibrillation

10.127
Regularity: regular
Rate: atrial rate 300 beats per minute;
ventricular rate 60 beats per minute
P Waves: characteristic sawtooth pattern
PRI: unable to determine
QRS: .08 seconds (slightly obscured by Flutter waves)
Interp: Atrial Flutter with 5:1 response

10.128
Regularity: irregular
Rate: approximately 110 beats per minute
P Waves: configuration varies from beat to beat
PRI: varies
QRS: .08 seconds
Interp: Wandering Pacemaker

10.129
Regularity: slightly irregular
Rate: approximately 48 beats per minute
P Waves: uniform; regular P–P interval
PRI: .16 seconds and constant
QRS: .10 seconds
Interp: Sinus Brady-Arrhythmia

10.130
Regularity: regular
Rate: 150 beats per minute
P Waves: none visible
PRI: none
QRS: .16 seconds
Interp: Ventricular Tachycardia

10.131
Regularity: slightly irregular
Rate: approximately 75 beats per minute
P Waves: shape changes from beat to beat
PRI: varies
QRS: .08 seconds
Interp: Wandering Pacemaker

10.132
Regularity: regular
Rate: 71 beats per minute
P Waves: uniform; regular P–P interval
PRI: .32 seconds and constant
QRS: .08 seconds
Interp: Sinus Rhythm with First Degree Heart Block

10.133
Regularity: regular underlying rhythm interrupted by ectopic
Rate: atrial rate 300 beats per minute;
ventricular rate 75 beats per minute

P Waves: characteristic sawtooth pattern
PRI: unable to determine
QRS: .08 seconds in underlying rhythm (slightly obscured by flutter waves); .16 seconds in ectopic
Interp: Atrial Flutter with 4:1 response, with one PVC

10.134   Regularity: regular underlying rhythm interrupted by ectopics in a pattern of grouped beating
Rate: approximately 70 beats per minute
P Waves: uniform; regular P–P interval; no P wave preceding ectopics
PRI: .16 seconds and constant
QRS: .10 seconds in underlying rhythm; .16 seconds in ectopics
Interp: Sinus Rhythm with bigeminy of PVCs

10.135   Regularity: irregular in a pattern of grouped beating
Rate: atrial rate 115 beats per minute; ventricular rate approximately 70 beats per minute
P Waves: uniform; regular P–P interval
PRI: varies; progressively lengthens until one P wave is not conducted
QRS: .10 seconds
Interp: Wenckebach

10.136   Regularity: regular underlying rhythm interrupted by ectopic
Rate: 103 beats per minute
P Waves: inverted preceding QRS complexes; no P waves preceding ectopics
PRI: .12 seconds and constant
QRS: .06 seconds in underlying rhythm; .12 seconds in ectopic
Interp: Junctional Tachycardia with PVC

10.137   Regularity: regular underlying rhythm interrupted by ectopics in a pattern of grouped beating
Rate: 79 beats per minute
P Waves: uniform in underlying rhythm; inverted P waves following QRS complexes of ectopics
PRI: .18 seconds and constant
QRS: .08 seconds in underlying rhythm; .08 seconds in ectopics
Interp: Sinus Rhythm with bigeminy of PJCs

10.138   Regularity: regular underlying rhythm interrupted by ectopic
Rate: 83 beats per minute
P Waves: uniform; regular P–P interval; ectopic is preceded by an upright P wave

PRI: .16 seconds and constant
QRS: .12 seconds in underlying rhythm;
              .12 seconds in ectopic
Interp: Sinus Rhythm (with wide QRS) with one PAC

10.139   Regularity: regular underlying rhythm interrupted by ectopics
          Rate: 94 beats per minute
          P Waves: uniform in underlying rhythm; no P waves preceding
                      ectopics
          PRI: .16 seconds and constant
          QRS: .08 seconds in underlying rhythm;
                      .16 seconds in ectopics
          Interp: NSR with bursts of Ventricular Tachycardia

10.140   Regularity: regular
          Rate: atrial rate 75 beats per minute;
                      ventricular rate 40 beats per minute
          P Waves: uniform; regular P–P interval
          PRI: none
          QRS: .08 seconds
          Interp: Third Degree Heart Block (CHB)

10.141   Regularity: regular
          Rate: 47 beats per minute
          P Waves: uniform; regular P–P interval
          PRI: .20 seconds and constant
          QRS: .08 seconds
          Interp: Sinus Bradycardia

10.142   Regularity: regular
          Rate: 125 beats per minute
          P Waves: none visible
          PRI: none
          QRS: .20 seconds
          Interp: slow Ventricular Tachycardia

10.143   Regularity: regular
          Rate: 94 beats per minute
          P Waves: inverted preceding QRS complex
          PRI: .12 seconds
          QRS: .12 seconds
          Interp: Accelerated Junctional Rhythm

10.144   Regularity: irregular
          Rate: atrial rate 300 beats per minute;
                      ventricular rate approximately 80 beats per minute
          P Waves: characteristic sawtooth pattern

	PRI:	unable to determine
	QRS:	.10 seconds
	Interp:	Atrial Flutter with variable response

10.145 Regularity: regular
        Rate: atrial rate 103 beats per minute;
                   ventricular rate 42 beats per minute
        P Waves: uniform; regular P–P interval
        PRI: none
        QRS: .16 seconds
        Interp: Third Degree Heart Block (CHB)

10.146 Regularity: regular underlying rhythm interrupted by ectopics
        Rate: approximately 80 beats per minute
        P Waves: uniform in underlying rhythm; morphology changes
                   with ectopics
        PRI: .14 seconds and constant
        QRS: .10 seconds in underlying rhythm;
                   .10 seconds in ectopics
        Interp: Normal Sinus Rhythm with three PACs

10.147 Regularity: regular
        Rate: 83 beats per minute
        P Waves: uniform; regular P–P interval
        PRI: .32 seconds and constant
        QRS: .10 seconds
        Interp: Sinus Rhythm with First Degree Heart Block

10.148 Regularity: regular
        Rate: 38 beats per minute
        P Waves: uniform; regular P–P interval
        PRI: .16 seconds and constant
        QRS: .14 seconds
        Interp: Sinus Bradycardia (with wide QRS)

10.149 Regularity: regular underlying rhythm interrupted by ectopic
        Rate: 115 beats per minute
        P Waves: uniform; regular P–P interval;
                   no P wave preceding ectopic
        PRI: .16 seconds and constant
        QRS: .06 seconds in underlying rhythm
                   .14 seconds in ectopic
        Interp: Sinus Tachycardia with PVC

10.150 Regularity: slightly irregular underlying rhythm interrupted by
                    ectopic
        Rate: approximately 55 beats per minute

	P Waves:	uniform in underlying rhythm; no P wave preceding ectopic
	PRI:	.16 seconds
	QRS:	.08 seconds in underlying rhythm; .12 seconds in ectopic
	Interp:	Sinus Bradycardia with PVC

10.151
Regularity: slightly irregular
Rate: approximately 250 beats per minute
P Waves: none visible
PRI: none
QRS: approximately .16 seconds
Interp: Ventricular Tachycardia

10.152
Regularity: no visible waves or complexes
Rate: unable to determine
P Waves: none visible
PRI: none
QRS: none
Interp: Asystole

10.153
Regularity: irregular
Rate: approximately 150 beats per minute
P Waves: none visible
PRI: none
QRS: .08 seconds
Interp: uncontrolled Atrial Fibrillation

10.154
Regularity: regular
Rate: 79 beats per minute
P Waves: uniform; regular P–P interval
PRI: .22 seconds and constant
QRS: .10 seconds
Interp: Sinus Rhythm with First Degree Heart Block

10.155
Regularity: regular
Rate: 25 beats per minute
P Waves: none visible
PRI: none
QRS: .12 seconds
Interp: Idioventricular Rhythm

10.156
Regularity: totally chaotic baseline
Rate: unable to determine
P Waves: none visible
PRI: none

QRS: unable to determine
Interp: Ventricular Fibrillation

10.157   Regularity: regular
Rate: 100 beats per minute
P Waves: uniform; regular P–P interval
PRI: .14 seconds and constant
QRS: .10 seconds
Interp: Sinus Tachycardia

10.158   Regularity: regular
Rate: 58 beats per minute
P Waves: uniform, regular P–P interval
PRI: .20 seconds and constant
QRS: .08 seconds
Interp: Sinus Bradycardia

10.159   Regularity: totally chaotic baseline
Rate: unable to determine
P Waves: none visible
PRI: none
QRS: unable to determine
Interp: Ventricular Fibrillation

10.160   Regularity: regular
Rate: 56 beats per minute
P Waves: uniform; regular P–P interval
PRI: .16 seconds and constant
QRS: .08 seconds
Interp: Sinus Bradycardia

10.161   Regularity: regular
Rate: atrial rate 63 beats per minute;
                 ventricular rate 32 beats per minute
P Waves: uniform; regular P–P interval; more P waves than QRS
                 complexes
PRI: none
QRS: .14 seconds
Interp: Third Degree Heart Block (CHB)

10.162   Regularity: regular
Rate: 38 beats per minute
P Waves: uniform; regular P–P interval
PRI: .16 seconds and constant
QRS: .10 seconds
Interp: Sinus Bradycardia

10.163
    Regularity: regular
    Rate: 79 beats per minute
    P Waves: uniform; regular P–P interval
    PRI: .20 seconds and constant
    QRS: .10 seconds
    Interp: Normal Sinus Rhythm

10.164
    Regularity: regular underlying rhythm interrupted by ectopics
    Rate: 63 beats per minute
    P Waves: uniform in underlying rhythm; no P waves preceding ectopics
    PRI: .20 seconds and constant
    QRS: .16 seconds in underlying rhythm;
               .16 seconds in ectopic
    Interp: Sinus Rhythm (with wide QRS) with PVC

10.165
    Regularity: regular underlying rhythm interrupted by ectopics
    Rate: 63 beats per minute
    P Waves: uniform in underlying rhythm; no P waves preceding ectopics
    PRI: .24 seconds and constant
    QRS: .10 seconds in underlying rhythm;
               .16 seconds in ectopics
    Interp: Sinus Rhythm with First Degree Heart Block with 2 unifocal PVCs

10.166
    Regularity: irregular
    Rate: approximately 110 beats per minute
    P Waves: none visible; undulations present
    PRI: none
    QRS: .06 seconds
    Interp: uncontrolled Atrial Fibrillation

10.167
    Regularity: irregular
    Rate: atrial rate 300 beats per minute; ventricular rate approximately 100 beats per minute
    P Waves: characteristic sawtooth pattern
    PRI: unable to determine
    QRS: .10 seconds
    Interp: Atrial Flutter with variable response

10.168
    Regularity: regular
    Rate: 107 beats per minute
    P Waves: uniform; regular P–P interval
    PRI: .14 seconds and constant
    QRS: .06 seconds
    Interp: Sinus Tachycardia

10.169   Regularity: regular underlying rhythm interrupted by ectopics
           Rate: 103 beats per minute
           P Waves: uniform in underlying rhythm; no P waves preceding
                       ectopics
           PRI: .14 seconds and constant
           QRS: .08 seconds in underlying rhythm;
                       .14 seconds in ectopics
           Interp: Sinus Tachycardia with frequent unifocal PVCs and
                       coupled PVCs

10.170   Regularity: regular underlying rhythm interrupted by ectopics in a
                       pattern of grouped beating
           Rate: visible sinus rate is 36 beats per minute; actual sinus
                       rate is probably 72 beats per minute
           P Waves: uniform in underlying rhythm; no P waves preceding
                       ectopics
           PRI: .16 seconds and constant
           QRS: .08 seconds in underlying rhythm;
                       .16 seconds in ectopics
           Interp: Sinus Rhythm with bigeminy of PVCs

10.171   Regularity: totally chaotic baseline
           Rate: unable to determine
           P Waves: none visible
           PRI: none
           QRS: unable to determine
           Interp: Ventricular Fibrillation (agonal rhythm)

10.172   Regularity: regular
           Rate: atrial rate 96 beats per minute;
                       ventricular rate 48 beats per minute
           P Waves: uniform; regular P–P interval; two P waves for every
                       QRS complex
           PRI: .20 seconds and constant
           QRS: .10 seconds
           Interp: Classical Second Degree Heart Block (2:1)

10.173   Regularity: regular underlying rhythm interrupted by ectopics
           Rate: 68 beats per minute
           P Waves: uniform in underlying rhythm; morphology changes in
                       ectopics
           PRI: .20 seconds and constant
           QRS: .08 seconds in underlying rhythm;
                       .10 seconds in ectopics
           Interp: Normal Sinus Rhythm with PACs

10.174   Regularity: irregular
           Rate: atrial rate 333 beats per minute; ventricular rate ap-
                       proximately 70 beats per minute

	P Waves:	characteristic sawtooth pattern
	PRI:	unable to determine
	QRS:	.08 seconds
	Interp:	Atrial Flutter with variable response

10.175
Regularity:	regular underlying rhythm interrupted by ectopics in a pattern of grouped beating
Rate:	83 beats per minute
P Waves:	uniform in underlying rhythm; morphology changes in ectopics
PRI:	.12 seconds and constant
QRS:	.10 seconds in underlying rhythm; .10 seconds in ectopics
Interp:	Sinus Rhythm with trigeminy of PVCs

10.176
Regularity:	regular underlying rhythm interrupted by ectopics
Rate:	75 beats per minute
P Waves:	uniform in underlying rhythm; no P waves preceding ectopics
PRI:	.20 seconds and constant
QRS:	.08 seconds in underlying rhythm; .12 seconds in ectopics
Interp:	Normal Sinus Rhythm with two unifocal PVCs

10.177
Regularity:	regular
Rate:	60 beats per minute
P Waves:	uniform; regular P–P interval
PRI:	.24 seconds and constant
QRS:	.08 seconds
Interp:	Sinus Rhythm with First Degree Heart Block

10.178
Regularity:	irregular
Rate:	approximately 80 beats per minute
P Waves:	morphology changes with each beat
PRI:	varies
QRS:	.12 seconds
Interp:	Wandering Pacemaker (with wide QRS)

10.179
Regularity:	regular underlying rhythm interrupted by ectopics in a pattern of grouped beating
Rate:	approximately 80 beats per minute
P Waves:	uniform in underlying rhythm; no P waves preceding ectopics
PRI:	.14 seconds and constant in underlying rhythm
QRS:	.08 seconds in underlying rhythm; .14 seconds in ectopics
Interp:	Sinus Rhythm with bigeminy of PVCs

10.180   Regularity: regular
          Rate: 115 beats per minute
          P Waves: none visible
          PRI: none
          QRS: .08 seconds
          Interp: Junctional Tachycardia

10.181   Regularity: irregular in a pattern of grouped beating
          Rate: approximately 60 beats per minute
          P Waves: uniform; regular P–P interval; some P waves are not
                      followed by QRS complexes
          PRI: varies; progressively lengthens until a beat is not con-
                      ducted
          QRS: .10 seconds
          Interp: Wenckebach

10.182   Regularity: regular underlying rhythm interrupted by ectopics
          Rate: 107 beats per minute
          P Waves: uniform in underlying rhythm; no P wave preceding
                      ectopics
          PRI: .12 seconds and constant
          QRS: .08 seconds in underlying rhythm;
                      .14 seconds in ectopics
          Interp: Sinus Tachycardia with PVC and coupled PVCs

10.183   Regularity: no visible complexes; essentially straight line
          Rate: not discernible
          P Waves: none
          PRI: none
          QRS: none
          Interp: Asystole (agonal rhythm)

10.184   Regularity: slightly irregular
          Rate: approximately 70 beats per minute
          P Waves: morphology changes from beat to beat
          PRI: varies slightly (.18–.20 seconds)
          QRS: .08 seconds
          Interp: Wandering Pacemaker

10.185   Regularity: regular underlying rhythm interrupted by ectopics in a
                      pattern of grouped beating
          Rate: 120 beats per minute
          P Waves: uniform in underlying rhythm; no P waves preceding
                      ectopics
          PRI: .12 seconds and constant
          QRS: .08 seconds in underlying rhythm;
                      .12 seconds in ectopics
          Interp: Sinus Tachycardia with bigeminy of PVCs

10.186   Regularity: regular
          Rate: 54 beats per minute
          P Waves: inverted in front of QRS complexes
          PRI: .12 seconds and constant
          QRS: .08 seconds
          Interp: Junctional Escape Rhythm

10.187   Regularity: regular
          Rate: atrial rate 100 beats per minute; ventricular rate 35
                      beats per minute
          P Waves: uniform; regular P–P interval; more P waves than QRS
                      complexes
          PRI: none
          QRS: .20 seconds
          Interp: Third Degree Heart Block (CHB)

10.188   Regularity: irregular
          Rate: approximately 100 beats per minute
          P Waves: none visible; undulations present
          PRI: none
          QRS: .08 seconds
          Interp: controlled Atrial Fibrillation

10.189   Regularity: totally chaotic baseline
          Rate: unable to determine
          P Waves: none visible
          PRI: none
          QRS: none
          Interp: Ventricular Fibrillation

10.190   Regularity: irregular
          Rate: approximately 90 beats per minute
          P Waves: none visible; undulations present
          PRI: none
          QRS: .08 seconds
          Interp: controlled Atrial Fibrillation

10.191   Regularity: irregular
          Rate: approximately 80 beats per minute
          P Waves: none discernible; undulations present
          PRI: none
          QRS: .16 seconds
          Interp: controlled Atrial Fibrillation (with wide QRS)

10.192   Regularity: regular underlying rhythm interrupted by ectopics in a
                      pattern of grouped beating
          Rate: 100 beats per minute

P Waves: uniform in underlying rhythm; no P waves preceding ectopics
PRI: .14 seconds and constant
QRS: .08 seconds in underlying rhythm;
           .14 seconds in ectopics
Interp: Sinus Tachycardia with trigeminy of PVCs

10.193
Regularity: slightly irregular
Rate: approximately 136 beats per minute
P Waves: none visible
PRI: none
QRS: .16 seconds
Interp: Ventricular Tachycardia

10.194
Regularity: regular underlying rhythm interrupted by ectopics
Rate: 83 beats per minute
P Waves: uniform in underlying rhythm; no P waves preceding ectopics
PRI: .16 seconds and constant
QRS: .12 seconds in underlying rhythm;
            .16 seconds in ectopics
Interp: Sinus Rhythm (with wide QRS) with multifocal PVCs

10.195
Regularity: regular
Rate: atrial rate 125 beats per minute;
            ventricular rate 22 beats per minute
P Waves: uniform; regular P–P interval
PRI: none
QRS: .12 seconds
Interp: Third Degree Heart Block (CHB)
Note: You might also want to note that the atria are being depolarized at a faster-than-normal rate. You could call this a CHB with an underlying Sinus Tachycardia.

10.196
Regularity: regular
Rate: 125 beats per minute
P Waves: uniform; regular P–P interval
PRI: .16 seconds and constant
QRS: .10 seconds
Interp: Sinus Tachycardia

10.197
Regularity: regular
Rate: 94 beats per minute
P Waves: uniform; regular P–P interval
PRI: .24 seconds and constant
QRS: .10 seconds
Interp: Sinus Rhythm with First Degree Heart Block

10.198   Regularity: regular
         Rate: atrial rate 300 beats per minute;
                      ventricular rate 88 beats per minute
         P Waves: characteristic sawtooth pattern
         PRI: unable to determine
         QRS: .12 seconds
         Interp: Atrial Flutter (with wide QRS)

10.199   Regularity: regular underlying rhythm interrupted by ectopic
         Rate: 71 beats per minute
         P Waves: uniform; regular P-P interval; no P wave preceding
                      ectopic
         PRI: .16 seconds and constant
         QRS: .08 seconds in underlying rhythm;
                      .14 seconds in ectopic
         Interp: Normal Sinus Rhythm with one PVC

10.200   Regularity: regular
         Rate: 167 beats per minute
         P Waves: none visible
         PRI: none
         QRS: .16 seconds
         Interp: Ventricular Tachycardia

10.201   Regularity: totally chaotic baseline
         Rate: unable to determine
         P Waves: none visible
         PRI: none
         QRS: none
         Interp: Ventricular Fibrillation (agonal rhythm)

10.202   Regularity: regular
         Rate: approximately 48 beats per minute
         P Waves: uniform; regular P-P interval
         PRI: .20 seconds and constant
         QRS: .10 seconds
         Interp: Sinus Bradycardia

10.203   Regularity: regular underlying rhythm interrupted by frequent ec-
                      topics
         Rate: 107 beats per minute
         P Waves: uniform in underlying rhythm; no P waves preceding
                      ectopics
         PRI: .12 seconds and constant
         QRS: .08 seconds in underlying rhythm;
                      .14 seconds in ectopics
         Interp: Sinus Tachycardia with frequent unifocal PVCs and
                      coupled PVCs

10.204
Regularity: regular
Rate: 115 beats per minute
P Waves: uniform; regular P–P interval
PRI: .14 seconds and constant
QRS: .08 seconds
Interp: Sinus Tachycardia

10.205
Regularity: irregular
Rate: approximately 100 beats per minute
P Waves: none visible; undulations present
PRI: none
QRS: .08 seconds
Interp: controlled Atrial Fibrillation

10.206
Regularity: regular
Rate: 43 beats per minute
P Waves: uniform; regular P–P interval
PRI: .20 seconds and constant
QRS: .06 seconds
Interp: Sinus Bradycardia

10.207
Regularity: irregular
Rate: approximately 60 beats per minute
P Waves: none visible; undulations present
PRI: none
QRS: .08 seconds
Interp: controlled Atrial Fibrillation

10.208
Regularity: regular underlying rhythm interrupted by ectopics in a
            pattern of grouped beating
Rate: 94 beats per minute
P Waves: uniform in underlying rhythm; no P waves preceding
            ectopics
PRI: .16 seconds and constant
QRS: .08 seconds in underlying rhythm;
            .14 seconds in ectopics
Interp: Normal Sinus Rhythm with possible quadrigeminy of
            PVCs

10.209
Regularity: regular
Rate: 143 beats per minute
P Waves: uniform; regular P–P interval
PRI: .14 seconds and constant
QRS: .08 seconds
Interp: Sinus Tachycardia

10.210
Regularity: regular
Rate: 47 beats per minute

P Waves: uniform; regular P–P interval
PRI: .28 seconds and constant
QRS: .10 seconds
Interp: Sinus Bradycardia with First Degree Heart Block

10.211   Regularity: irregular
Rate: approximately 150 beats per minute
P Waves: none visible; undulations present
PRI: none
QRS: .12 seconds
Interp: uncontrolled Atrial Fibrillation (with wide QRS)

10.212   Regularity: irregular initially, then totally chaotic
Rate: unable to determine
P Waves: none visible
PRI: none
QRS: approximately .16 seconds in initial rhythm; unable to
             measure in terminal pattern
Interp: Ventricular Tachycardia into Ventricular Fibrillation

10.213   Regularity: irregular
Rate: approximately 130 beats per minute
P Waves: none visible; undulations present
PRI: unable to determine
QRS: .10 seconds
Interp: uncontrolled Atrial Fibrillation

10.214   Regularity: regular underlying rhythm interrupted by ectopic
Rate: 84 beats per minute
P Waves: uniform in underlying rhythm; no P wave preceding
             ectopic
PRI: .24 seconds and constant
QRS: .08 seconds in underlying rhythm;
             .12 seconds in ectopic
Interp: Sinus Rhythm with First Degree Heart Block with one
             PVC

10.215   Regularity: irregular
Rate: approximately 110 beats per minute
P Waves: none visible; undulations present
PRI: none
QRS: .08 seconds
Interp: uncontrolled Atrial Fibrillation

10.216   Regularity: irregular
Rate: atrial rate 250 beats per minute;
             ventricular rate 70 beats per minute

	P Waves:	characteristic sawtooth pattern
	PRI:	unable to determine
	QRS:	.08 seconds
	Interp:	Atrial Flutter with variable response

10.217
Regularity:	regular
Rate:	125 beats per minute
P Waves:	uniform; regular P–P interval
PRI:	.16 seconds and constant
QRS:	.14 seconds
Interp:	Sinus Tachycardia (with wide QRS)

10.218
Regularity:	regular
Rate:	atrial rate 167 beats per minute; ventricular rate 22 beats per minute
P Waves:	uniform; regular P–P interval
PRI:	none
QRS:	.14 seconds
Interp:	Third Degree Heart Block (CHB)
Note:	You might also want to note that the atria are being depolarized at a faster-than-normal rate. You could call this a CHB with an underlying Sinus Tachycardia.

10.219
Regularity:	regular
Rate:	167 beats per minute
P Waves:	none visible
PRI:	unable to determine
QRS:	.08 seconds
Interp:	Supraventricular Tachycardia

10.220
Regularity:	irregular
Rate:	approximately 120 beats per minute
P Waves:	none visible; undulations present
PRI:	none
QRS:	.10 seconds
Interp:	uncontrolled Atrial Fibrillation

Appendix A
Clinical Effects of Arrhythmias

- The primary function of the heart is to maintain a constant flow of blood (with the oxygen and nutrients it carries) to the rest of the body.

- The volume of blood pumped by the heart is called cardiac output. Cardiac output is defined as the total volume of blood pumped by the left ventricle in one minute. If you measured the volume of blood pumped during each ventricular contraction (called stroke volume) and multiplied that by the number of contractions (heart beats) per minute, you would have a measured cardiac output. The formula for a measured cardiac output is:

  Heart Rate × Stroke Volume = Cardiac Output

- Anything that alters either heart rate or stroke volume will also affect cardiac output.

- Three groups of arrhythmias are known to interfere with cardiac output:

  BRADYCARDIAS (heart rate is too slow to maintain adequate cardiac output)

  TACHYCARDIAS (heart rate is too fast to allow ventricles to fill completely before contraction)

  VENTRICULAR IRRITABILITY (the erratic ventricular contraction isn't effective enough to maintain stroke volume)

- When cardiac output is diminished, it produces symptoms in the patient. These include:

  anxiety
  chest pain
  shortness of breath
  diaphoresis
  hypotension
  cool clammy skin
  cyanosis
  decreased level of consciousness

- If untreated, the patient can become unconscious and eventually go into respiratory and cardiac arrest.

Appendix B
Treatment Concepts

GENERAL PRINCIPLES

- Any patient with arrhythmias *or the potential for them* should be monitored and receive a keep-open IV as a precaution.

- If arrhythmias do occur, assess the patient for the various perfusion parameters (BP, pulses, skin, etc.) to determine impact on cardiac output.

- If an arrhythmia is causing signs/symptoms of decreased cardiac output, institute treatment immediately.

- All patients should have a keep-open IV, oxygen, and a monitor.

- To enhance conversion of an arrhythmia, try to identify and correct the underlying cause, i.e., if acidotic, give bicarbonate; if hypovolemic, give fluids; if hypoxic, give oxygen; if dig-toxic, withhold digitalis, etc.

- In addition to treating the specific presenting arrhythmia, it may be also necessary to provide general supportive measures such as CPR to support circulation and dopamine to maintain blood pressure.

TREATMENT MODALITIES

Bradycardias

Treatment Objective: Speed up rate.
Treatment Options:
    Atropine
    Isuprel
    Epinephrine
    Pacemaker
The decision as to which of these is used for which bradycardia depends in large part on the severity of the bradycardia, the pacemaker site, and the personal preference of the treating clinician.
NOTE: When faced with a bradycardia interrupted by PVCs, treat the bradycardia first (speed up rate); PVCs should be eliminated as rate increases.

Tachycardias (other than those caused by ventricular irritability)

Treatment Objective: Slow down heart rate.
Treatment Options:
   Mechanical
   Valsalva's Maneuver
   Carotid Sinus Massage
   Cardioversion

   Pharmaceutical
   Digitalis
   Inderal
   Verapamil

The order of intervention is often progressive, i.e., the ordering clinician may first try vagotonic maneuvers, then cardioversion and/or drugs if the rhythm fails to convert. In other situations the treatment may be specific to the presenting arrhythmia.

Ventricular Irritability

Treatment Objective: Suppress irritable ventricular focus
Treatment Options:
   Abortive (when you catch the arrhythmia before it has a chance to interfere with cardiac output)
      Lidocaine
      Pronestyl
   Aggressive (when the patient is already losing perfusion)
      Cardioversion/Defibrillation
      Lidocaine

The American Heart Association's current recommendation for drug treatment of ventricular fibrillation includes:
   Epinephrine
   Sodium Bicarbonate
   Atropine
   Calcium Chloride
   Isuprel

For recurrent or refractory ventricular fibrillation, AHA recommends:
   Atropine
   Lidocaine
   Pronestyl
   Bretylium

Once ventricular irritability is suppressed and a viable rhythm restored, a lidocaine drip should be started to maintain therapeutic blood levels of the drug.

Appendix C
Arrhythmia Significance and Treatments

RHYTHM	SIGNIFICANCE	CLINICAL PICTURE	TREATMENT
NSR	• Normal cardiac pattern.	• Does not produce symptoms.	• None required.
Sinus Bradycardia	• Can precede blocks or asystole. • Can precipitate escape rhythms or ventricular irritability. • Can be caused by AMI, vagal stimulation, increased ICP. • Can reflect normal, athletic heart.	• Slow, regular pulse. • Can cause s/s of decreased c.o.	• If symptomatic, increase rate with Isuprel, Epinephrine, or pacemaker. • In presence of MI, do not increase rate unless patient is symptomatic.
Sinus Tachycardia	• Usually a normal compensatory response to fever, activity, pain, anxiety, hypovolemia, heart failure, etc. • Dangerous in AMI (can extend infarct).	• Rapid, regular pulse. • Probably asymptomatic. • Possibly palpitations, dyspnea.	• Treat cause. • Propranalol, Verapamil
Sinus Arrhythmia	• Common in children and young adults.	• Irregular pulse. • Rarely causes symptoms.	• None required.

RHYTHM	SIGNIFICANCE	CLINICAL PICTURE	TREATMENT
Premature Atrial Contractions	• Usually benign. • Can be early sign of CHF. • Can lead to other atrial tachyarrhythmias. • Causes include fatigue, hypoxia, dig-toxicity, caffeine, ischemia, CHF, alcohol.	• Irregular pulse. • Rarely causes symptoms.	• Treat underlying cause. • Digitalis, Procainamide, Quinidine
Wandering Pacemaker	• Normal; often seen in very old or very young, or in athletes. • Persistence of junctional rhythm can indicate heart disease.	• Rarely causes symptoms.	• Usually unnecessary.
Atrial Tachycardia	• Very dangerous in AMI or heart disease. • Commonly caused by dig-toxicity.	• Rapid regular pulse. • May show s/s of drop in c.o. • Can cause pulmonary edema, CHF, & shock.	• Vagotonic Maneuvers • Digitalis, Propranalol, Aramine, Tensilon • Cardioversion • Atrial Pacing
Atrial Flutter	• Rapid ventricular rate and loss of atrial kick can drop c.o.	• Rapid ventricular rate can cause s/s of low c.o.	• Only treated if rate is too fast.

RHYTHM	SIGNIFICANCE	CLINICAL PICTURE	TREATMENT
	• Risk of pulmonary and cerebral emboli. • Can cause CHF or myocardial ischemia. • Seen in CAD, rheumatic heart disease.	• Pulse can be regular or irregular.	• Quinidine, Procainamide, Propranolol • Cardioversion • Digitalization • CSM rarely works.
Atrial Fibrillation	• Very rapid rate can lead to CHF or myocardial ischemia. • Threat of pulmonary or cerebral emboli. • Commonly caused by dig-toxicity.	• Irregular pulse. • Can have pulse deficit. • If ventricular rate is rapid, can cause s/s of low c.o.	• Only treated if rate is too fast. • Cardioversion • Digitalization
Premature Junctional Contractions	• May precede AV block.	• Rarely causes s/s.	• Quinidine, Procainamide
Junctional Escape Rhythm	• Fail-safe mechanism. • Can be normal, as with athletes.	• Slow pulse. • If rate is slow enough can cause s/s of low c.o.	• Atropine, Isuprel • Pacemaker may be necessary.
Accelerated Junctional Rhythm	• Indicates irritable junction overriding normal pacemaker. • Often caused by AMI, open-heart surgery, myocarditis, dig-toxicity.	• Usually asymptomatic.	• Treatment not usually necessary.
Junctional Tachycardia	• Same as Accelerated Junctional Rhythm (above).	• Rapid rate can cause s/s of low c.o.	• Vagotonic maneuvers • Tensilon, Metaraminal,

RHYTHM	SIGNIFICANCE	CLINICAL PICTURE	TREATMENT
First Degree AV Block	• Can be caused by anoxia, ischemia, AV node malfunction, edema following open heart surgery, dig-toxicity. • Can lead to more serious AV block.	• Usually asymptomatic.	Digitalis, Propranalol, Pronestyl • Cardioversion • Watch for progression.
Second Degree AV Block (Wenckebach, Mobitz I)	• Common following inferior MI. • Can progress to more serious AV block.	• Usually asymptomatic.	• Watch for progression. • If symptomatic: Atropine, Isuprel, Pacemaker
Second Degree AV Block (Classical, Mobitz II)	• Can be caused by anoxia, edema after open heart surgery, dig-toxicity, hyperkalemia, anterior MI.	• Slow rate can cause s/s of low c.o.	• If symptomatic, increase rate: Atropine, Isuprel • Pacemaker may be necessary.
Third Degree AV Block (Complete Heart Block)	• Can progress to ventricular standstill.	• Very slow rate and abnormal pacemaker site severely impair cardiac output. • Patients will frequently be unconscious from poor perfusion. • Cardiac failure can quickly follow.	• Atropine, Isuprel • Pacemaker may be necessary. • Be prepared for CPR.

RHYTHM	SIGNIFICANCE	CLINICAL PICTURE	TREATMENT
Premature Ventricular Contractions	• Indicate ventricular irritability; increasing frequency indicates increasing irritability. • Causes include ischemia/infarction, hypoxia, acidosis, hypovolemia, electrolyte imbalance, caffeine, smoking, alcohol. • PVCs which are considered to be extremely dangerous include: – more than 5/min – patterns (bigeminy, trigeminy, etc.) – couplets – runs – R on T – multifocal – any PVC in the presence of AMI	• Patients feel PVCs and are distressed by them. • Pulse is irregular. • Perfusion is generally not impaired unless PVCs become quite frequent. • Many adults have chronic PVCs from underlying respiratory disease, smoking, caffeine intake, etc.	• Lidocaine (bolus and drip) • Procainamide. Quinidine, Phenytoin, Bretylium, Propranolol • Treat cause. • In bradycardia, give Atropine first.
Ventricular Tachycardia	• Will quickly progress to ventricular fibrillation.	• Patient will begin to lose consciousness as perfusion drops.	*If Patient IS Perfusing:* • Lidocaine, Pronestyl, *If Patient IS NOT Perfusing:* • cardiovert/defibrillate • Lidocaine, Bretylium

443

RHYTHM	SIGNIFICANCE	CLINICAL PICTURE	TREATMENT
Ventricular Fibrillation	• Lethal arrhythmia. • Indicative of extreme myocardial irritability.	• Patient is clinically dead.	• Precordial thump (if monitored) • CPR • Defibrillate • Epinephrine, Bicarbonate • Defibrillate again • Atropine, Calcium Chloride, Isoproterenol *If Recurrent:* • Atropine • Lidocaine (slow bolus), Procainamide, Bretylium *After Conversion:* • Lidocaine (bolus and drip)
Idioventricular Rhythm	• Associated with poor prognosis. • Often associated with large MI and damage to large amount of ventricular muscle mass.	• Patient is clinically dead.	• Atropine, Isuprel • Fluid challenge • Pacemaker • Open chest massage
Asystole	• Mortality exceeds 95%. • Often seen after patient has been in arrest for some time.	• Patient is clinically dead.	• CPR • Epinephrine, Bicarbonate, Calcium, Atropine, Isuprel • Pacemaker

Glossary

Artifact: Electrical activity displayed on graph paper which is superimposed on cardiac tracings, interfering with interpretation of the rhythm; can be caused by outside electrical sources, muscle tremors, patient movement; also called interference.

Asystole: The absence of any cardiac electrical activity; appears as a straight line on graph paper.

Atria: The upper two chambers of the heart.

Atrial Arrhythmia: A cardiac arrhythmia originating from the conduction system within the atria.

Atrial Fibrillation: The cardiac arrhythmia in which the atria are controlled by numerous irritable foci, thereby causing ineffectual, chaotic atrial activity and irregular ventricular response.

Atrial Flutter: The cardiac arrhythmia in which an irritable focus in the atria produces a rapid, repetitive discharge, resulting in rhythmic atrial depolarizations at a rate of 150–250 beats per minute, some of which are usually blocked by the AV node to keep the ventricular rate in a more normal range.

Atrial Tachycardia: The cardiac arrhythmia in which a single irritable focus takes over control of the heart to produce a rate of 150–250 beats per minute; this arrhythmia is often paroxysmal in nature, that is, it starts and stops suddenly—in that instance it is called Paroxysmal Atrial Tachycardia (PAT).

Atrioventricular Dissociation: A conduction defect which causes the atria and ventricles to depolarize and function independently; AV Dissociation.

Automaticity: The unique ability of cardiac pacemaker cells to initiate spontaneous excitation impulses.

Autonomic Nervous System: The system responsible for control of involuntary bodily functions, including cardiac and vascular activity; branches are Sympathetic Nervous System and Parasympathetic Nervous System.

AV: Atrioventricular.

AV Heart Block: Arrhythmias caused by disturbances in conduction through the AV node.

AV Junction: That part of the cardiac conduction system that connects the atria and the ventricles; contains the AV node and the non-branching part of the Bundle of His.

AV Node: A part of the cardiac conduction system located within the AV Junction; does not contain pacemaking cells; its purpose is to slow conduction of impulses through the AV junction.

Baseline: The isoelectric line; that line on EKG graph paper which indicates lack of electrical activity, and from which all other cardiac wave impulses deviate.

Bigeminy: A pattern of cardiac electrical activity in which every other beat is an ectopic, usually a PVC.

Biological Death: The second phase of death, following clinical death; defined by brain death, usually following 4–6 minutes of cardiac arrest if no resuscitation is instituted.

Block: A defect in conduction within the heart's electrical system.

Bolus: A single loading dose of a drug; used to achieve a rapid high therapeutic blood level prior to instituting IV drip therapy.

Bradyarrhythmia: Any cardiac arrhythmia with a rate below 60 beats per minute.

Bradycardia: A heart rate less than 60 beats per minute.

Bundle Branches: The portion of the cardiac conduction system within the ventricles that conducts impulses from the Bundle of His to the Purkinje fibers; consists of right and left bundle branches.

Bundle Branch Block: A conduction disturbance which prevents or delays passage of impulses from the Bundle of His through to the Purkinje network; can involve the right or left bundle, or less frequently, both.

Bundle of His: That part of the cardiac conduction system that conducts impulses from the AV junction through to the bundle branches.

Calibration: The act of standardizing the graphic display of electrical activity; the calibration mark should measure 1 millivolt on the graph paper.

Capture: The act of responding to an electrical stimulus with depolarization; generally refers to an arrhythmia's response to an artificial pacemaker.

Cardiac Arrest: Cessation of cardiac function, resulting in sudden drop in perfusion and resultant clinical death.

Cardiac Cycle: The interval from the beginning of one heartbeat to the beginning of the next; on the EKG it encompasses the PQRST complex.

Cardiac Output: The amount of blood pumped by the left ventricle in one minute; it is calculated by multiplying the stroke volume by the heart rate, and is measured in liters per minute.

Cardioversion: A maneuver used to convert various tachyarrhythmias to more viable rhythms; consists of application of electrical countershock (DC current) to the chest wall; the electrical discharge is usually synchronized to fall on the R wave, thus avoiding the relative refractory period.

Carotid Sinus Massage: A maneuver used to convert various supraventricular tachycardias to a more viable rhythm; consists of gentle massage with fingertips over the carotid sinus in the neck.

Classical Second Degree Heart Block: The form of AV heart block in which the AV node intermittently blocks sinus impulses, preventing them from being conducted through to the ventricles; the EKG shows more P waves than QRS complexes, but some (usually every other or every third) are conducted normally through to the ventricles.

Clinical Death: Absence of pulse and blood pressure; occurs immediately following cardiac arrest.

Compensatory Pause: The time lag following an ectopic beat before the next normal beat occurs; is identified by measuring the interval from the R wave immediately preceding the ectopic to the R wave immediately following it; a fully compensatory pause (such as occurs following most PVCs) will be exactly two times the normal R–R interval.

Complete Heart Block: Third degree AV block, a form of AV dissociation.

Conduction System: The pathways of conductive tissues within the heart that facilitate passage of electrical impulses throughout the myocardium.

Conductivity: The property of some cardiac cells that enables them to transmit electrical impulses.

Contractility: The ability of heart muscle to contract in response to electrical simulation.

Defibrillation: Application of electrical countershock (DC current) to the chest wall to terminate ventricular tachyarrhythmias.

Depolarization: The electrical process of discharging polarized cells, usually resulting in muscle contraction.

Dissociation: Independent function of two parts, generally the atria and ventricles.

Dysrhythmia: Arrhythmia.

ECG: Electrocargiogram; EKG.

Ectopic: Originating from a focus other than the primary pacemaker.

EKG: Electrocardiogram; ECG.

Electrode: Metal wire attached to the patient's body for the purpose of conveying electrical impulses to a machine for recording or displaying.

Electrocardiogram: EKG; graphic representation of the electrical activity in the heart.

Escape: The mechanism that allows a lower pacemaker site to assume pacemaking responsibilities when a higher site fails.

Fibrillation: Chaotic, ineffective movement of the heart muscle.

First Degree Heart Block: A type of AV heart block characterized by prolonged but consistent conduction of atrial impulses through to the ventricles.

Flutter: Rhythmic, rapid beating of the heart muscle.

Heart Block: AV heart block.

Heart Rate: Number of heartbeats per minute.

His-Purkinje System: The lower part of the cardiac conduction system that transmits impulses throughout the ventricles; located in the interventricular septum and ventricular walls.

Idioventricular Rhythm: A ventricular escape rhythm; characterized by a rate less than 40 beats per minute.

Interference: See artifact.

Interpolation: The placement of an ectopic (especially PVCs) between two normal beats without disturbing the regularity of the underlying rhythm.

Interval: Distance between two points on an EKG tracing.

Interventricular Septum: The muscular wall dividing the right and left ventricles.

Intraatrial Pathways: Branches of the cardiac conduction system that service the atria.

Isoelectric Line: The line created on EKG graph paper when no electrical current is flowing; see Baseline.

Junction: See AV Junction.

Junctional Escape Rhythm: An arrhythmia resulting from failure of a higher pacemaker site, allowing the AV junction to pace the heart at a bradycardia rate.

Junctional Tachycardia: A rapid arrhythmia originating in the AV junction.

Lead: An electrocardiographic view of the heart, gained by recording the electrical activity between two or more electrodes.

Millivolts: A measure of electricity; one volt equals one thousand millivolts.

Monitor: The machine on which electrocardiographic impulses are displayed; oscilloscope.

Mobitz I: A type of second degree heart block in which sinus impulses are delayed at the AV node for increasingly long periods, until conduction is blocked completely, then the cycle repeats itself; Wenckebach.

Mobitz II: A type of second degree heart block in which the AV node selectively blocks every second, third, fourth, etc., beat; Classical Second Degree Heart Block.

Multifocal: Term used to describe ectopic beats that originate from more than one irritable focus.

Myocardium: Heart muscle.

Noise: Electrical interference displayed on graph paper which interferes with interpretation of the underlying arrhythmia.

Normal Sinus Rhythm: The usual cardiac electrical pattern of healthy people.

Oscilloscope: Display device with a screen for viewing EKG and other physiological information.

PAC: Premature Atrial Contraction; an ectopic beat created when an irritable focus in the atrium assumes pacemaking responsibility for a single beat.

Pacemaker: The source of electrical stimulation for cardiac rhythm.

Pacemaker Site: The site of origin of the electrical stimulation that is causing the cardiac rhythm.

Palpitations: The feeling the patient senses when the heart is beating abnormally.

PAT: Paroxysmal Atrial Tachycardia; the term used to describe an Atrial Tachycardia which is characterized by abrupt onset and cessation.

Parasympathetic Nervous System: A branch of the autonomic nervous system involved in control of involuntary bodily functions; depresses cardiac activity in opposition to the sympathetic branch of the ANS; effects include slowing of heart rate and conduction, and diminished myocardial irritability.

PJC: Premature Junctional Contraction; an ectopic beat originating from an irritable focus in the AV Junction.

Paroxysmal: Sudden onset and cessation; often used to describe Atrial Tachycardia if it is characterized by abrupt onset and termination.

Premature Atrial Contraction: An ectopic beat originating from an irritable focus in the atria.

Premature Junctional Contraction: An ectopic beat originating from an irritable focus in the AV Junction.

Premature Ventricular Contraction: An ectopic beat originating from an irritable focus in the ventricles.

PQRST: A single cardiac cycle on the EKG graph paper; includes the P wave, QRS complex, and T wave, and any segments and intervals between.

PRI: See PR Interval.

PR Interval: The time interval on EKG graph paper measured from the beginning of the P wave to the beginning of the R wave; includes both the P wave and the PR segment; indicates time of atrial depolarization.

PR Segment: The time interval on EKG graph paper measured from the end of the P wave to the beginning of the R wave; indicates delay in the AV node.

Pump (Sodium-Potassium): The chemical phenomenon that takes place at a cellular level within the cardiac electrical conduction system, in which sodium and potassium trade places across the cell wall, thereby initiating the flow of electrical current within the heart.

Purkinje System: The part of the cardiac conduction system that transmits impulses from the bundle branches to the myocardial cells in the ventricles; consists of Purkinje fibers and terminal branches.

PVC: Premature Ventricular Contraction; an ectopic beat originating from an irritable focus in the ventricles.

P Wave: The first wave form in the normal cardiac cycle; indicates atrial depolarization.

QRS Complex: The wave form on an EKG that represents ventricular depolarization; includes the Q, R, and S waves.

Quadrigeminy: A cardiac rhythm in which ectopics replace every fourth normal beat, resulting in a cycle of three normal beats and one ectopic, repeated continuously.

Q Wave: The first negative deflection following the P wave, but before the R wave.

QT Interval: The time interval from the beginning of the QRS complex to the end of the T wave; varies with heart rate.

Relative Refractory Period: The terminal portion of the cardiac refractory period, during which a strong enough electrical stimulus could discharge the heart, resulting in inefficient and potentially dangerous arrhythmias; located on the downslope of the P wave.

Refractory: The state wherein the electrical cells are unable to respond to electrical stimulation because they are still not recovered from the previous discharge.

Refractory Period: That portion of the cardiac cycle in which the heart is unable to respond to electrical stimulation because it has not yet recovered from the preceding depolarization; consists of the Absolute Refractory Period (QRS Complex and upslope of the T wave) and the Relative Refractory Period (downslope of the T wave).

Repolarization: The process of recharging depolarized cells back to their "ready" (polarized) state.

Rhythm: The regularity of a cardiac pattern; generally used to refer to the arrhythmia itself, rather than its rhythmicity, i.e., "The patient's rhythm is Atrial Fibrillation," even though atrial fibrillation is an irregular arrhythmia; synonymous with arrhythmia.

"R on T" Phenomenon: The situation in which the R wave of a PVC occurs on or near the downslope of the preceding T wave, thereby falling in the vulnerable phase of the cardiac cycle, the Relative Refractory Period, and threatening to cause premature discharge and result in an ineffective pattern such as Ventricular Tachycardia or Ventricular Fibrillation.

R Wave: The first upright deflection following the P wave, or the first positive wave of the QRS complex.

Sinus Arrhythmia: The arrhythmia in which the pacemaker is located in the SA Node but discharges irregularly, usually correlated with respirations; rate increases on inspiration and decreases on expiration.

Sinus Bradycardia: The arrhythmia in which the pacemaker is located in the SA Node but discharges at a rate less than 60 beats per minute.

Sinus Tachycardia: The arrhythmia in which the pacemaker is located in the SA Node but discharges at a rate greater than 100 beats per minute.

Sinus Node: The normal pacemaker of the heart; located at the junction of the superior vena cava and the right atrium; SA Node; Sino-Atrial Node.

Sinus Rhythm: Any rhythm that originates in the Sinus (SA) Node; used loosely to refer to normal sinus rhythm.

Second Degree Heart Block: The grade of AV heart block characterized by intermittent conduction disturbances at the AV node; includes Mobitz Type I (Wenckebach) and Mobitz Type II (Classical Second Degree Heart Block).

Standardization: The act of calibrating the EKG machine or oscilloscope to a standard (1 mv).

Stroke Volume: The amount of blood ejected with each contraction of the left ventricle.

ST Segment: The portion of the cardiac cycle between the S wave and the T wave.

Supraventricular: Originating above the ventricles.

Supraventricular Tachycardia: Term used to describe a rapid arrhythmia that is regular, has no visible P waves, and has a rate range common to other arrhythmias, thereby making more accurate identification impossible; commonly applied to atrial tachycardia, junctional tachycardia, sinus tachycardia, and atrial flutter with 1:1 response; loosely used to refer to any tachycardia that originated above the ventricles.

S Wave: The second negative deflection following the P wave, or the first negative deflection following the R wave.

Sympathetic Nervous System: One of the two main branches of the autonomic nervous system, which controls involuntary bodily functions; stimulates cardiac activity in opposition to parasympathetic branch; effects include increased heart rate and conduction, and increased myocardial irritability.

Tachyarrhythmia: Any cardiac arrhythmia with a ventricular rate greater than 100 beats per minute.

Tachycardia: Heart rate greater than 100 beats per minute.

Third Degree Heart Block: The arrhythmia in which all atrial impulses are prevented from reaching the ventricles because of a complete block at the AV node; constitutes a form of AV dissociation because atria and ventricles function totally independent of each other; Complete Heart Block (CHB).

Trigeminy: A pattern in which ectopics occur every third beat, producing a repetitive cycle of two normal beats and one ectopic.

Ventricles: The lower two chambers of the heart.

Ventricular Depolarization: Discharge of electrical activity throughout the ventricles to stimulate ventricular contraction; produces the QRS complex on an EKG.

Ventricular Fibrillation: The arrhythmia in which the ventricles are controlled by numerous irritable foci, producing chaotic, ineffective muscle activity rather than the normal contraction.

Ventricular Flutter: The arrhythmia in which a single irritable focus in the ventricles depolarizes the heart at a rate of 250–350 beats per minute; usually considered to be a rapid form of Ventricular Tachycardia.

Ventricular Tachycardia: The arrhythmia in which a single irritable focus in the ventricles depolarizes the heart at a rate of 150–250 beats per minute.

Ventricular Standstill: The arrhythmia in which the ventricles are not depolarized by any electrical stimulation, and therefore do not contract; if atrial activity is present it is not conducted through the AV node; if no atrial activity is present it is called Asystole.

Vulnerable Period: The period in the cardiac cycle when the heart is most susceptible to premature discharge with a resultant ineffective pattern if it receives a strong enough electrical stimulus; the Relative Refractory Period; corresponds with the downslope of the T wave.

Wandering Pacemaker: The arrhythmia in which the pacemaker site shifts from the SA node to the atrium and back again, sometimes dropping as low as the AV junction.

Waves: Deflections on the electrocardiograph caused by changes in electrical activity in the heart.

Wenckebach: The form of Second Degree AV block in which the node progressively holds each impulse longer until one is eventually not conducted, then the cycle starts over; Mobitz I.

Index

Accelerated junctional rhythm, 144–146
  rules for determining, 145, 148
  significance and treatments of, 439
Agonal, 222
Arrhythmia,
  approach to interpretation, 56
  defined, 3
Arrhythmias,
  accelerated junctional rhythm, 144–146
    rules for determining, 145, 148
    significance and treatments of, 439
  asystole, 222
    rules for determining, 222, 224
    significance and treatments, 442
  atrial fibrillation, 111–113
    rules for determining, 113, 114
    significance and treatments of, 441
  atrial flutter, 109–111
    rules for determining, 111, 112
    significance and treatments of, 440–441
  atrial tachycardia, 107–109
    rules for determining, 107, 109
    significance and treatments of, 440
  clinical effects of, 436
  ectopic beat, 103–104, 106
  idioventricular rhythm, 220–222
    rules for determining, 221, 222
    significance and treatments of, 444
  junctional, 135–166
    rules for determining, 142–143
  junctional escape rhythm, 142–144
    rules for determining, 143–144, 145
    significance and treatments of, 441
  junctional tachycardia, 144, 146–147
    rules for determining, 146, 149
    significance and treatments of, 441
  premature atrial contraction (PAC), 104–107
    rules for determining, 107, 108
    significance and treatment, 440
  premature junctional contraction (PJC), 141–142
    rules for determining, 142, 143
    significance and treatment, 441
  premature ventricular contraction (PVC), 207–216
    rules for determining, 216, 217
    significance and treatments of, 443
  significance and treatments of:
    accelerated junctional rhythm, 441
    asystole, 444
    atrial fibrillation, 441
    atrial flutter, 440–441
    atrial tachycardia, 440
    first degree AV block, 442
    idioventricular rhythm, 444
    junctional tachycardia, 441–442
    premature atrial contractions, 440
    premature junctional contractions, 441
    premature ventricular contractions, 443
    second degree AV block, 442
    sinus arrhythmia, 439
    sinus bradycardia, 439
    sinus tachycardia, 439
    third degree AV block, 442

ventricular fibrillation, 444
    wandering pacemaker, 440
  sinus, 82–84
    rules for determining, 84
    significance and treatments of, 439
  supraventricular, 206
  supraventricular tachycardia, 148–149
  treatment concepts, 437
  ventricular fibrillation, 218–20
    rules for determining, 220–221
    significance and treatments, 444
  ventricular tachycardia, 216–218
    rules for determining, 215, 216, 218, 219
    significance and treatments of, 443
  wandering pacemaker, 103, 104
    rules for, 103, 105
    significance and treatments of, 440
Artifact, 33
  types of, 34, 35
Asystole, 222
  rules for determining, 222, 223
  significance and treatments of, 444
Atria, 6, 10, 51
Atrial arrhythmias, 102
  ectopic beat, 103–104, 106
  fibrillation, 111–113
    rules for determining, 113, 114
    significance and treatments of, 441
  flutter, 109–111
    rules for determining, 111, 112
    significance and treatments of, 440–441
  premature contractions (PAC), 104–107
    rules for determining, 107, 108
    significance and treatments of, 440
  tachycardia, 107–109
    rules for determining, 107, 109
    significance and treatments of, 440
  wandering pacemaker, 103, 104
    rules for determining, 103, 105
    significance and treatments of, 440
Atrial contractions, premature (PAC), 104–107
  rules for determining, 107, 108
  significance and treatments of, 440
Atrial fibrillation, 111–113
  rules for determining, 113, 114
  significance and treatments of, 441
Atrial flutter, 109–111
  rules for determining, 111, 112
  significance and treatments of, 440–441
Atrial rhythms, 101–133
Atrial tachycardia, 107–109
  rules for determining, 107, 109
  significance and treatments of, 440
Atrioventricular junction see AV junction
AV blocks, 167–203
  first degree, 168, 169–170, 171, 185
  mechanisms of, 169
  rules for determining, 170–172
  significance and treatments of, 442
second degree, 168, 169, 171–178, 185
  mechanisms of, 169
  rules for determining, 174
  significance and treatments of, 442

third degree, 168–169, 178–184, 186
  mechanisms, 169
    rules for determining, 181, 184
    significance and treatments of, 442
AV junction, 6–10, 136
  beats per minute, 8
AV node, 6–10, 62, 109, 136

Bigeminy, 214–215, 216
Bradycardia, 80, 81–82
  rules for determining, 82
  sinus, 80, 81–82
    rules for determining, 82
    significance and treatments, 439
  treatment of, 437
Bundle of His, 6

Cardiac cell, electrical charges and, 3
Cardiac cycle, 19, 54
Classical heart block, 168, 169, 173–175, 186
  rules for determining, 177
Complete heart block, 168–169, 178–184, 186
  mechanisms of, 169
  rules for determining, 181, 184
  significance and treatments of, 442
Condition system, 6
  illustration of, 7–13

Depolarization, defined, 4
Dysrhythmia see Arrhythmia

Ectopic beat, 103–104, 106
EKG,
  analyzing rhythm strips, 53–75
  complex illustrated, 20
  defined, 3
  electrode placement for monitoring, 138
  graph paper used, 49–52
  interpreting, 55–65
  lead II, 47–48
    positioning of, 49
  leads, 47
  MCL_1, 47–48
  pattern recognition, 54
  positioning of electrodes, 47
  tracing, 2–3
Electrical charges, cardiac cells and, 3
Electrical flow, rule of, 47
  illustrated, 48
Electrocardiogram see EKG
Electrode,
  defined, 46
  insuring contact with skin, 46
  positioning of, 47
    lead II, 49
Electrophysiology, 1–15

"F" waves, 109
"f" waves, 111

Fibrillation,
  atrial, 111–113
    rules for determining, 113, 114
    significance and treatments of, 441
  ventricular, 218–220
    rules for determining, 220–221
    significance and treatments of, 444
Flutter, atrial, 109–111
  rules for determining, 111, 112

Glossary, 445–451
Graph paper, EKG, 49–52

Heart,
  "fail safe" mechanism, 62
  function of, 2
Heart blocks, 167–203
  first degree, 168, 169, 170, 171, 185
    mechanisms of, 169
    rules for determining, 170–172
    significance and treatments, 442
  second degree (classical), 168, 169, 173–175, 186
    mechanisms of, 169
    rules for determining, 174
  second degree (Wenckebach), 168, 169, 175–178
    mechanisms of, 169
    rules for determining, 178, 180
  third degree, 168–169, 178–184, 186
    mechanisms of, 169
    rules for determining, 181, 184
    significance and treatments, 442
Heart rate, calculating, 56, 57–59

Idioventricular rhythm, 220–222
  rules for determining, 221, 222
  significance and treatments of, 444
Impulse formation, chemical basis for, 3, 4
  illustrated, 5
Interference, 24
  types of, 25–26
Isoelectric line, 46

Junctional arrhythmias, 135–166
  accelerated, 144–146
    rules for determining, 145, 148
    significance and treatments of, 444
  electrical flow in, 137
  junctional escape rhythm, 142–144
    rules for determining, 143–144, 145
    significance and treatments, 441
  premature junctional contraction (PJC), 139–140
    rules for determining, 141, 142
    significance and treatments of, 441
  supraventricular tachycardia, 148–149
  tachycardia, 144, 146–147
    rules for determining, 146, 149
    significance and treatments, 441
Junctional escape rhythm, 142–144

rules for determining, 143–144, 145
significance and treatments of, 441
Junctional rhythms, 135–166
P wave placement in, 140
Junctional tachycardia, 144, 146–147
rules for determining, 146, 149
significance and treatments of, 441
Junction, AV, 6–10
beats per minute, 8

Lead II, 47–48, 136
positioning of, 49

MCL₁, 47–48
Mobitz I see Wenckebach heart block
Mobitz II see Classical heart block
Modified chest lead (see MCL₁)

Nodes,
AV, 6–10, 62, 109, 136
SA, 6–10, 54
beats per minute, 8
Normal sinus rhythm, 54–55
rules for determining, 79–80
significance and treatments, 439

P wave, 19, 56, 59–61
atrial, 102
interpreting, 56, 59–61
inverted, 138–140
placement in junctional rhythms, 140
sinus, 101, 102
Pacemaker sites, 54
Parasympathetic branch, 10, 11, 13
"Passive" junctional rhythm, 142–144
rules for determining, 143–144, 145
Pattern recognition, 54
Polarization, defined, 3–4
Potassium, 3
PR interval, 20, 23
interpreting, 56
PR segment, 29
Practice rhythm strips, 254–364
Premature atrial contraction (PAC), 104–107
rules for determining, 107, 108
significance and treatments of, 440
Premature junctional contraction (PJC), 141–142
rules for determining, 142, 143
significance and treatments of, 441
Premature ventricular contractions (PVC), 207–216
rules for determining, 216, 217
significance and treatments of, 443
PRI, 62
Purkinje, 6

Q wave, 21
QRS complex, 20–21, 23, 62–63, 136
configurations of, 22
interpreting, 56

Quadrigeminy, 211, 212, 213

R wave, 55
R-to-R interval (RRI), 57–58
Rate, see heart rate
Refractory period, 25, 26–27
absolute, 27
related, 27
Regularity, interpreting, 56, 57
Repolarization, defined, 4
Rhythm strips,
analyzing, 53–69
practice, 254–364
Rhythms,
accelerated junctional, 144–146
rules for determining, 145, 148
atrial, 90–133
interpreting, 56, 57
junctional, 135–166
sinus, 77–89
ventricular, 205–226

S wave, 23
SA node, 6–10
beats per minute, 8
Sinus arrhythmia, 82–84
rules for determining, 84
significance and treatments of, 439
Sinus bradycardia, 80, 81–82
rules for determining, 82
significance and treatments, 439
Sinus rhythms, 77–99
arrhythmia, 82–84
rules for determining, 8–24
significance and treatments of, 439
bradycardia, 80, 81–82
rules for determining, 82
significance and treatments, 439
normal (NSR), 78–80
rules for determining, 79, 80, 81
significance and treatments, 439
tachycardia, 80–81, 82
rules for determining, 80–81, 82
significance and treatments, 439
Sodium, 3
Sodium pump, 4
ST segment, 23
Supraventricular arrhythmias, 206
Supraventricular tachycardia, 148–149

T wave, 21, 23, 37, 61
Tachycardia,
atrial, 107–109
significance and treatments, 439
junctional, 144, 146–147
rules for determining, 146, 149
significance and treatments, 441
sinus, 80–81, 82
rules for determining, 83
significance and treatments, 439
supraventricular, 148–149

treatment of, 439
  ventricular, 216–218
    rules for determining, 218, 219
    significance and treatment of, 443
Trigeminy, 214, 215, 216

Vagus nerve, 11, 13
Ventricle, 51
  beats per minute, 8
Ventricular arrhythmias,
  fibrillation, 218–220
    rules for determining, 220–221
    significance and treatments of, 444
  idioventricular rhythm, 220–222
    rules for determining, 221, 222
    significance and treatments, 444
  premature ventricular contraction (PVC), 207–216
    rules for determining, 213, 214
    significance and treatments, 443
  tachycardia, 216–218
    rules for determining, 218, 219
    significance and treatments of, 443
Ventricular depolarization, 20
Ventricular fibrillation, 218, 220
  rules for determining, 220–221
  significance and treatments of, 444

Ventricular irritability, treatment of, 436
Ventricular rhythms, 205–252
Ventricular tachycardia, 216–218
  rules for determining, 218, 219
  significance and treatments of, 443

Wandering pacemaker arrhythmia, 103, 104
  rules for determining, 103, 105
  significance and treatments of, 440
Wave patterns, interpreting, 59–64
Waves,
  "F", 109
  "f", 111
  P, 51, 56, 59–61
    atrial, 102
    inverted, 138–140
    sinus, 102
  Q, 21
  R, 55
  S, 23
  T, 21, 27, 33, 61
Waves and measurements, 19–52
Wenckebach heart block, 168, 169, 175–178
  conduction pattern in, 179
  rules for determining, 178, 180

Flash Cards

Inherent Rates

The inherent rate ranges of the major sites are

SA Node	60–100 beats per minute
AV Junction	40–60 beats per minute
Ventricle	20–40 beats per minute

Electrical Conduction through the Heart

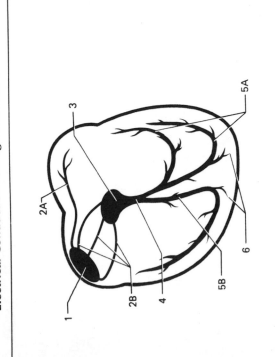

1. Sinoatrial (SA) node
2A. Intraatrial pathway
2B. Internodal pathways
3. Atrioventricular (AV) junction
4. Bundle of His
5A. Left bundle branches (2 divisions)
5B. Right bundle branch
6. Purkinje fibers

Rate Calculation

METHOD	DIRECTIONS	FEATURES
A	Count the number of R waves in a 6-second strip and multiply by 10.	• not very accurate • used only with very quick estimate
B	Count the number of large squares between 2 consecutive R waves and divide into 300. –OR– *Memorize this Scale:* 1 large square = 300 bpm 2 " " " = 150 " 3 " " " = 100 " 4 " " " = 75 " 5 " " " = 60 " 6 " " " = 50 "	• very quick • not very accurate with fast rates • only used with regular rhythms
C	Count the number of small squares between 2 consecutive R waves and divide into 1500.	• most accurate • used only with regular rhythms • time consuming

EKG Wave Patterns

Electrical Activity	Associated Pattern	Graphic Depiction
Atrial Depolarization	P Wave	
Delay at AV Node	PR Segment	
Ventricular Depolarization	QRS Complex	
Ventricular Repolarization	T Wave	
No Electrical Activity	Isolectric Line	

Normal EKG Measurements

PRI: .12–.20 seconds
QRS: < .12 seconds

EKG Complex

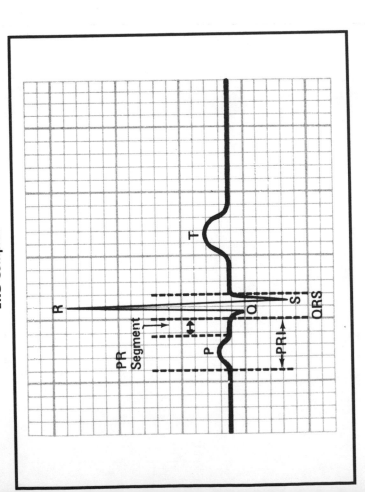

Sinus Bradycardia

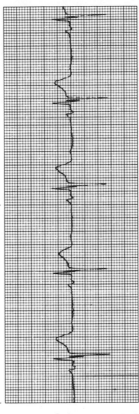

SINUS node is the pacemaker, firing regularly at a rate of less than 60 times per minute. Each impulse is conducted normally through to the ventricles.

REGULARITY: The R–R intervals are constant; the rhythm is regular.
RATE: The atrial and ventricular rates are equal; heart rate is less than 60 beats per minute.
P WAVE: There is a uniform P wave in front of every QRS complex.
PRI: The PR interval measures between .12 and .20 seconds; the PRI measurement is constant across the strip.
QRS: The QRS complex measures less than .12 seconds.

Normal Sinus Rhythm

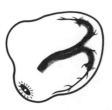

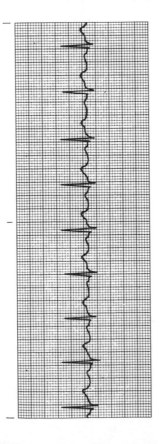

SINUS node is the pacemaker, firing at a regular rate of 60–100 times per minute. Each beat is conducted normally through to the ventricles.

REGULARITY: The R–R intervals are constant; the rhythm is regular.
RATE: The atrial and ventricular rates are equal; heart rate is between 60 and 100 beats per minute.
P WAVE: The P waves are uniform. There is one P wave in front of every QRS complex.
PRI: The PR interval measures between .12 and .20 seconds; the PRI measurement is constant across the strip.
QRS: The QRS complex measures less than .12 seconds.

Sinus Tachycardia

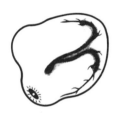

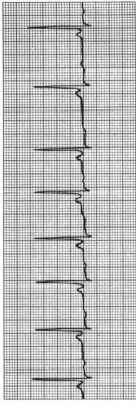

SINUS node is the pacemaker, firing regularly at a rate of greater than 100 times per minute. Each impulse is conducted normally through to the ventricles.

REGULARITY: The R–R intervals are constant; the rhythm is regular.
RATE: The atrial and ventricular rates are equal; the heart rate is greater than 100 beats per minute (usually between 100 and 160 beats per minute).
P WAVE: There is a uniform P wave in front of every QRS complex.
PRI: The PR interval measures between .12 and .20 seconds; the PRI measurement is constant across the strip.
QRS: The QRS complex measures less than .12 seconds.

Sinus Arrhythmia

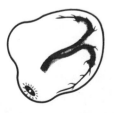

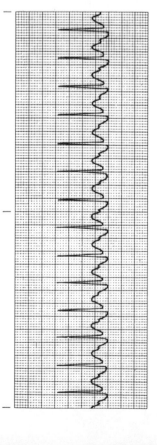

SINUS node is the pacemaker, but impulses are initiated in an irregular pattern. The rate increases as the patient breathes in and decreases as the patient breathes out. Each beat is conducted normally through to the ventricles.

REGULARITY: The R–R intervals vary; the rate changes with the patient's respirations.
RATE: The atrial and ventricular rates are equal; heart rate is usually in a normal range (60–100 beats per minute), but can be slower.
P WAVE: There is a uniform P wave in front of every QRS complex.
PRI: The PR interval measures between .12 and .20 seconds; the PRI measurement is constant across the strip.
QRS: The QRS complex measures less than .12 seconds.

Premature Ventricular Contraction

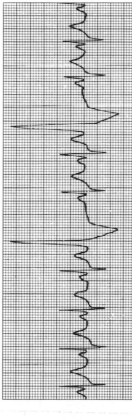

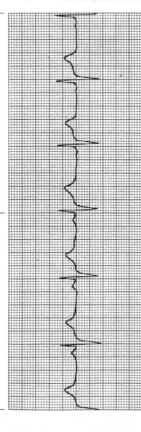

The pacemaker is an irritable focus within the ATRIUM which fires prematurely and produces a single ectopic beat. Conduction through to the ventricles is normal.

REGULARITY: Since this is a single premature ectopic beat, it will interrupt the regularity of the underlying rhythm.

RATE: The overall heart rate will depend on the rate of the underlying rhythm.

P WAVE: The P wave of the premature beat will have a different morphology than the P waves of the rest of the strip. The ectopic beat will have a P wave, but it can be flattened, notched, or otherwise unusual. It may be hidden within the T wave of the preceding complex.

PRI: The PRI should measure between .12 and .20 seconds, but can be prolonged; the PRI of the ectopic will probably be different from the PRI measurements of the other complexes.

QRS: The QRS complex measurement will be less than .12 seconds.

Wandering Pacemaker

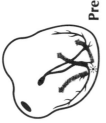

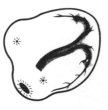

The pacemaker site wanders between the SINUS node, the ATRIA, and the AV JUNCTION. Although each beat originates from a different focus, the rate usually remains within a normal range, but can be slower. Conduction through to the ventricles is normal.

REGULARITY: The R–R intervals vary slightly as the pacemaker site changes; the rhythm can be slightly irregular.

RATE: The atrial and ventricular rates are equal; heart rate is usually within a normal range (60–100 beats per minute) but can be slower.

P WAVE: The morphology of the P wave changes as the pacemaker site changes. There is one P wave in front of every QRS complex, although some may be difficult to see depending on the pacemaker site.

PRI: The PRI measurement will vary slightly as the pacemaker site changes. All PRI measurements should be less than .20 seconds; some may be less than .12 seconds.

QRS: The QRS complex measures less than .12 seconds.

Atrial Flutter

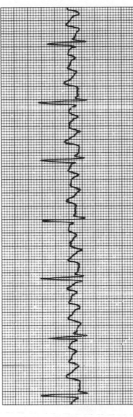

A single irritable focus within the ATRIA issues an impulse that is conducted in a rapid, repetitive fashion. To protect the ventricles from receiving too many impulses, the AV node blocks some of the impulses from being conducted through to the ventricles.

REGULARITY: The atrial rhythm is regular. The ventricular rhythm will be regular if the AV node conducts impulses through in a consistent pattern. If the pattern varies, the ventricular rate will be irregular.

RATE: Atrial rate is between 250 and 350 beats per minute. Ventricular rate will depend on the ratio of impulses conducted through to the ventricles.

P WAVE: When the atria flutter they produce a series of well-defined P waves. When seen together, these "Flutter" waves have a saw-tooth appearance.

PRI: Because of the unusual configuration of the P wave (Flutter wave) and the proximity of the wave to the QRS complex, it is often impossible to determine a PRI in this arrhythmia. Therefore, the PRI is not measured in Atrial Flutter.

QRS: The QRS complex measures less than .12 seconds; measurement can be difficult if one or more Flutter waves is concealed within the QRS complex.

Atrial Tachycardia

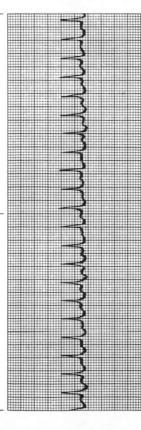

The pacemaker is a single irritable site within the ATRIUM which fires repetitively at a very rapid rate. Conduction through to the ventricles is normal.

REGULARITY: The R–R intervals are constant; the rhythm is regular.

RATE: The atrial and ventricular rates are equal; the heart rate is usually 150–250 beats per minute.

P WAVE: There is one P wave in front of every QRS complex. The configuration of the P wave will be different than that of sinus P waves; they may be flattened or notched. Because of the rapid rate, the P waves can be hidden in the T waves of the preceding beats.

PRI: The PRI is between .12 and .20 seconds and constant across the strip. The PRI may be difficult to measure if the P wave is obscured by the T wave.

QRS: The QRS complex measures less than .12 seconds.

Premature Junctional Contraction

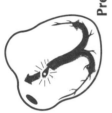

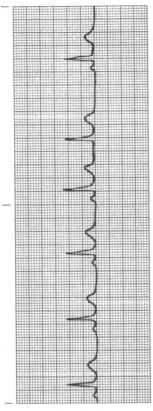

The pacemaker is an irritable focus within the AV JUNCTION which fires prematurely and produces a single ectopic beat. The atria are depolarized via retrograde conduction. Conduction through the ventricles is normal.

REGULARITY: Since this is a single premature ectopic beat, it will interrupt the regularity of the underlying rhythm. The R–R interval will be irregular.

RATE: The overall heart rate will depend on the rate of the underlying rhythm.

P WAVES: The P wave can come before or after the QRS complex, or it can be lost entirely within the QRS complex. If visible, the P wave will be inverted.

PRI: If the P wave precedes the QRS complex, the PRI will be less than .12 seconds. If the P wave falls within the QRS complex or following it, there will be no PRI.

QRS: The QRS complex measurement will be less than .12 seconds.

Atrial Fibrillation

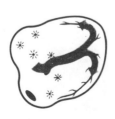

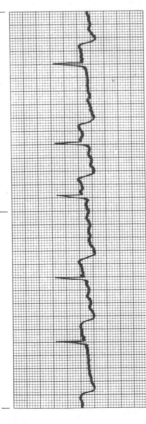

The ATRIA are so irritable that a multitude of foci initiate impulses, causing the atria to depolarize repeatedly in a fibrillatory manner. The AV node blocks most of the impulses, allowing only a limited number through to the ventricles.

REGULARITY: The atrial rhythm is unmeasurable; all atrial activity is chaotic. The ventricular rhythm is grossly irregular having no pattern to its irregularity.

RATE: The atrial rate cannot be measured because it is so chaotic: research indicates that it exceeds 350 beats per minute. The ventricular rate is significantly slower because the AV node blocks most of the impulses. If the ventricular rate is below 100 beats per minute the rhythm is said to be "controlled"; if it is over 100 beats per minute it is considered to have a "rapid ventricular response."

P WAVE: In this arrhythmia the atria are not depolarizing in an effective way; instead, they are fibrillating. Thus, no P wave is produced. All atrial activity is depicted as "fibrillatory" waves, or grossly chaotic undulations of the baseline.

PRI: Since no P waves are visible, no PRI can be measured.

QRS: The QRS complex measurement should be less than .12 seconds.

Junctional Escape Rhythm

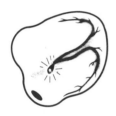

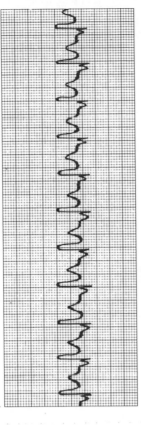

When higher pacemaker sites fail, the AV JUNCTION is left with pacemaking responsibility. The atria are depolarized via retrograde conduction. Ventricular conduction is normal.

REGULARITY: The R–R intervals are constant. The rhythm is regular.
RATE: Atrial and ventricular rates are equal. The inherent rate of the AV Junction is 40–60 beats per minute.
P WAVES: The P wave can come before or after the QRS complex, or it can be lost entirely within the QRS complex. If visible, the P wave will be inverted.
PRI: If the P wave precedes the QRS complex, the PRI will be less than .12 seconds. If the P wave falls within the QRS complex or following it, there will be no PRI.
QRS: The QRS complex measurement will be less than .12 seconds.

Junctional Tachycardia

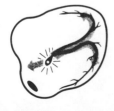

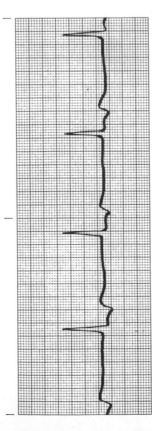

An irritable focus in the AV JUNCTION speeds up to override the SA node for control of the heart. The atria are depolarized via retrograde conduction. Conduction through the ventricles is normal.

REGULARITY: The R–R intervals are constant. The rhythm is regular.
RATE: Atrial and ventricular rates are equal. The rate will be in the tachycardia range, but does not usually exceed 180 beats per minute. Usual range is 100–180 beats per minute.
P WAVES: The P wave can come before or after the QRS complex, or it can be lost entirely within the QRS complex. If visible, the P wave will be inverted.
PRI: If the P wave precedes the QRS complex, the PRI will be less than .12 seconds. If the P wave falls within the QRS complex or following it, there will be no PRI.
QRS: The QRS complex measurement will be less than .12 seconds.

First Degree Heart Block

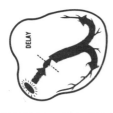

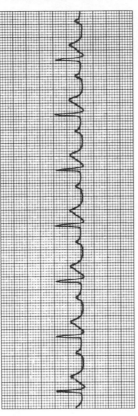

The AV NODE holds each sinus impulse longer than normal before conducting it through the ventricles. Each impulse is eventually conducted. Once into the ventricles, conduction proceeds normally.

REGULARITY: This will depend on the regularity of the underlying rhythm.

RATE: The rate will depend on the rate of the underlying rhythm.

P WAVES: The P waves will be upright and uniform. Each P wave will be followed by a QRS complex.

PRI: The PRI will be constant across the entire strip, but it will always be greater than .20 seconds.

QRS: The QRS complex measurement will be less than .12 seconds.

Accelerated Junctional Rhythm

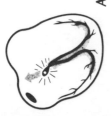

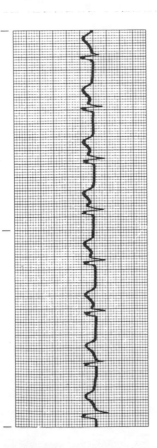

An irritable focus in the AV JUNCTION speeds up to override the SA node for control of the heart. The atria are depolarized via retrograde conduction. Conduction through the ventricles is normal.

REGULARITY: The R-R intervals are constant. The rhythm is regular.

RATE: Atrial and ventricular rates are equal. The rate will be faster than the AV Junction's inherent rate, but not yet into a true tachycardia range. Usually in the 60–100 beats per minute range.

P WAVES: The P wave can come before or after the QRS complex, or it can be lost entirely within the QRS complex. If visible, the P wave will be inverted.

PRI: If the P wave precedes the QRS complex, the PRI will be less than .12 seconds. If the P wave falls within the QRS complex or following it, there will be no PRI.

QRS: The QRS complex will be less than .12 seconds.

Wenckebach

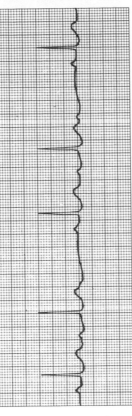

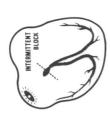

As the sinus node initiates impulses, each one is delayed in the AV NODE a little longer than the preceding one, until one is eventually blocked completely. Those impulses that are conducted travel normally through the ventricles.

REGULARITY: The R–R interval is irregular in a pattern of grouped beating. The R–R interval gets progressively shorter as the PRI gets progressively longer.

RATE: Since some beats are not conducted, the ventricular rate is usually slightly slower than normal. The atrial rate is normal.

P WAVES: The P waves are upright and uniform. Some P waves are not followed by QRS complexes.

PRI: The PR intervals get progressively longer, until one P wave is not followed by a QRS complex. After the blocked beat, the cycle starts again.

QRS: The QRS complex measurement will be less than .12 seconds.

Classical Second Degree Heart Block

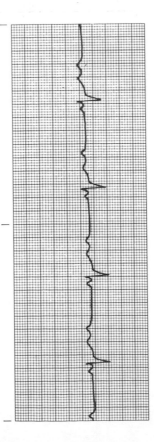

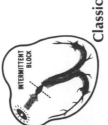

The AV NODE selectively conducts some beats while blocking others. Those that are not blocked are conducted through to the ventricles, although they may encounter a slight delay in the node. Once in the ventricles, conduction proceeds normally.

REGULARITY: If the conduction ratio is consistent, the R–R interval will be constant, and the rhythm will be regular. If the conduction ratio varies, the R–R will be irregular.

RATE: The atrial rate is usually normal. Since many of the atrial impulses are blocked, the ventricular rate will usually be in the bradycardia range, often one half, one third, or one fourth of the atrial rate.

P WAVES: P waves are upright and uniform. There are always more P waves than QRS complexes.

PRI: The PRI on conducted beats will be constant across the strip, although it might be longer than a normal PRI measurement.

QRS: The QRS complex measurement will be less than .12 seconds.

Premature Atrial Contraction

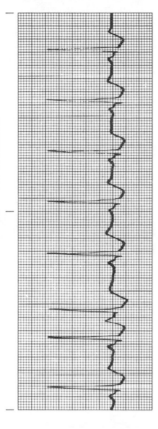

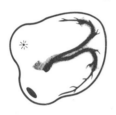

A PVC is a single irritable focus within the VENTRICLES that fires prematurely to initiate an ectopic complex.

REGULARITY: The underlying rhythm can be regular or irregular. The ectopic PVC will interrupt the regularity of the underlying rhythm (unless the PVC is interpolated).

RATE: The rate will be determined by the underlying rhythm. PVCs are not usually included in the rate determination because they frequently do not produce a pulse.

P WAVES: The ectopic is not preceded by a P wave. You may see a coincidental P wave near the PVC, but it is dissociated.

PRI: Since the ectopic comes from a lower focus, there will be no PRI.

QRS: The QRS complex will be wide and bizarre, measuring at least .12 seconds. The configuration will differ from the configuration of the underlying QRS complexes. The T wave is frequently in the opposite direction from the QRS complex.

Complete Heart Block

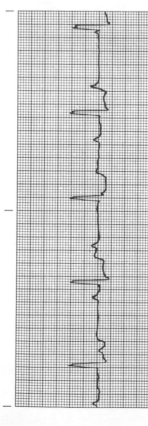

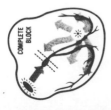

The block at the AV NODE is complete. The sinus beats cannot penetrate the node, and thus, are not conducted through to the ventricles. An escape mechanism from either the junction or the ventricles will take over to pace the ventricles. The atria and the ventricles function in a totally dissociated fashion.

REGULARITY: Both the atrial and the ventricular foci are firing regularly, thus the P–P intervals and the R–R intervals are regular.

RATE: The atrial rate will usually be in a normal range. The ventricular rate will be slower. If a junctional focus is controlling the ventricles, the rate will be 40–60 beats per minute. If the focus is ventricular, the rate will be 20–40 beats per minute.

P WAVES: The P waves are upright and uniform. There are more P waves than QRS complexes.

PRI: Since the block at the AV node is complete, none of the atrial impulses is conducted through to the ventricles. There is no PRI. The P waves have no relationship to the QRS complexes. You may occasionally see a P wave superimposed on the QRS complex.

QRS: If the ventricles are being controlled by a junctional focus, the QRS complex will measure less than .12 seconds. If the focus is ventricular, the QRS will measure .12 seconds or greater.

Ventricular Tachycardia

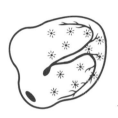

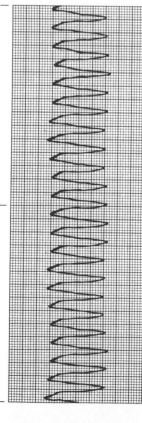

An irritable focus in the VENTRICLES fires regularly at a rate of 150–250 beats per minute to override higher sites for control of the heart.

REGULARITY: This rhythm is usually regular, although it can be slightly irregular.

RATE: Atrial rate cannot be determined. The ventricular rate range is 150–250 beats per minute. If the rate is below 150 beats per minute it is considered a slow VT. If the rate exceeds 250 beats per minute it's called Ventricular Flutter.

P WAVES: None of the QRS complexes will be preceded by P waves. You may see dissociated P waves intermittently across the strip.

PRI: Since the rhythm originates in the ventricles, there will be no PRI.

QRS: The QRS complexes will be wide and bizarre, measuring at least .12 seconds. It is often difficult to differentiate between the QRS and the T wave.

Ventricular Fibrillation

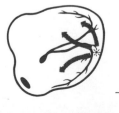

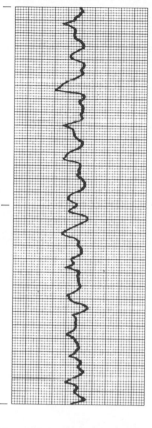

Multiple foci in the ventricles become irritable and generate uncoordinated, chaotic impulses that cause the heart to fibrillate rather than contract.

REGULARITY: There are no waves or complexes that can be analyzed to determine regularity. The baseline is totally chaotic.

RATE: The rate cannot be determined since there are no discernible waves or complexes to measure.

P WAVES: There are no discernible P waves.

PRI: There is no PRI.

QRS: There are no discernible QRS complexes.